Praise for

Cancer-Free with Food

"Cancer-Free with Food *is an extraordinarily relevant book as Liana Werner-Gray writes about the latest scientific discoveries on the role of specific ingredients in making the body an inhospitable environment for cancer. Given that 70 percent of all cancers are related to diet, Liana points us in the right direction in showing us that food can be used as medicine. Cancer-Free with Food is medicine for the 21st century."*

— **Mark Hyman, M.D.**, #1 *New York Times* best-selling author and director, Cleveland Clinic Center for Functional Medicine

"In Cancer-Free with Food, *Liana Werner-Gray shows how to turn your kitchen into a pharmacy so that you can take care of your health at the most fundamental and important level. Whether you are looking to boost your immunity to prevent or beat cancer, to find ways to cope with the unwanted side effects of chemotherapy and radiation treatment, or to repair your tissues after surgery, the nutritional keys Liana has identified will make you feel better."*

— **Ty M. Bollinger**, *New York Times* best-selling author of *The Truth about Cancer*

"This book is an essential guide for anyone diagnosed with cancer. Cancer is recognized worldwide to be a major health problem affecting millions of people each year. One extremely important way to prevent and or treat cancer is by getting the proper nutrition. Cancer-Free with Food *is part of the solution, and includes a plethora of recipes that are nutritionally rich."*

— **Dr. Josh Axe, DNM, DC, CNS**, best-selling author of *Eat Dirt*

"Cancer-Free with Food *is a guidebook for anyone looking to heal their body from the inside out. Every time I enjoy foods like sprouts, kale, and turmeric, I notice a huge burst in energy. The nutrient content in these foods is incredibly high and they increase the alkalinity of your body. An alkaline body helps prevent diseases like cancer."*

— **Vani Hari**, *New York Times* best-selling author of
The Food Babe Way and *Feeding You Lies*

"An excellent resource for those serious about preventing and treating cancer. The meal planning will reduce your stress and supercharge your immune system!"

— **Dr. Mark Stengler**, co-author of *Outside the Box Cancer Therapies*

"As a cancer survivor who literally overcame a ticking time bomb, Liana brings her direct experience into the many healing protocols in Cancer-Free with Food. *The cancer-healing foods, nutritional recommendations, and immune-supportive recipes in this book will help to uplift and rejuvenate so many people. She radiates confidence, joyfulness, and a deep well of expertise as she highlights the delicious, myriad possibilities for using food as medicine."*

— **Jason Wrobel**, celebrity chef, wellness wizard, cooking channel TV host, and author of *Eaternity*

CANCER-
FREE
WITH
FOOD

ALSO BY LIANA WERNER-GRAY

The Earth Diet: Your Complete Guide to Living Using Earth's Natural Ingredients

10-Minute Recipes: Fast Food, Clean Ingredients, Natural Health

All of the above are available at your local bookstore,
or may be ordered by visiting:

Hay House USA: www.hayhouse.com®
Hay House Australia: www.hayhouse.com.au
Hay House UK: www.hayhouse.co.uk
Hay House India: www.hayhouse.co.in

CANCER-FREE WITH FOOD

A Step-by-Step Plan
with 100+ Recipes to Fight Disease,
Nourish Your Body & Restore Your Health

Liana Werner-Gray

HAY HOUSE, INC.
Carlsbad, California • New York City
London • Sydney • New Delhi

Published in the United States by: Hay House, Inc.: www.hayhouse
.com® • *Published in Australia by:* Hay House Australia Pty. Ltd.: www.hayhouse.
com.au • *Published in the United Kingdom by:* Hay House UK, Ltd.: www.hayhouse.
co.uk • *Published in India by:* Hay House Publishers India: www.hayhouse.co.in

Indexer: Joan Shapiro
Cover design: Kathleen Lynch • *Interior design:* Nick C. Welch

Library of Congress Cataloging-in-Publication Data

Names: Werner-Gray, Liana.
Title: Cancer-free with food : heal the disease and support your immune
  system with the right foods for you / Liana Werner Gray.
Description: Carlsbad, California : Hay House, Inc., [2019] | Includes
  bibliographical references and index.
Identifiers: LCCN 2019000136 | ISBN 9781401956424 (paperback)
Subjects: LCSH: Cancer--Alternative treatment. | Natural foods--Therapeutic
  use. | Cooking (Natural foods) | Self-care, Health. | BISAC: HEALTH &
  FITNESS / Diseases / Cancer. | HEALTH & FITNESS / Alternative Therapies.
Classification: LCC RC271.A62 W47 2019 | DDC 616.99/40654--dc23 LC record
available at https://lccn.loc.gov/2019000136

Tradepaper ISBN: 978-1-4019-5642-4
E-book ISBN: 978-1-4019-5643-1

10 9 8 7 6 5 4 3 2 1
1st edition, April 2019

Printed in the United States of America

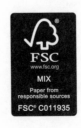
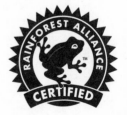

*To everyone whose life
has been touched by cancer*

CONTENTS

FOREWORD

Cancer-Free with Food is an outstanding book that provides delicious recipes, health tips, advice from doctors and other experts, and an empowering perspective that you can easily adopt to help you prevent and heal from cancer and manage the unpleasant side effects of treatment. Liana Werner-Gray writes about the latest scientific discoveries on the role of specific ingredients in making the body an inhospitable environment for cancer and highlights the shift the medical community is making toward a more functional, systems-based, and environmental approach to treatment. This is an extraordinarily relevant book given the poor quality of what most people eat. By teaching us that food can be used as medicine, Liana is pointing us in the right direction. It's the new medicine for the 21st century.

In my oncology rotation in medical school, I asked my professor what percentage of cancer was related to diet. Expecting a gracious, but insignificant nod to the role of diet as a cause of cancer, I was surprised when he said that 70 percent of all cancers are related to diet. Given this, in her book Liana answers the incredibly important question: *If I've got or want to avoid cancer, what should I eat?*

Ultimately, *Cancer-Free with Food* is a recipe book that answers this question—one that is also filled with an abundance of evidence that diet, exercise, thoughts, feelings, and environmental toxins can all play a role in the initiation, growth, and progression of cancer. We are not at the mercy of our genetic predispositions. There is a lot we can do to stay healthy. If a nutrient-poor diet full of sugar and chemicals, lack of exercise, chronic stress, and persistent exposure to pollutants like heavy metals can cause cancer, doesn't it make sense that a nutrient-dense, plant-based diet, physical activity, changing thoughts and reactions to stress, and detoxification can prevent and help heal cancer? To me, it does.

I love that this book is full of great-tasting recipes that are quick and easy to make while packed with high doses of antioxidants and protein, two of the foundational elements of any eating plan whose aim is preventing and treating cancer. Liana's genius is finding satisfying ways to enhance immune function and facilitate the body's elimination of cancer-causing compounds. For years, I've been preaching the dangers of the typical contemporary refined-carbohydrate diet: Out-of-control inflammation and hormonal imbalance are just two that are leading reasons people get cancer. By following Liana's advice and using her wholesome recipes, you can avoid these and other dangers.

One of the key principles for overcoming cancer offered in *Cancer-Free with Food* is never to consume white or refined sugar or artificial sweeteners again. Small amounts of real sugar, as found in ingredients like fruit, honey, and maple syrup, are fine to eat, but not the 152 pounds a year per person averaged in America. Liana admits that she formerly thought of sugar as a kind of recreational drug. But then she developed fulfilling recipes that satisfied her sweet tooth and was able to stop making herself sick. Cancer loves sugar. You can learn from Liana's example how to get off it and stay off it by responding to your cravings with genuine nourishment. And if sugar isn't your "drug" of choice, she shows how to satisfy other types of cravings you may have that could potentially lead you into trouble health-wise. Liana is a real person who has traveled the path before you. You can trust her insights.

Food is just the tip of the iceberg when it comes to making us prone to developing cancer. The 2008 to 2009 report from the President's Cancer Panel found that as a society we have grossly underestimated the link between environmental toxins, plastics, chemicals, and cancer risk. And the authorities have yet to acknowledge how thoughts, emotions, and overall stress also impact and add to the risk—but acknowledgment is sure to come. Liana is ahead of her time in presenting facts that should motivate us all to take a deeper look at how we nourish ourselves mentally, emotionally, and spiritually, as well as physically. Her approach to nourishment is comprehensive.

— Mark Hyman, M.D.,

Director of the Cleveland Clinic Center for Functional Medicine

INTRODUCTION

The literal meaning of healing is "becoming whole."

— ANDREW WEIL, M.D.

It was important for me to write this book for many reasons. The statistics on cancer are alarming. Cancer will affect one in two men and one in three women in the United States at some point in their lifetime, and the number of new cases of cancer is set to nearly double by the year 2050. Both predictions are based on statistics collected by the Surveillance, Epidemiology, and End Results (SEER) program at the National Cancer Institute (NCI).[1] None of us can afford to ignore these statistics.

My personal reason for writing this book is that cancer has been prevalent in my family and circle of friends. The first time I lost someone to this disease was at age nine, when one of my grandfathers died from colon cancer. Then at 11, my friend Danielle was diagnosed with a brain tumor. I vividly remember my sister and I visiting her at the hospital after her surgery. After a yearlong battle, she passed away. Next, when I was 12 years old, my second grandfather died from cancer. It started in his stomach and ended up spreading everywhere. A few years ago, my mum was diagnosed with breast cancer.

Cancer just sucks. Learning that our nutritional choices affect whether or not we get cancer and can help us heal has given me a sense of control over my health destiny that I believe everyone should feel. That's the ultimate reason this book exists. I wanted to put together a resource that would ensure that my younger sisters, my friends, and you and your friends and family never have to go through this same pain. Once we know what to eat and what not to eat, everything is easier.

My family is not unique and lots of people have similar stories to tell. Here's mine . . .

In 2009, I had a major wakeup call. Although I was only 21, I ended up in the hospital with a golf ball–size lump sticking out of the right side of my neck. At first, I thought it was just a swollen gland, so I went to see my holistic therapist, Mae Rose O'Connell. She told me to immediately go to the hospital and get it checked out further. A biopsy revealed I had a 3.7-centimeter (1.45-inch) solid mass in my neck.

Looking for appropriate guidance, I saw three doctors for the diagnosis. The first doctor told me I had stage I cancer, while the second said I had stage 0 cancer. Both doctors offered me conventional medical treatment, beginning with surgery. The third doctor told me the lump was precancerous and benign, suggested it was the symptom of a cat allergy—even though I've never been allergic to cats before or since—and offered me a prescription for allergy pills. I was also offered a cervical cancer vaccination, which I declined.

The whole diagnostic experience was confusing: I saw three different doctors and had three different diagnoses, with three different treatment options. This made me skeptical about the medical industry; it seemed as if the job of the doctors I was meeting was to sell me on surgery, chemotherapy, vaccinations, and pharmaceutical drugs. I knew my situation was serious—I remember thinking *I need to get this tumor out of my body!*—but I didn't want to do surgery or any other conventional treatments unless I absolutely had no other option.

I was devastated to have this ticking time bomb in my neck. Following the third doctor visit, I made a bold decision about my course of action. None of the doctors' proposed treatments sounded appealing. In fact, to me they sounded like torture; I didn't want to aggravate my condition. I had already put my body through five years of agony by engaging in a self-destructive cycle of binge eating toxic junk food followed by starvation. I had no doubt that my sickness was related to my disordered eating, which had spiraled out of control when I left home. So, I decided to opt out of conventional treatments—at least for several months. Instead I would heal myself using all-natural methods because that was what intuitively felt right for me to do. And that is just what I did.

Something in my background gave me confidence that I could heal the tumor on my own. I had grown up in Alice Springs, Australia, an area that's home to a large community of Aborigines who eat in a manner that's unlike the modern Western diet: with more plants, less meat, and very little processed food. They taught me that food is medicine. Knowing it was possible for food to be a source of healing, even as the doctors were giving me conflicting opinions, my mind was on the lookout for an alternative approach.

At this point, I felt so sick, so sluggish, and so fatigued. I went back to my holistic therapist, Mae, who was the main guide during my healing journey. She sent me to a naturopath, who did a live blood analysis for me that showed how my blood was riddled with parasites. It made me feel so sick to see these critters taking over my body. Based on my high white blood cell count and abnormally low number of red blood cells, this doctor said I was on the verge of developing leukemia! Mae kept me from being discouraged by this news by reminding me, "You need to make more of your own meals with your own healing hands and not eat out." She had confidence that I could heal the lump by detoxifying my body, especially my gut.

One of the things I did to create accountability for my new lifestyle was to start a daily blog. I studied nutrition and learned how to turn my kitchen into a pharmacy, publishing recipes on the blog. At the end of a year, I collected these recipes and published them in a book, *The Earth Diet*. This opened doors for me with thought leaders—integrative doctors, nutritionists, healers, natural food purveyors, restaurateurs, and other authors—who welcomed me as a fellow traveler and were generous in sharing their expertise.

Since then, I've interviewed these cutting-edge thinkers. I've done research. I wrote a second book, *10-Minute Recipes*.

I've lectured and done cooking demonstrations at conferences around the world. And I've coached many, many people on their eating plans. The best of what I learned and know as it pertains to cellular health, disease prevention, healing, and supporting the body to cope with the side effects of cancer treatment is included in this book.

Let me be clear. In this book, I am not suggesting that you refuse conventional treatments for cancer if they are warranted, only that you eat healthily and are proactive in deciding what is right for your body and condition. As a health and nutrition coach, my aim is to help people improve their eating habits. On many occasions, the people I've counseled about food have undergone surgery for cancer or done rounds of chemotherapy or radiation. I've also worked with people who, like me, took an exclusively natural approach to healing cancer. What you decide to do is really up to you and should be based on your physical condition, your personal beliefs, the professional medical advice you get, and your intuition about what is the right protocol for you.

No matter what you decide to do, you should think of food as your original medicine. If you choose to undergo one or more conventional treatments for cancer, the recipes in *Cancer-Free with Food* can be a great adjunct to those treatments. It will complement them. Good nutrition is the foundation of good health. Science is constantly revealing incredible insights on this.

In *Cancer-Free with Food*, I am not promising you a "miracle cure" for a serious health issue. My goal is to offer you comfort, inspiration, and hope that you can reverse or slow the progression of cancer in your body or prevent cancer from taking root in the first place. The delicious recipes in this book are so nutrient-rich and wholesome that by eating them you'll boost your immunity and resilience, as well as reduce your exposure to toxins, steering your body toward optimal health.

Frequently, I am asked *exactly* how I healed my body. In a nutshell, I avoided chemotherapy, radiation, surgery, and pharmaceutical medication. This strategy was my choice because I wanted to address the deeper causes of my tumor, not just react to the surface-level symptoms. I saw the illness as an opportunity to heal myself and become healthy on every level—mind, body, and spirit—in a way I had forgotten or lost.

So what *was* involved in my recovery? Instead of conventional treatment, I:

- changed my diet and consumed a lot of nutrients.
- juiced up to six times a day.
- bathed in bentonite clay, used it as a plaster to draw out toxins, and drank it.
- had sessions of integrative-health therapies, like reflexology and massage.
- received a colonic or a coffee enema every day for two months.
- rested, relaxed, and did everything I could to reduce stress.

The lump in my neck started to noticeably get smaller and smaller, and within three months of commencing this regimen, it had completely broken down and dissolved. I have been tumor-free and cancer-free for 10 years as of this moment.

How This Book Is Organized

This book is structured in a supersimple way so that you can read the sections that are relevant to your situation and learn what foods you need to eat and what to avoid in a day—just in case you got diagnosed with cancer today. My heart goes out to you, if that's the case. But you should know, I have confidence in you and your ability to heal. You are powerful!

In Part I, "Food as Medicine," I will teach you the exact things to eat to strengthen your immune system, foods like vibrantly colored plants with antioxidant properties and cold-water fish high in omega-3 fatty acids. Also, I'll explain what not to eat because it will weaken your immune system.

In Chapter 1, "Seven Key Nutritional Principles for Preventing and Overcoming Cancer," I sum up the seven principles that all the leading experts, doctors, naturopaths, and nutritionists are saying will increase our chances of beating cancer. One extremely important way to prevent and/or treat cancer is through eating a nutrient-dense diet. Unfortunately, until food manufacturers are forced to clean up the ingredients they use in their products, it's up to us to avoid the worst kinds and to choose cancer-preventing foods. It's also up to us to reduce our exposure to chemicals and things known to increase our cancer risk, like sugar, alcohol, and drugs.

To relieve some of the confusion you may feel about what to eat, in Chapter 2, "Top 15 Cancer-Healing Foods," I'll give you a breakdown of the science behind my recommendations for the most healing ingredients—everything from broccoli sprouts and turmeric, to blueberries, quinoa, cacao, and flaxseed. I had no idea before starting my research how potent broccoli sprouts are! And I have long eaten cacao pretty much every day for the past nine years, but I didn't know there had been countless studies on its positive health effects and for exactly what until putting this book together. The science is overwhelming! You'll learn how much and how often to eat each ingredient and the types of cancer it is especially useful for.

One of the things you'll hear me repeat time and again is that you want to make your body inhospitable to cancer. These foods will help with that.

In Chapter 3, "Anticancer Supplements," I sum up the top supplements you could get and always keep on hand to prevent cancer or even kill cancer cells. Some are concentrated forms of the foods you are introduced to in Chapter 1. For instance, you could eat turmeric in a curry recipe you prepare, or you could take a turmeric or curcumin capsule. You have options.

In Chapter 4, "Avoid the Most Toxic Foods on the Planet," you'll learn which crazily toxic foods and substances to cut out of your life beginning today—and why they drain your energy and affect your nervous system, leaving you feeling anxious and tired.

In Chapter 5, "Living the Food Upgrades Mind-Set," I'll teach you the mind-set I adopted that changed everything for me. You will learn how to fulfill every single craving you have.

Then, in Chapter 6, "Healing Guide for Common Specific Cancers," I'll give you quick tips on what foods are best to eat when you have one of the 10 most prevalent cancers (for instance, breast cancer, prostate cancer, lung cancer, colon cancer). Beyond the nutritional science, we'll look at a few complementary treatments you might want to consider. Throughout the book you will find sidebars detailing the real-life stories from individuals who shared their cancer journey with me.

And this is all easier than you think, so don't be overwhelmed. You are in the right place right now to receive the support you need! If you ever feel overwhelmed as you read this book, repeat the following affirmation to help bring you back to peace immediately: *I am peaceful. I feel peaceful. All is well in my world. All is well with my soul.*

And finally, in Part II, "Cancer-Free with Food Recipes," you'll find more than 200 recipes for immune-boosting juices, brain-protecting smoothies, life-extending lunches and dinners, comforting soups and broths, alkalizing vegetable dishes, nutrient-rich desserts and sweet snacks (my favorite), strength-building meals, delicious sides, sauces, condiments, and much more.

KNOWING WHAT FOOD OR TREATMENT IS RIGHT FOR YOU

As I share what natural remedies and foods worked for me, keep in mind that there are literally hundreds of different ingredients that would be appropriate for healing cancer, if not thousands. You have tons of options when it comes to choosing healing, delicious foods.

My intention in this book is to provide you with sufficient knowledge to pick which ingredients will work best for you based on your condition and your preferences. For example, tomatoes might be better than mushrooms, or cacao could accelerate your healing. Pretend you are opening a cancer-healing catalog as you're picking the recipes you want to eat. The guidelines of this approach are super simple, and the recipes are easy to prepare.

I also encourage you to go within and trust your intuition, just as I did when I was healing my lump. And pray for guidance—you can probably never pray enough! Your soul will tell you if a particular healing tool or food is right for you. You might also get goose bumps while reading a description of a certain food or when you're standing in the produce aisle holding it. Trust your sense that this is the right food for you. Our bodies are intelligent in ways our conscious minds cannot comprehend. We evolved in nature and nature evolved to provide for us. We just have to open up to its wisdom.

Trusting her intuition is what my mum did when I presented her with all the options available to her. She always picked the ingredients that resonated with her, and it worked. She made it through breast cancer treatment a few years ago and is now living cancer-free. My mum had surgery and then opted out of chemotherapy and radiation. She had confidence that she would beat cancer if she quit smoking and changed her diet. And she did.

What to Expect When You Follow Cancer-Free with Food

Most people who improve their dietary habits by flooding their bodies with nutrients begin to feel better almost immediately. You can expect the same. These nutrients will come mainly from plant foods like vegetables, fruits, leaves, roots, nuts, and seeds, with the addition of lean protein sourced exclusively from beans, if you're vegetarian, and from eggs, fish, poultry, and modest amounts of red meat, if you're a meat eater.

Similarly, when people stop eating the wrong foods—those that are toxic to their bodies, like refined sugar (you'll notice I repeat this a lot)—most feel better almost immediately. If you reduce your levels of stress, spend time with friends and family, increase the hours you sleep, avoid exposure to pollution, and nourish yourself emotionally and spiritually, healing is promoted.

You can expect your mind to clear and your thoughts and mood to become more positive moving forward. I encourage you to embrace the initial discomforts and celebrate your progress.

That said, healing is always a process. It can take time for the body to overcome cancer—weeks, months, possibly years. But please feel encouraged. Healing is possible!

PART I

FOOD AS MEDICINE

CHAPTER 1

SEVEN KEY NUTRITIONAL PRINCIPLES FOR PREVENTING AND OVERCOMING CANCER

In recent years, scientists have come to realize that it's not just our genes that decide whether we get cancer. From the emerging science of epigenetics, we know that we can influence the way our genes express themselves through the lifestyles we lead and the foods we choose to eat. Describing a study conducted by the acclaimed cardiologist Dean Ornish, Mark Hyman, M.D., writes: "After just three months on an intensive lifestyle program including a whole-foods, plant-based diet, over 500 genes that regulate cancer were beneficially affected, either turning off the cancer-causing genes or turning on the cancer-protective genes. No medication can do that."[1]

Through lifestyle modification alone, we can literally rewrite our genetic code. Just because your parents, grandparents, or siblings had cancer doesn't mean you have to!

TOXICITY AND STRESS

There are two main underlying reasons affecting whether we get cancer: toxicity and stress.

When we have been exposed to too many toxins, this creates an unhealthily acidic environment in the body that weakens the immune system and causes our organs to stop working up to their full potential. Acidity creates a breeding ground for cancer because the cells in the human body can survive only in the slightly alkaline range of 7.35 to 7.45 pH. (Acidity and alkalinity are polar opposites on the pH scale.) We can promote a healthy state within our bodies by eating more alkalizing foods and avoiding inflammatory and acid-forming foods, like sugar and alcohol.

When we are put under stress for a short period, our bodies can recover from it reasonably quickly. But when the pressure is unrelenting, our resources eventually become depleted; we are less resilient and cannot counteract the effects of stress as easily. Stress can be mental, emotional, or physical.

- *Physical stress* can come from chemical exposure, lack of sleep, and overworking for an extended period. These things make the body vulnerable to illness.

- *Mental stress* includes negative thoughts, whether your own self-talk based on your belief system or ongoing exposure to outside criticism. Sadness and anxiety make us more vulnerable to illness.

- *Emotional stress* includes wounds from traumas in your past that haven't healed yet. If you had a car crash, lost your job, are mourning a loss, or are in the middle of a divorce, this could be an emotional stress factor.

Whatever the source, the impact of chronic stress can be reduced by eating nutritious foods, implementing new thought processes, praying, getting adequate sleep, and spending time talking and having fun with people you care about.

Do your best to avoid toxins. We are often exposed to carcinogenic chemicals in our environment, including our workplace or household, or pollution in the air. Even medical treatments that suppress the immune system can be considered carcinogenic. We can turn off the genes that are likely to develop into cancer by making some lifestyle shifts—by reducing our chemical intake from food and from the products we use and put on our skin. Through a few simple steps, we can make our bodies inhospitable environments for cancer cells to grow.

GOING BACK TO NATURE

From what I have learned from the past decade of studying the healing power of nutrition on the immune system, inflammation, and cancer from medical experts, the most fundamental common thread I am finding is increasing our consumption of vegetables. It's as simple as that. In general, experts advocate that we need to cut way back on our toxic consumption and go back to eating foods straight from nature.

It is obvious that foods that God and nature have created are the ones we are intended to eat to survive, thrive, and heal. It is also obvious that consuming a huge amount of chemicals and ingredients we can't even pronounce is dangerous for the chemistry of our bodies. Always remember to use common sense when it comes to eating and nutrition. At the end of the day, experts can help explain things and point you to focus on certain things, but ultimately your natural instincts will be your best guide.

If I were diagnosed with cancer today, the first thing I would do is commit to eating a majority whole-food, plant-based diet as much as possible, incorporating fruits, nuts, seeds, organic dairy, grass-fed beef, pasture-raised eggs, and herbal remedies. We never go wrong by adding nutrient-rich foods to our diets. All the recipes in Part II of this book are healing in this way.

Second, I would look at ways to quickly switch out any refined sugar with more natural sugars. If you are like me, with a liking for or addiction to sugar, this step is critical. When you have cancer, every time you put something unhealthy into your body you are essentially feeding the cancer—and cancer loves sugar.

Of course, I don't want you to feel guilty or put extra mental stress on you if you have cancer and feel attached to eating processed foods and sweet foods right now. There are tools you can use to help break the stranglehold of a sugar addiction. One of these is to feed yourself ultra-nutritious and delicious meals to reduce your cravings. In the next chapter, I'll teach you the Upgrade Mind-Set, which will help you continuously improve your choices.

THE SEVEN KEY NUTRITIONAL PRINCIPLES

In summarizing the work of experts with comprehensive, authoritative knowledge of nutrition in relation to cancer, I can report the conclusions they unanimously draw:

- Nutrition matters when it comes to preventing and healing cancer.
- Certain nutrients are most effective for fighting cancer overall, as well as for healing certain types of cancer.

To increase your chances of preventing and overcoming cancer at any stage, here are the seven key nutritional principles that have proven to be most effective. Basically, if you embrace these strategies for establishing a healthful diet and lifestyle, you will have a way higher chance of healing cancer—simply banishing it from your life so that it never comes back again.

#1. Eat More Whole Foods

Freshly picked whole food is the most healthful. When we can go out to our backyard and pick a fruit, vegetable, leaf, or herb straight from the bush, tree, or vine it grows on, as it comes to the table it's still alive with the vital energy we need to thrive and is extremely nutrient-rich.

Most of us don't have gardens of our own anymore—more than 50 percent of the world's population now lives in cities. The next best way to eat fresh produce after picking it is to obtain our produce from a local farm or a farmers market and eat as many seasonal and as local foods as possible. When food is shipped to a supermarket, whether it travels around the world or across the nation, it loses some of its nutritional value and energy. Do a test for yourself, if you can: It's fascinating to observe the difference in taste and energy between a local vegetable and a vegetable shipped in from another country.

Hidden malnourishment is one of the reasons people overeat. Nutrient deficiency is an epidemic right now. Because of hunger that is not being assuaged, people respond by eating more processed foods. They fill up on calories and crave sugar and fat. Their hunger and dietary choices are in a vicious cycle that can only be interrupted by consumption of nutrient-dense food.

Another reason to eat fresh whole foods is because they are replete with antioxidants, which are anti-inflammatory. Renowned physician Deepak Chopra, M.D., F.A.C.P., says: "Because cancer is so strongly associated with chronic inflammation, eating foods that fight inflammation can have a chemoprotective effect."[2]

Incorporate the top 15 cancer-healing foods into your daily diet. These ingredients are filled with many antioxidants, vitamins, minerals, and phytochemicals that inhibit tumor growth and help make the body inhospitable to cancer. See Chapter 2 for more details about:

- Blueberries
- Broccoli
- Broccoli sprouts
- Cacao
- Dark leafy greens (bok choy, cilantro, kale, parsley, spinach, and watercress)
- Flaxseed (aka linseed)
- Garlic

- Ginger
- Grapes
- Lemon
- Mushrooms
- Quinoa
- Tigernuts
- Tomatoes
- Turmeric

You may also wish to take dietary supplements of certain healing nutrients (see Chapter 3).

#2. Drink at Least One Juice Daily

When I committed myself to healing, I researched ways to put high amounts of nutrition in my body as quickly as possible. I knew that to support my immune system so that it could play its role in healing my body, I would have to essentially feast on nutrients. Having deprived my body of proper foods for many years, I knew my body didn't have the resources it needed to function properly and keep me well.

I learned that an extremely fast way to get the vitamins and phytochemicals we need is to drink fresh juices. An alternative method of healing is for a qualified health-care practitioner to give an antioxidant-rich vitamin drip from an IV. However, I knew that wasn't for me. (I don't like needles and the cost was prohibitive.) Intuitively, I knew that through daily juicing, my cells would be nourished and detoxified.

Every time I had a juice, I imagined it as liquid medicine going into my bloodstream and pumping energy straight into my cells. I visualized cancer cells and my cravings for junk food being forced out of my body. I knew that the nutrients I was taking in were helping me create new cells and build a new body.

When I was focused on healing my precancerous tumor, I drank up to six juices a day. I wanted to heal my body quickly. My original intention was to detox. Mostly I alternated between Green Lemonade (page 150), which is a combination of apple, cucumber, celery, ginger, and lemon, and any dark leafy green, like kale or spinach; and Beet Juice (page 147), which is made from beet, apple, and carrot.

Your situation is unique. As was mine. But there is something that everyone who wants to fight or prevent cancer has in common, which is a desire to take excellent care of ourselves. Juicing can give us peace of mind about our nutrition, easing some of our mental and emotional distress. It gives us a chance to focus on something better and positive, like life and healing.

As soon as we drink a juice, we can't help but feel better. Fresh juice instantly provides us with a high dose of vitamins, like nothing else on the planet can! A morning juice is a powerful way to start each day. Taking this one step, we can know that we already got a good, foundational level of nutrition for the day.

If you have been feeling guilty about not taking care of yourself properly, you can begin to erase that by basically loading up your body nutritionally through juicing. If you are like me and for years deprived yourself of proper nutrition, nourishment, and love, I believe juicing is the quickest, most effective way to restore your body to the healthy state it wants to be in. The body is super intelligent. It will take the nutrients it needs and use them wisely. We don't need to micromanage its many processes. We just need to give it nutrients and it does the rest itself.

For 10 years I have drunk at least one juice per day, and I consider this my ultimate nutritional secret.

#3. Buy Organic, Non-GMO Foods

Foods that may be consumed whole in their natural state, like fruits, vegetables, nuts, and seeds, provide the body with vitamins, minerals, and other nutrients that are healthy, unless we add chemicals to them. Something that should be healthy to eat, like a carrot, for example, if it is grown on a farm where the farmers spray it with pesticides and herbicides, becomes carcinogenic.

We want to avoid all toxic chemicals in our food, so it's important to buy organic produce that has not been genetically modified. Farmers grow a lot of foods these days with pesticides, so loads of chemicals are being absorbed by fruits and vegetables through their roots as well as through their leaves and peels when they are being sprayed. These chemicals deplete them of their nutrients and also make them toxic. Whether you buy organic produce or not, always wash your produce thoroughly in clean water to get rid of any possible chemical residue on it.

Chemicals in processed foods, like preservatives, additives, and artificial flavorings, can be considered carcinogens—substances capable of causing cancer to grow in living tissue. When you follow the Cancer-Free with Food model, sticking to an organic, whole-food, plant-rich diet, you won't be consuming any of these.

This principle applies to fish and meat as well. Joseph Mercola, D.O., author of a blog on complementary and alternative therapies, writes: "I'm convinced that most cancers are preventable through proper diet and nutrition, and besides optimizing your nutrient ratios, avoiding toxic exposures is another important factor. This is one reason why I recommend eating organic foods, especially grass-fed or pastured meats and animal products, whenever possible."[3]

Buy foods that are labeled non-GMO too. To receive this designation the supplier has to prove that the food meets certain quality requirements. You can read more about why this is important in Chapter 4, "Avoid the Most Toxic Foods on the Planet."

I believe when you go to your refrigerator it should make you excited and happy. Eating should always be nourishing, a source of joy, and never be a source of anxiety and alarm.

#4. Cut Out Refined Sugars

Is there ever a need for refined sugar in our diets? No. It causes far too many health problems for us to accept it in our food. Sugar feeds cancer and supports its growth. According to Dr. Mark Hyman, author of *The Blood Sugar Solution*: "The number one thing you can do to prevent or control cancer is to control insulin levels with a high-fiber diet rich in real, fresh, whole foods and minimize or eliminate sugary, processed, insulin-raising foods."[4]

I've come across two types of people with cancer. When they get diagnosed, one type feels the need to give up sugars altogether, including fruits, while the other type prefers to adopt my upgrade system. Here are the sweet foods that I advise my clients are safe to eat (because they are nutrient-dense) and unsafe to eat (because they only contain empty calories or they are made with chemicals).

SAFE LIST:

- Fruits
- Dates
- Figs
- Maple syrup
- Honey
- Stevia
- Monk fruit sweetener

UNSAFE LIST:

- Refined white sugar (cane or beet sugar)
- Raw sugar (cane sugar)
- Brown sugar
- Corn syrup (regular and high-fructose corn syrup)
- Artificial sweeteners
- Acesulfame potassium (Sunett, Sweet One)
- Neotame
- Saccharin (Sugar Twin, Sweet'N Low)
- Sucralose

#5. Avoid Refined Carbs; Eat High-Fiber Carbs

Processed foods such as conventional breads, pastas, cakes, cookies, and the like are made with refined carbohydrates. These break down in the body into sugar, which we know feeds cancer cells. Because they're low in nutrients, they're considered "empty calories."

There are more natural versions of most of these foods—for instance, high-protein pasta is made with lentils, black beans, or red beans. My view is that God made foods in nature that are ideal for us, but it's up to us to stick to principle #1 and eat those foods. That includes potatoes and rice. While potatoes are starchy, they are high in nutrients like vitamin C. Rice and beans together compose a whole protein—a combination that has been sustaining us for millennia in numerous countries, Mexico and India to name two.

The beauty of the Cancer-Free with Food plan is that by eating a wide variety of nutritious plant-based foods, a rainbow of vegetables and fruits, you are getting healthy carbs you need, which are life-sustaining, cancer-preventive, and also high in fiber. In fact, fiber is one of the top seven nutrients that fight cancer, according to the American Institute for Cancer Research.[5]

If you're going to have carbs, eating high-fiber carbs is the way to go. Fiber is an essential nutrient. It has these benefits:

- Slows the absorption of sugar during digestion.
- Cleans the colon, acting like a scrub brush.
- Reduces constipation.
- Increases satiety. And remember, you can't live a full life on an empty stomach!

Good sources of high-fiber carbs include chia seeds, psyllium seed husks, peas, brussels sprouts, and root and tuber crops (beets, parsnips, potatoes, sweet potatoes, radishes).

A lot of us have digestive systems that are not absorbing all the nutrition they could be. This certainly was the case for me in my teens and early 20s. After years of eating processed foods and taking laxatives instead of eating fiber, I had compacted waste stuck to the walls of my gut that was inhibiting me from absorbing nutrients from the fruits and vegetables I ate. When I switched to eating whole foods—tons of high-fiber veggies and fruits—my gut was healed.

If you're unused to eating fiber, be on notice that it will bulk up your stools. It's not a bad idea to take a digestive enzyme with your meals (see Resources) to assist your body with its adaptation to this new way of eating. In time, it will seem normal.

#6. Cultivate a Healthy Gut

Mehmet Oz, M.D., is a board-certified cardiothoracic surgeon and professor in the department of surgery at Columbia University in New York City. He is also famous, of course, for his daytime television program, *The Dr. Oz Show*. His blog provided an alarming statistic about how natural it is to have cancer cells in our bodies: "Disturbing new research suggests that microscopic cancer, small cancer cells that can only been seen under a microscope, is widely prevalent. A recent study of women in their 40s indicated that 40 percent of them had microscopic breast cancer. Even more shocking, almost 100 percent of people in their 70s will have microscopic cancer in their thyroid glands."[6] The lesson in sharing this is how critical is it to bolster our immune systems.

On his blog, Dr. Mark Hyman explains his belief that cancer is a result of an imbalance of the immune system that makes it unable to fight off tumors—and that our goal should be to make the body inhospitable to cancer. An advocate for prevention, he says we should think of ourselves as farmers cultivating the land in which we want to grow our crops.[7] Cancer, in this analogy, is like root rot or an infestation of locusts. Healthy soil is a body so resilient and healthy that pests and pestilence like these can't take hold in it.

The place to begin boosting your immunity is in the gut. If your gut is not working correctly—for example, you're experiencing bloating, cramps, constipation, diarrhea—then you need to intervene. In addition to eating high-fiber foods, consider establishing a cleansing regimen of juicing with beet juice and green juices, and colonics to get things moving. Also, take prebiotic and probiotic supplements (see Chapter 3) to repopulate the beneficial bacteria that help us with absorption of vitamins and other nutrients.

#7. Hydrate with Purified Water

Clean drinking water is so important! Tap water is filled with toxic pollutants, including chlorine and even pharmaceutical drugs, so invest in a water filter. Your body needs to stay well hydrated to function at its best.

It's easy to become dehydrated, so drink copious amounts of filtered water at staggered intervals, approximately a cup an hour. Good hydration will contribute to the body's natural process of eliminating toxins. The idea is to be well-hydrated on a continuous basis, not to drown yourself.

In her book *Quench*, integrative physician Dana Cohen, M.D., describes how she began to notice a trend among her patients of dehydration and connected the dots between this and many of their health complaints. She says that drinking water at regular intervals throughout the day is good, but we must also eat fruits and vegetables with high water content. Drinking too much plain water can flush nutrients out of our tissues. High water content produce infuses us with valuable electrolytes and the fiber in the plants helps us achieve deep hydration.[8]

A Word about a Vegan Diet vs. a Meat-Inclusive Diet for Healing Cancer

The subject of whether a vegan (or vegetarian) diet or an omnivorous diet is the best for healing cancer is controversial. There are many who advocate for either position. I strongly advise you to use your inner guidance system to determine what works best for you in boosting your immune system and strengthening your body.

Sometimes physicians will specifically recommend that individuals undergoing treatment for cancer add some red meat to their diets. This usually happens if they have identified a deficiency of iron or a need for a surge of protein. However, there are numerous sources of quick protein other than red meat, should you choose to avoid it.

Christiane Northrup, M.D., whose advice has been followed by women around the world, recommends eating a lean protein (poultry, egg, beans, as you prefer) at every meal when healing cancer.

The diet that works for me personally is 80 percent plant-based and 20 percent meat (inclusive of grass-fed beef, game meat, organic free-range chicken, and wild-caught fish). However, I avoid dairy and gluten.

Some people are truly able to thrive from a completely plant-based diet. There are plenty of vegan healing diet advocates who swear their 100 percent approach helped them heal: Kris Carr, author of *Crazy Sexy Cancer* and other books, who now has been living happily and productively with vascular cancer for more than 15 years, for one. Chris Wark, author of *Chris Beat Cancer*, who survived stage IIIC colon cancer at age 26 and declined to take physician-recommended chemotherapy after surgery, is another. He eats fish but advocates for a vegan diet when healing cancer. Other well-respected individuals say the same.

The key question for you to answer is: Does eating meat, poultry, or fish make you feel stronger and more energized or does it seem to drain your energy? Either way, you'll mainly be feasting on plant-based foods and changing the environment in which your cells are grown.

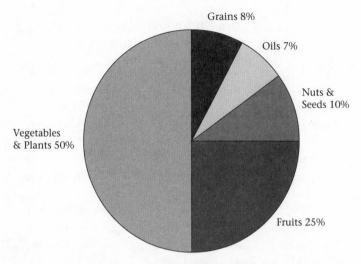

Figure 1. Cancer-Free with Food Healing Garden

Cancer-Free with Food

Grains 8%	Fruits 25%
Oils 7%	Vegetables & Plants 50%
Nuts & Seeds 10%	

Ideally all organic, without pesticide and herbicides
+ then add options (your choice for what fits your body)
MEAT: Must be organic, grass-fed beef, free-range chicken
& wild-caught fish
DAIRY: Must be organic, from a farm you trust

Welcome to the cancer-healing garden. It's a great place for a picnic. This garden is abundant with nutrient-rich, brightly colored, and vibrant produce—fruits, vegetables, herbs, seeds, and nuts. It has spiritual and energetic properties too. Remember, food is more than its individual components. There is more to food than the fats, protein, and vitamins it contains. When you make food at home, be sure to add love to the recipe. Can you pick the ingredients you'll cook with yourself? Can you practice feeling gratitude while you're stirring the pot? Can you farm the ingredients in your backyard? There's tremendous healing energy in raising and picking your own produce.

CHAPTER 2

THE TOP 15 CANCER-HEALING FOODS

The doctors and nutritional experts with whom I have spoken, and the articles and research studies I have spent almost a decade reading, all point to the same information: As much as 75 percent of cancer can be linked to our choices. The good news, however, is that we also have proof that specific foods are useful for preventing *and* healing cancer.

Woo-hoo! We've got this! Habits can be broken. Choices can be changed. As the proverb states, "No matter how far you have gone on the wrong road, you can always turn back."

HIGH-NUTRIENT SUPERFOODS

Researchers studying dietary factors associated with cancer have learned that there are significant associations between cancer risk and the low intakes of specific nutrients. This fact is important to more than just residents of impoverished areas and inhabitants of famine-stricken nations. In the West, we overeat but are undernourished. And when we are nutrient-deficient, we are at risk for cancer.

Cancer cells are distorted versions of healthy cells. Knowing this, we can focus on feeding the body the nutrients that support healthy cellular function. The fastest way to promote healing is to put a high number of nutritious compounds into the body so it has what it needs to kill aggressive cancer cells. Superfoods—foods rich in compounds that are considered especially beneficial for our health and well-being—are much more powerful than cancer. These foods, which are the foundation of the Cancer-Free with Food plan, help kill cancer cells before they take up residence in our bodies and stop existing tumors from growing any further.

It is up to you to put these foods into your body to make it impossible for cancer to find a home. Higher intakes of nutrients like vitamin C, carotenoids, retinol, and alpha-tocopherol (a vitamin found in olive and sunflower oils, whole grains, nuts, and leafy green vegetables), as well as fiber, lower our overall risk. Many studies show that those who eat a Mediterranean-style diet have the most protection against colorectal, prostate, aerodigestive tract (mouth, esophagus, pharynx, and larynx), and breast cancer. And it improves cancer mortality rates. In countries like Greece and Italy, people regularly consume foods like vegetables, olive oil, nuts, seeds, fruit, fish, and fiber.

The Cancer-Free with Food recipes contain all of these ingredients. It's about filling up your body on the good stuff from the foods in the list to come.

FILL UP YOUR BODY WITH THE GOOD STUFF

Never forget that food can be powerful medicine. The food you choose to eat can either assist you in healing your body or in destroying it. So, every day from now on, I want you to ask yourself: "Am I eating enough cancer-fighting foods?"

Fueling your body on real, wholesome ingredients is fulfilling, so it satisfies urges you might have previously experienced for sugar, fat, and fried foods. For example, if you eat enough good, healthy fats like the ones from avocados and flaxseeds, your cravings for fried foods should diminish.

When you alkalize your body with broccoli sprouts and dark green, leafy vegetables, you will be less likely to binge on highly acidic foods, especially once you get some momentum going. And when you are eating a sufficient amount of fresh fruits, especially blueberries, it can satisfy your sweet tooth.

What exactly makes some foods cancer *causing* and others cancer *healing*? The following foods are incredibly high in antioxidants, so they reduce inflammation. They are also more alkaline than other foods. And they have been proven in studies to kill cancer cells and stop tumor growth. If you are going through cancer treatment right now, these will assist your healing because they contain potent, cancer- killing compounds. If you want to prevent cancer, they will help you stay healthy.

#1 CANCER-HEALING FOOD: BROCCOLI SPROUTS

I became absolutely fascinated with broccoli sprouts when I discovered they are incredibly potent killers of cancer cells because of their unusually high sulforaphane content.[1] Sulforaphane is also found in broccoli, spinach, kale, cauliflower, bok choy, cabbage, and brussels sprouts. But broccoli sprouts contain the most of any other vegetable on the planet.

Paul Talalay, M.D., a professor of pharmacology and molecular sciences at the Johns Hopkins University School of Medicine, who has done research for 25 years on vegetable compounds, is a major advocate of broccoli spouts. He says: "Three-day-old broccoli sprouts consistently contain 20 to 50 times the amount of chemoprotective compounds found in mature broccoli heads and may offer a simple dietary means of chemically reducing cancer risk."[2] In 1992, Talalay and his research team found that sulforaphane has the ability to reinforce the body's natural defenses against oxidative stress, inflammation, and DNA damage.[3]

Over the years, many studies by other researchers have supported Dr. Talalay's conclusions.[4] One by Jed Fahey, Sc.D., director of the Cullman Chemoprotection Center at Johns Hopkins University, proved that broccoli sprouts provide "dramatic protection" against digestive issues, including stomach cancer, ulcers, gastritis, and overgrowths of Helicobacter pylori, a bacterium "strongly associated with inflammation related to digestive cancers."[5]

During an experiment involving 48 patients with H. pylori infections in which half the volunteers ate 2.5 ounces of broccoli sprouts per day for two months, and half ate the equivalent amount of alfalfa sprouts, which do not contain sulforaphane, biomarkers of infection dropped for the volunteers eating the broccoli sprouts.[6]

Broccoli Sprouts Are Good for All Cancer, and Especially Useful for . . .

- Stomach cancer
- Colon cancer
- Prostate cancer
- Bladder cancer[7]
- Breast cancer[8]
- Liver cancer
- Brain cancer

If you are doing chemo, radiation, and surgery, you may have a higher risk of developing an infection, so I would strongly advise incorporating broccoli sprouts into your diet at this time.

Suggested "Dosage"

- To heal cancer: 2.5 ounces of broccoli sprouts per day
- To prevent cancer: 2.5 ounces of broccoli sprouts every third day

Cancer-Free with Food Recipes with Broccoli Sprouts

- Anticancer Omelet (page 205)
- Superpowerful Green Juice (page 148)

- The Big 3: Anti-Inflammatory Blueberry Broccoli Sprouts Turmeric Juice (page 149)
- Zucchini Pasta with Broccoli Sprouts Pesto (page 212)
- Broccoli Sprout Guacamole (page 298)

Ways of Incorporating Broccoli Sprouts in Your Cancer-Healing Kitchen

Since reading all the studies, I have made broccoli sprouts a weekly staple on my shopping list. I pick up a small container once a week and add sprouts to my juices and smoothies, and use them as garnishes on soups, salads, and gluten-free pasta. To save money, consider growing broccoli sprouts in your own kitchen!

Dr. Mehmet Oz says, "Broccoli sprouts are best when eaten raw in order to absorb the full nutrient and cancer-fighting properties including glucosinolates, which can prevent cancer."[9] Ways to incorporate broccoli sprouts into your diet include:

- Eat them raw by the handful.
- Juice them.
- Add them to your salads, soups, and smoothies.

#2 Cancer-Healing Food: Turmeric

Turmeric root is perhaps the most studied and talked about food for preventing and fighting cancer. In fact, it is so powerful that MD Anderson Cancer Center formed a Center for Cancer Prevention by Dietary Botanicals specifically to evaluate the efficacy of using ginger, black pepper, and turmeric—a trio of spices routinely used in Indian food—to heal and prevent colorectal cancer.[10]

Okay, so we hear about turmeric all the time, but why is it *so* good? To break it down, turmeric is an anti-inflammatory, antioxidant, anticancer, and brain-protecting superfood. The spice made from turmeric root gives curry its bright-yellow color. It has its superpowers because it contains three potent compounds: curcumin, demethoxycurcumin, and bisdemethoxycurcumin.[11]

No matter how you do it, consuming turmeric is a no-brainer! The curcuminoid compounds in turmeric have been shown to decrease tumor size in cases of colon, prostate, and breast cancer.

Memorial Sloan Kettering Cancer Center published a study with rats who were exposed to cancer-causing substances. They then treated them with turmeric and found they were protected from colon, stomach, and skin cancers. How amazing is that? Furthermore, in this same study, the replication of tumor cells stopped when turmeric was applied directly to them in the laboratory.[12]

Other laboratory experiments have shown that curcuminoids protect the body in a few more ways: They enhance the activity of a crucial detoxifying enzyme and act as antioxidants by neutralizing free radicals (which cause DNA damage).[13] Detoxifying the body is one of the beneficial healing strategies discussed in Chapter 5.

There is hope for healing colon cancer with turmeric. Functional medicine expert Dr. Mark Hyman recommends turmeric root to reduce gut-based inflammation.[14] Michael Greger, M.D., founding member of the American College of Lifestyle Medicine and author of *How Not to Die*, states that the low incidence of bowel cancer in India is often attributed to natural antioxidants such as curcumin (the yellow pigment in the spice turmeric used in curry powder), which the majority of Indians consume on a daily basis.[15] And in one small study in 2006, patients at high risk for colon cancer who received 480 milligrams of curcumin and 20 milligrams of quercetin (found in red onions and grapes) three times a day realized a decrease in the number and size of polyps in their colons.[16]

If you are undergoing a course of radiation treatment, it may interest you to know that turmeric may help to reduce skin irritation and damage from radiation, according to the National Center for Complementary and Integrative Health and Mayo Clinic.[17,18]

Turmeric Is Especially Good for . . .

- Breast cancer[19]
- Prostate cancer
- Stomach cancer
- Skin cancer
- Pancreatic cancer[20]
- Colon cancer[21]

- Lung cancer[22]
- Bladder cancer[23]
- Ovarian cancer[24]
- Cervical cancer[25]
- Lymphoma[26]
- Oral cancer[27]

Suggested "Dosage"

- Consume 2 teaspoons of turmeric powder per day in curry or as a supplement.
- If using a curcumin powder supplement, follow the package instructions.

Caution: If you are undergoing a course of chemotherapy, please check with your doctor. There is some conflicting advice regarding turmeric; some reports say it may interfere with chemotherapy drugs and others say it can make chemo even more effective.[28]

Turmeric can stain the teeth. To avoid staining, swish and spit out water with activated charcoal toothpaste after eating.

Cancer-Free with Food Recipes with Turmeric

- Golden Milk (page 161)
- Sick-Kick Smoothie (page 169)
- Pain-Relieving Tea (page 187)

- Almond Turmeric Crusted Chicken Tenders (page 287)
- Turmeric Rice (page 237)

Ways of Incorporating Turmeric in Your Cancer-Healing Kitchen

- Turmeric can be used in its whole, raw form (it's a root that looks similar to ginger but smaller) or in its powdered form.

- Incorporate more curry powder into your foods; it always contains turmeric as one of the ingredients.

- Add turmeric powder to water, juice, smoothies, eggs, salads, soups, or veggie stir-fry. You can incorporate this daily, especially if you do have cancer.

- Make a big batch of soothing curry with chickpeas and quinoa.

- Make a turmeric paste with 1 teaspoon turmeric, ¼ teaspoon black pepper, and 2 teaspoons of water (though it may not be tasty).You can store the paste in the fridge and stir it into a recipe like a vegetable stir-fry, quinoa, or add to a smoothie.

- To enhance absorption, try cooking your turmeric in a bit of extra-virgin olive oil. Also add black pepper at a ratio of ¼ teaspoon black pepper for every teaspoon of turmeric.

- Boil turmeric root and make a tea.

- Add a smidgen of turmeric powder to green tea or ginger tea.

- Buy turmeric or curcumin supplements.

#3 CANCER-HEALING FOOD: BLUEBERRIES

Blueberries are a powerful anticancer superfruit. When tested among 20 fruits, guess which one ranked first for antioxidant capacity? Blueberries! The reason? Mainly their many phytochemicals, including anthocyanins, catechins, quercetin, kaempferol, and other flavonoids (these are antibacterial); ellagitannins and ellagic acid; and pterostilbene and resveratrol.[29] They also contain vitamins C and K, manganese, and fiber.

The American Cancer Society writes: "Anthocyanidins, as well as other molecules present in blueberry, would slow the progression of cancer by blocking the development of blood vessels feeding the malignant cells. This antiangiogenic process deprives cancer cells of their supply of oxygen and nutrient molecules needed to reproduce, which makes it a powerful anticancer food."[30]

Blueberries are definitely my berry of choice. While they are sweet enough to satisfy my sweet tooth, they don't spike blood sugar or create an acid-forming environment in which cancer cells can grow. If you're not as big a fan as I am, cranberries, blackberries, raspberries, strawberries, golden berries, and goji berries closely follow blueberries in their antioxidant capacity. Try one type, or try them all. Berries can help you introduce plenty of variety to your meals.

Studies show that blueberries protect the brain, prevent damage to our DNA, and inhibit cancer cell development.[31] Basically, you can imagine that the blueberries you eat are little (beneficial) bombs that go off in your body and increase the pace of natural programmed cancer cell death (apoptosis). They have been proven to kill cancer cells and reduce tumor size—how cool is this! Where's my bowl?

Blueberries Are Especially Good for . . .

- Breast cancer [32]
- Colon cancer
- Bladder cancer
- Lung cancer
- Esophageal cancer
- Skin cancer
- Prostate cancer
- Leukemia
- Cervical cancer[33]

Suggested "Dosage"

- If you have cancer, enjoy 1 ½ cups of blueberries per day—in one or two servings. (This amount is based on findings from a Rutgers University animal study of pterostilbene extract, an antioxidant that comes from blueberry. The animals that ate blueberry extract reduced precancerous lesions in their colons by 57 percent more than animals that didn't.)[34]
- To prevent cancer, have ½ cup per day, or every few days.

Cancer-Free with Food Recipes with Blueberries

- The Big 3: Anti-inflammatory Blueberry Broccoli Sprouts Turmeric Juice (page 149)
- Berry Green Juice (page 154)
- Chocolate Nut Berry Smoothie (page 176)
- Liana's Favorite Smoothie Bowl (page 182)
- Blueberry Chia Seed Pudding (page 334)

Ways of Incorporating Blueberries in Your Cancer-Healing Kitchen

Because blueberries are such a wonderful source of vitamin C, MD Anderson Cancer Center put them on its list of the top five foods to reduce cancer risk.[35] Add blueberries wherever you can! Get creative. I add blueberries to juices, smoothies, cereal, and desserts. I'm fond of adding them to the Chocolate Block. In addition:

- You may eat blueberries fresh, frozen, dried, or powdered—all forms are good.
- Eat blueberries as a stand-alone snack.
- Freeze fresh blueberries for an icy treat.

#4 CANCER-HEALING FOOD: BROCCOLI

I love when studies are done to show that vegetables have anticancer properties. Broccoli is, of course, one of the most studied among the vegetable family. Broccoli gets its own section here, separate from broccoli sprouts, because they have vast nutritional differences. They are completely different ingredients, both beneficial in their own right. Research shows that broccoli contains "compounds that may protect the body from stomach cancer, as well as cancers of the mouth, pharynx, larynx, and esophagus."[36] And when we break down broccoli, we can see why.

This mighty, green, treelike veg is in the cruciferous vegetable family, along with cauliflower, cabbage, brussels sprouts, bok choy, and kale. They are all excellent or good sources of immune-boosting vitamins, nutrients, and phytochemicals: vitamin C, sulforaphane, manganese, vitamin K, folate, vitamin B, potassium, fiber, magnesium, and carotenoids, such as beta-carotene. Carotenoids inhibit cancer growth, support the immune system, and aid vision and skin health.[37] Broccoli is also rich in glucosinolates, a compound found in all cruciferous vegetables. Glucosinolates form isothiocyanates and indoles, which are known to prevent tumor growth and decrease the production of cancer cells, which stop cancer from being able to survive in the body.[38]

In a five-year study of patients in Spanish hospitals, researchers observed a reduced risk of cancer by those who consumed broccoli and pumpkin. They concluded that the frequent consumption of leafy greens and other vegetables might be associated with a reduced risk of lung cancer.[39]

Broccoli Is Especially Good for . . .

- Lung cancer
- Stomach cancer
- Breast cancer
- Oral cancer
- Pharynx cancer
- Larynx cancer
- Esophageal cancer
- Prostate cancer[40]

Suggested "Dosage"

- If you have cancer, eat 1 to 2 cups of broccoli per day.
- To prevent cancer, eat ½ cup at least every third day.

The National Cancer Institute reports that three or more servings of cruciferous vegetables (broccoli, cauliflower, cabbage, bok choy, brussels sprouts) a week may reduce prostate cancer risk by nearly 50 percent.[41] Empowering info!

Cancer-Free with Food Recipes with Broccoli

- Broccoli Popcorn (page 224)
- Anticancer Veggie Stir-Fry (page 238)
- Pasta Primavera (page 230)
- Mason Jar Salad (page 256)
- Energy Soup (page 268)

Ways of Incorporating Broccoli in Your Cancer-Healing Kitchen

There are so many ways to eat broccoli! You can eat it raw, steamed, or roasted with some olive oil, garlic, and sea salt. My favorite way to eat broccoli is roasted and sprinkled with some nutritional yeast so it tastes a bit like cheesy popcorn. It makes a great side dish or even an entire meal. You could:

- Puree steamed broccoli with avocado, garlic, and hemp or tigernut milk for a refreshing cold soup.
- Dip raw broccoli into guacamole or hummus for a snack.
- Add broccoli to soups or vegetable and bone broths.
- Add broccoli to smoothies or juices.

#5 Cancer-Healing Food: Flaxseed

Flaxseed (also known as linseed) can be ground into a flour called flax meal and cold-pressed into an oil. Flaxseed is one of the top anticancer foods due to the alpha-linolenic acid (ALA) it contains, which is a prime source of omega-3 fatty acids. ALA protects the kidneys from damage.

Flaxseed and flaxseed oil are great vegan sources of omega-3s. Having a sufficient amount of omega-3 in the body is good for the brain, and can help prevent the depressive moods that are a common symptom of a cancer diagnosis.[42]

- Adding more flax to your diet is an incredibly promising action for reducing cancer risk. Flaxseed also contain lignans, a type of phytoestrogen that changes estrogen metabolism because it binds to some of the same receptors.[43] Animal studies have shown that the lignans in flaxseed oil reduce breast cancer growth and spread.[44] Cancer prevention studies of postmenopausal women showed that flaxseed supplementation improved the ratio of hormones in women's bodies, making them less hospitable environments for cancer to occur.[45] One study with mice shows it may work well alone or as an adjunct to Tamoxifen, a drug used to prevent breast cancer recurrence.[46]

Flaxseed Is Especially Good for . . .

- Breast cancer[47]
- Colon cancer[48]
- Skin cancer[49]
- Colorectal cancer
- Endometrial cancer

- Lung cancer
- Prostate cancer[50]
- Side effects of radiation therapy[51]

Cancer-Free with Food Recipes with Flaxseed

- Flax Milk
- Superfood Kale Salad
- A Splash of Sunshine Smoothie

- Bean Burgers
- Chocolate Hazelnut Cake

Ways of Incorporating Flaxseed in Your Cancer-Healing Kitchen

- Add flaxseed or flax meal to your cereal, oatmeal, smoothies, and salads.

- Grind up flaxseeds yourself at home to make a meal or flax flour, or buy flax meal and add to cereals and oatmeal.

- You can use flax meal instead of eggs in baking. Just mix 3 teaspoons of flax meal and 4 teaspoons of water, then let the mixture sit for 10 minutes and it will get gummy, like eggs.

- Add to grass-fed beef meatballs and lentil loaf.

- Add flax oil to your eggs, smoothies, salads, and soups.

#6 CANCER-HEALING FOOD: DARK LEAFY GREENS

Darky leafy greens play a crucial role in overall health. Many compounds in dark leafy vegetables are praiseworthy, including isothiocyanates (in this case, sulforaphane and erucin), which help the body detox at the cellular level.[52] Dark leafy greens have antibacterial and antiviral properties, inactivate carcinogens, and help reprogram cancer cells to die off! This prevents tumor formation and metastasis. One research group isolated a compound from spinach, and after testing, concluded it has great potential for development as an effective clinical anticancer chemotherapy.[53]

Greens are loaded with vitamins, minerals, flavonoids, and chlorophyll.[54] Some people have even gone so far as to say that drinking a green juice made with dark leafy greens—especially mixed with coconut water—is the equivalent of a blood transfusion. This is why I've drunk a green juice every day for the past nine years. Make your new motto "A dark leafy green juice a day can keep cancer far, far away!"

Dark leafy greens must be purchased organic, as they are highly absorbent to pesticides and herbicides. Dark leafy greens include:

- Arugula
- Bok choy
- Cilantro
- Collard greens
- Kale
- Parsley
- Romaine (not as dark as some greens, but certainly highly nutritious)

- Spinach
- Watercress, which some believe is a more potent superfood than kale![55]

Dark Leafy Greens Are Good for All Cancer, and Especially Useful for . . .

- Lung cancer
- Leukemia

- Lymphatic cancers
- Brain Cancer

Suggested "Dosage"

- If you have cancer, eat up to 8 cups of leafy greens daily.
- To prevent cancer, eat at least 1 cup of leafy greens daily in a salad, soup, or juice.

Cancer-Free with Food Recipes with Dark Leafy Greens

- Superfood Kale Salad (page 245)
- Super Powerful Green Juice (page 148)
- Classic Green Smoothie (page 174)
- Five-Ingredient Green Salad (page 244)
- Super Detox Broccoli Sprout Green Salad (page 245)

Ways of Incorporating Dark Leafy Greens in Your Cancer-Healing Kitchen

- Add leafy greens to your smoothie or juice.
- Make a salad out of a mixture of them.
- Add a handful of leafy greens to your lunch and dinner to increase your nutrient intake.

#7 Cancer-Healing Food: Garlic

Garlic has many medicinal properties that have benefited people from cultures around the world for centuries. Delicious as well as healthful, garlic's close relatives include the onion, shallot, leek, and chive.

Garlic boosts the functions of the immune system. One study found that it elicits anti-inflammatory and antioxidant responses that prime our bodies to eradicate emerging tumors.[56]

Epidemiologic studies indicate that garlic consumption is associated with decreased risk of cancer at every stage of its development, particularly for cancers of the gastrointestinal tract.[57] And an extract of garlic has also been investigated for its potential as a nontoxic treatment for breast cancer tumors with significant preliminary results in a study on mice.[58]

Garlic Is Especially Good for . . .

- Esophageal cancer
- Stomach cancer
- Throat cancer
- Brain cancer
- Colon cancer

- Breast cancer[59]
- Lymphatic cancer
- Blood cancer, including leukemia
- Bladder cancer[60]

Suggested "Dosage"

- If you have cancer, consume 1 to 2 cloves (10 to 20 grams) daily.
- To prevent cancer, consume 1 clove (10 grams) daily.

Cancer-Free with Food Recipes with Garlic

- Tangy Ginger-Garlic Dressing (page 259)
- Chickpea Burgers (page 220)

- Dr. Oz's Sautéed Portobello Mushrooms (page 218)
- Lentil Soup (page 275)
- Mediterranean Omelet (page 206)

Ways of Incorporating Garlic in Your Cancer-Healing Kitchen

- Add a raw garlic clove to smoothies and juices.
- Roast an entire garlic bulb with some olive oil and sea salt.
- Take garlic supplements.
- Swallow an entire garlic clove.

- Buy garlic powder and/or garlic salt (or make your own with garlic powder and sea salt).

- Add garlic to your eggs.

- Buy crushed garlic (packaged in olive oil, no other preservatives) and always keep it on hand in your fridge in case you need to quickly add it to salad dressings, soups, stir-fry, meat dishes, or eggs.

- You must buy organic garlic! Unfortunately, much of the world's supply of garlic is bleached white.

- Grow your own garlic by adding a bulb to some water. Once it grows roots, you can place it in the ground or potted soil! Mmm, what is better than your own fresh garlic?!

#8 Cancer-Healing Food: Mushrooms

Mushrooms have mega-medicinal properties! They are among the few edible sources of vitamin D. There are thousands of mushroom species to choose from; however, not all are cancer preventative or healing.

Reishi, cordyceps, and maitake are known to be packed with anti-inflammatory and immune-boosting compounds. These types have been used to fight cancer for centuries.[61] They inhibit tumor growth and also help the body create new healthy cells, so definitely consider including them in your diet if you're undergoing chemo and radiation. Beta-glucan, a naturally occurring chemical in mushrooms, stimulates cell healing and improves immune function.[62]

For breast cancer, try Ganoderma mushrooms, which suppress tumor growth by altering lipid metabolism and triggering cell death.[63]

For colorectal cancer, try chaga mushrooms.[64] Please follow the recommended dosages on the back of the package in which you buy it.

I interviewed Ocean Robbins, founder of Food Revolution Network, for this book and he pointed me to a study done in Australia that indicates we should all be eating mushrooms regularly and in conjunction with green tea. In his book *31-Day*

Food Revolution, he highlights a 2004 study of 2,000 Chinese women, roughly half with breast cancer, conducted by the University of Western Australia, Perth.[65] He writes:

> The scientists reviewed the women's eating habits and factored out other variables that contribute to cancer, such as being overweight, lack of exercise, and smoking. They came to a startling conclusion about mushrooms.[66]

Women who consumed at least a third of an ounce of fresh mushrooms per day (less than one typical-size mushroom) were 64 percent less likely to develop breast cancer. Dried mushrooms had a slightly less protective effect, reducing the risk by around half. What was even more impressive is that women who combined eating mushrooms with regular consumption of green tea saw an even greater benefit—they reduced their breast cancer risk by an astounding 89 percent.

Why are mushrooms so powerful? They are thought to protect against breast and other hormone-related cancers because they inhibit an enzyme called aromatase, which produces estrogen.[67] Mushrooms also contain specialized lectins that recognize cancer cells and prevent these cells from growing and dividing. (Lectins, a type of carbohydrate-binding protein, have gotten a bad reputation in some circles, but some of them, such as the ones in mushrooms, can be beneficial.)

Mushrooms Are Especially Good for . . .

- Breast cancer
- Prostate cancer
- Colorectal cancer
- Brain cancer
- Suppressing tumor growth

Suggested "Dosage"

- If you have cancer, try adding ¾ cup of shiitake or maitake mushrooms—fresh sliced and sautéed—to your main dishes.
- To prevent cancer, have the same quantity 2 to 3 times per week.

Caution: Mushrooms are not for everyone and some body types are intolerant to mushrooms. You can take a DNA or food allergy test to see if mushrooms are healthy for your body.

Cancer-Free with Food Recipes with Mushrooms

- Mushroom Soup (page 276)
- Dr. Oz's Sautéed Portobello Mushrooms (page 218)
- Roasted Hazelnut Chocolate Block (page 331)

Ways of Incorporating Mushrooms in Your Cancer-Healing Kitchen

- Cook with fresh mushrooms at home and add them to your stir-fries and soups.
- Add raw mushrooms to your salads.
- You can take mushrooms in capsule form as a supplement.
- Check out mushroom-infused tea, coffee, and hot chocolate!
- Get a mushroom powder and add it to smoothies and even to desserts like chocolate.

#9 CANCER-HEALING FOOD: CACAO

I am a strong advocate for the healing power of cacao. Cacao is the main ingredient in pure chocolate before it is made into the treat as we know it. Usually, after cacao is harvested, it is taken and heat-processed to make it into cocoa powder. Because of the heat, cocoa does not have as many nutrients as a raw cacao powder. Raw cacao powder is very high in nutrients and minerals.

Cacao is superhigh in magnesium, a mineral that relaxes our muscles and eases pain in the body; it's no wonder that we crave chocolate! Cacao contains polyphenolic compounds that are highly beneficial to our health. It has also been proven by the science community to be an anti-inflammatory with anti-tumor activities.[68] Cacao has been shown to have many potential anticancer compounds because of its high antioxidant count (40 times that of blueberries!). It has the ability to reduce inflammation, reduce the risk of obesity, and improve cardiovascular circulation.[69]

By the way, chocolate can be healthy so long as it's eaten in a "clean" form—without all the crazy ingredients that are usually added, like GMO dairy, soy lecithin, and refined white sugar. Raw cacao powder is a glorious gift from God, but it's not for everyone because it is high in caffeine. If you want the antioxidant goodness of cacao in chocolate form, purchase a clean chocolate. (I offer a brand on my website.)

The physiological effects of caffeine and theobromine, the most abundant methylxanthines in cacao, are notable. Theobromine is a heart stimulant and vasodilator—meaning, it widens blood vessels. It is used to treat high blood pressure and is also a diuretic. All these benefits assist in keeping the body in a state less hospitable to cancer. A study showed that theobromine might be extremely effective in preventing human glioblastoma (brain tumors).[70]

Caffeine from tea or coffee helps increase stamina and focus, and has a positive effect on memory, which can help you if you are experiencing "chemo brain," the foggy thinking that is a side effect of chemotherapy. It also has many other known health benefits (as long as consumed in moderation) and has been observed to decrease risk of certain cancers, including endometrial cancer.[71,72]

These health-promoting benefits are so remarkable that chocolate is being explored as a functional food, useful for improving cardiovascular health.[73] Research is currently being done on the effects of cacao on aging, oxidative stress, blood pressure regulation, and atherosclerosis.[74] It appears to have the potential for lowering the risk of cardiovascular disease-related hypercoagulation due to hypercholesterolemia.[75] One study revealed that cacao can help with significant reduction of body weight and body mass index (BMI).[76] Along with a lower rate of obesity comes a lower risk of developing cancer.

Researchers investigating colitis-associated cancer found that a cacao treatment reduced inflammation, increased enzyme activity, and upped the presence of antioxidants. Although not definitive yet, the results suggest that cacao may prevent the development of colon cancer in humans.[77]

Patients with inflammatory bowel disease are at risk for developing ulcerative colitis–associated with colorectal cancer. However, another study of mice found that cacao significantly decreased tumor incidence and size. In addition to inhibiting proliferation of tumor epithelial cells, the findings also demonstrated that a cacao-rich diet suppresses the formation and growth of tumors.[78]

Cacao Is Especially Good for . . .

- Most cancers
- Breast cancer
- Cervical cancer
- Endometrial cancer
- Ovarian cancer
- Brain cancer

- Colon cancer
- For reducing the pain, depression, and anxiety side effects of cancer or from undergoing conventional treatments

Suggested "Dosage"

- If you have cancer, consume 26 to 60 grams of cacao per day, which is roughly 1 to 2 average-size "clean" chocolate bars or 1 to 2 tablespoons cacao powder.

- To prevent cancer, have 26 to 40 grams per day, about one "clean" chocolate bar. Or eat ½ to 1 tablespoon cacao powder.

Caution: Cacao contains natural caffeine, just like coffee and tea. Caffeine is not for everyone, especially if you have overconsumed it for years or have adrenal burnout.

Make sure to buy organic cacao that is labeled "fair trade." Chocolate is a huge industry, and major corporations associated with it have been found to use slave labor. You don't want to support that industry or consume the energy of that.

Cancer-Free with Food Recipes with Cacao

- Classic Three-Ingredient Chocolate Balls (page 324)
- Cashew Ice Cream with Chocolate Sauce (page 329)
- Chocolate Almond Butter Cups (page 332)
- Roasted Hazelnut Chocolate Block (page 331)
- Chocolate Avocado Mousse (page 328)

Ways of Incorporating Cacao in Your Cancer-Healing Kitchen

- The quickest way to satisfy a chocolate craving is to add 1 to 3 teaspoons cacao to a nut milk (for example, almond milk or tigernut milk) with some ice and dates (remove the seed), then blend it into a refreshing chocolate shake! You can also add superfoods like chia seed, hemp seed, or flaxseed, which pair well with banana, almond butter or peanut butter, and some honey. Absolutely delicious!

- For a hot chocolate, simply boil some water, add a couple tablespoonfuls of cacao powder, and then some nut milk.

- Use cacao when making desserts. In traditional recipes that call for cocoa powder, you can replace the cocoa with cacao for a more nutrient-rich preparation.

- Sprinkle cacao powder on oatmeal, Chia Seed Cereal, or fruit.

- Make a Chocolate Mousse by blending avocado and adding cacao powder and some maple syrup.

- Health benefits of cacao can also be accrued from smelling the aroma of cacao powder. Always make a point to take a good whiff of the cacao before you add it to a recipe.

#10 CANCER-HEALING FOOD: TIGERNUTS

A tigernut is a root vegetable—a tuber. It is called a tiger "nut" simply because of its appearance. (Once you see one, you'll know what I mean.) Tigernut is a vegetable our ancestors discovered a long time ago and would have relied on as a source of iron and prebiotic starch. A prebiotic starch is a substance that promotes health by encouraging the growth of probiotics, which are "friendly" gut flora (bacteria) such as bifidobacteria and lactobacilli.

Believe it or not, tigernut has the same amount of iron as red meat. Because tigernut is such an excellent source of iron, it is a vegetarian's best friend! People are just learning about tigernuts as they begin to surface in the mainstream. Every household should be stocked with tigernuts, tigernut flour, and tigernut milk because of their incredible health benefits, which include their anticancer properties.

One of my favorite root vegetables, tigernuts are high in fiber and resistant starch. Resistant starch has a similar physiologic effect as dietary fiber and can function as a milk laxative. Tigernuts are a viscous starch that is highly valued as a component in some functional foods.[79] They won me over as soon as I heard about them.

It's easy to grow your own tigernuts. When you purchase a bag of them, simply plant some in soil and water them every couple of days. Soon you will start to see grass-like shoots come up, and after about a month, you can pull up a whole cluster of new tigernuts. These low-maintenance plants grow like weeds, independently, without pesticides.

Eating tigernuts is good for the environment as well as your body. Tigernut milk can be made simply by tossing a quarter cup of tigernuts in four cups of water and giving them a spin in a blender. By contrast, almond trees require a lot of water and are often farmed using pesticides. Plus, store-bought almond milk is often pasteurized, which changes its nutritional value. Tigernut milk is naturally sweet—no cane sugar is generally added to the store-bought variety, like it is to many brands of nut milk.

One study showed that tigernut milk can be useful for preventing liver damage from the pain reliever acetaminophen! Researchers concluded that the phytochemicals in tigernut milk significantly prevented liver injury.[80] So drink tigernut milk for its liver-protecting properties during chemotherapy, when your liver is in danger of being overwhelmed with toxins.

Tigernuts Are Especially Good for...

- Breast cancer
- Prostate cancer
- Ovarian cancer
- Liver cancer

Suggested "Dosage"

- If you have cancer, consume 50 tigernuts (30 grams) daily. This amount could come from one serving of Tigernut milk.
- To prevent cancer, have the same dosage, but every 2 to 3 days.

Cancer-Free with Food Recipes with Tigernuts

- Iron-Boosting Tigernut Milk (page 162)
- Chocolate Tigernut Milk (page 162)
- Use tigernut flour in the Cookie Dough recipe (page 326) instead of almond flour.

Ways of Incorporating Tigernuts in Your Cancer-Healing Kitchen

- Soak tigernuts to make them easier to chew, and then add them to oatmeal and cereal. Tigernuts are extremely tough, so you want to soak them at least overnight, or buy the "peeled" variety.
- Use tigernut flour to make brownies and cookies.
- Eat them as a naturally sweet, filling snack when you crave sugar.
- Make Tigernut Milk instead of almond milk! It's so easy. Put ¼ cup tigernuts and 4 cups of water in a blender and combine—then add a dash of sea salt and/or vanilla, to taste (optional). I also add cacao powder to make it a Chocolate Tigernut Milk.

#11 CANCER-HEALING FOOD: GINGER ROOT

Ginger root contains gingerol, a natural chemical that kills and starves cancer cells. It also aids the body in detoxification by helping drain the lymphatic system and boosting the function of the digestive tract. Raw ginger is composed of 79 percent water and contains vitamin B_6 and the essential dietary minerals magnesium and manganese.

Ginger Root Is Especially Good for . . .

- Colon cancer[81]
- Gastrointestinal cancer[82]
- Skin cancer
- Lymphatic cancer
- Thyroid cancer
- Breast cancer
- Ovarian cancer[83]
- Prostate cancer[84]
- Relieving pain

- Easing nausea that is the side effect of chemo or radiation
- Treating dysentery, heartburn, flatulence, diarrhea, loss of appetite, infections, cough, and bronchitis— all of which are possible side effects of conventional cancer treatments

Suggested "Dosage"

- If you have cancer, consume 1 to 2 teaspoons fresh ginger root daily.
- To prevent cancer, include 2 to 3 grams of powdered ginger per day, in divided doses, or 1 teaspoon fresh grated ginger root.

Caution: If you are taking powdered ginger, Andrew Weil, M.D., suggests not taking more than 4 grams per day.[85]

If you are planning to undergo surgery, Memorial Sloan Kettering Cancer Center advises that you avoid ginger for two weeks prior to surgery and immediately afterward, due to its blood-thinning effects.[86]

Cancer-Free with Food Recipes with Ginger Root

- Lemon Ginger Shot (page 156)
- Digestion Helper Juice (page 153)
- Sick-Kick Smoothie (page 169)

- Vibrant Orange Carrot Ginger Juice (page 154)
- Turmeric Rice (page 237)

Ways of Incorporating Ginger Root in Your Cancer-Healing Kitchen

- Buy a whole raw ginger root from your local farmers market or an organic supermarket. Then chop it into chunks and boil it for a potent tea. I recommend drinking one cup of ginger tea every night before bed to help drain your lymphatic system.
- Grate raw ginger root and add it to salads, dressings, soups, meat, and/or stir-fries.
- Buy a premade dried ginger powder and use it as a spice in cooking and soups, or sprinkle it into boiling water for a quick ginger tea.
- Add ginger to your smoothies and juices.
- Buy a bottle of pure, therapeutic-grade essential oil and use a drop or two in 8 to 12 ounces of water or a green juice. Use ginger essential oil in place of raw or dried ginger elsewhere too, but add cautiously, tasting as you go so you do not overdo it.

#12 CANCER-HEALING FOOD: GRAPES

Grapes are a rich source of the antioxidant resveratrol, with red and purple grapes having significantly more than green grapes. Studies show that resveratrol has the potential to possibly stop cancer from starting in the breast, liver, stomach, and lymphatic system.[87] Be sure to leave the skin intact, as it has the most resveratrol.[88]

Grapes Are Especially Good for ...

- Breast cancer[89]
- Colorectal cancer[90]
- Skin cancer[91]

- Prostate cancer
- Ovarian cancer
- Brain cancer

Suggested "Dosage"

- If you have cancer, eat 1 cup (about 32 grapes) per day.
- To prevent cancer, eat ½ cup (about 16 grapes) per day.

Cancer-Free with Food Recipes with Grapes

- Grape Juice (page 146)
- Sweet Purple Grape Dressing (page 261)

Ways of Incorporating Grapes in Your Cancer-Healing Kitchen

- Grab a handful as a snack; one serving is about 16 grapes.
- Add grapes to a cold salad, especially one made with roasted chicken.
- Juice them to make Grape Juice.
- Freeze for a refreshing treat on a hot day.

#13 CANCER-HEALING FOOD: TOMATOES

Tomatoes are packed with lycopene, a powerful antioxidant that reduces the risk of skin cancer, breast cancer, and prostate cancer.[92] Men with prostate cancer who were surveyed reported eating fewer tomatoes than men who did not have prostate cancer.[93] Most fruits with red flesh, such as watermelon and pink grapefruit, contain lycopene.

Tomatoes are also high in vitamin C, which assists in boosting the immune system. They also have an impressive amount of vitamins A, K, and B_6, thiamin, and folate.

In one study, tomato extracts were investigated for their ability to induce cell death (apoptosis) in human cancer cells and normal cells. This is an important measure because cancer cells "forget" to die. The extracts strongly inhibited the perpetuation of human cancer cell lines that normally take up residence in the breast, colon, stomach, and liver.[94]

Tomatoes Are Especially Good for . . .

* Leukemia
* Prostate cancer[95]
* Breast cancer
* Lung cancer
* Colon cancer
* Liver cancer
* Skin cancer

Suggested "Dosage"

* If you have cancer, eat 1 cup of tomatoes, 2 small whole tomatoes, or about 20 cherry tomatoes per day.

* To prevent cancer, have the same dose as above, but every two to three days.

Caution: Tomatoes can sometimes irritate the mouth (particularly if you have canker sores or a wound) because of their acidity.

Cancer-Free with Food Recipes with Tomatoes

* Taco Salad (page 246)
* Tabbouleh (page 255)
* Immune-Boosting Soup (page 267)
* Tomato, Basil, and White Bean Soup (page 274)
* Zucchini Spaghetti with Tomato Sauce and Walnut "Meatballs" (page 213)

Ways of Incorporating Tomatoes in Your Cancer-Healing Kitchen

Cooking tomatoes boosts their powerful medicinal properties. According to Lindsey Wohlford, a wellness dietician at MD Anderson Cancer Center, "Processing the tomato ups its health-boosting power. This releases the lycopene, so it can be more easily absorbed by the body."[96]

- Eat tomatoes as they are, on their own, as a beautiful fruit.

- Make homemade Raw Tomato Sauce to go with organic and/or gluten-free pasta dishes. If the batch is doubled, you can freeze a few portions for future meals on days when you're resting.

- Add chopped or chunked tomatoes to guacamole.

- Make vibrant veggie platters with tomatoes.

- Juice some tomatoes for a fresh Tomato Juice to get a potent dose.

#14 CANCER-HEALING FOOD: LEMON

Lemon contains vitamin C and alkalizes the body, making it an inhospitable environment where cancer cells cannot survive. Lemon also contains hesperidin, which has been said to fight cancer by starving it. That means lemons cut off the blood supply to cancerous tumors. Water that has been infused with lemon helps to flush out the liver; this can be extremely helpful during a period of chemo treatment as the burden of the drugs taxes the liver.

There are a considerable amount of studies showing the health effects of citrus and the reduction of cancer risk and tumor growth. One study showed that bladder tumor growth was remarkably inhibited by lemon.[97] Studies included in a meta-analysis also showed an inverse association between citrus fruit intake and oral cancer. People with the highest citrus fruit intake had a 50 percent reduction in their risk of oral cavity and pharyngeal cancer.[98] And this study showed the role of pomegranate with citrus fruit juices for colon cancer prevention.[99] Another group of researchers showed that citrus intake may significantly reduce the risk of esophageal cancer.[100]

Lemon Is Especially Good for . . .

- Urinary bladder cancer
- Oral cancer
- Pharyngeal cancer
- Colon cancer
- Esophageal cancer

Suggested "Dosage"

- If you have cancer, consume 1 to 4 lemons per day.
- To prevent cancer, consume ½ to 1 lemon per day.

Caution: Lemon can erode tooth enamel, so be sure to rinse your mouth out after drinking it.

Cancer-Free with Food Recipes with Lemon

- Lemon Water (page 191)
- Sick-Kick Smoothie (page 169)
- Green Lemonade (page 150)
- Cashew Cheesecake (page 337)
- Five-Ingredient Green Salad (page 244)

Ways of Incorporating Lemon in Your Cancer-Healing Kitchen

- Drink Lemon Water upon waking in the morning and throughout the day by squeezing lemon into your water.
- Add a squeeze of lemon over your salads.
- Add a squeeze of lemon to soups and stir-fries.

- Add lemon to your juices and smoothies; you can even juice the rind for a more potent dose!

- For portability and ease, take your lemon in the form of lemon essential oil; made from the peels of lemon, one or two drops in a glass of water is refreshing and antioxidant.

#15 CANCER-HEALING FOOD: QUINOA

An ancient grain, quinoa is a whole food that is naturally loaded with fiber, vitamins, minerals, and plant compounds that reduce our cancer risk. It has more protein than any other grain, including rice, whole wheat, and oats. The fiber found in this whole grain helps immensely to keep blood sugar stable.[101] It is also great for the digestive tract because of compounds it contains that promote gastrointestinal health. One study shows how quinoa initiates a release of peptides in the gut that may have the potential to prevent or slow the development of cancer.

Quinoa is responsible for the antioxidant activity and peptides that show the greatest anticancer effects. Seventeen potentially bioactive peptides are derived from the protein in quinoa, which scientists believe might be utilized as new nutraceuticals with the aim of reducing diseases, like cancer, which are associated with oxidative stress.[102]

Quinoa Is Especially Good for...

- Ovarian cancer
- Brain cancer
- Prostate cancer
- Breast cancer
- Skin cancer
- Colon cancer[103]

Suggested "Dosage"

- If you have cancer, eat ½ cup to 1 cup of quinoa per day.
- To prevent cancer, eat ½ cup every other day.

Cancer-Free with Food Recipes with Quinoa

- Turmeric Cumin Quinoa Bowl (page 232)
- Black Bean Bowl with Sweet Potatoes and Roasted Chickpeas (page 216)
- Super Protein Powder (page 308)
- Anita Moorjani's Coconut Curry (page 222)

Ways of Incorporating Quinoa in Your Cancer-Healing Kitchen

- Serve with curries, soups, salads, meats, and stir-fries.
- Add a layer of quinoa to your Salad Jars.
- Serve with porridge, using half oats and half quinoa for more of a whole-grain option.

A Word about Sea Salt and Iodine

Sea salt is produced by the evaporation of seawater. Some is a residual of evaporation that happened long ago. For example, Himalayan salt, which is pink and comes from an inland mountain range, is harvested from terrain that was once covered in ocean water millions of years ago. The container may be labeled Celtic sea salt (aka sel gris, or "gray salt"), fleur de sel ("flower of salt"), or Hawaiian (black or red) salt. High-quality sea salts typically contain 60 to 84 trace minerals—zinc, iron, and potassium among them—making them healthful, and much better than bleached-white table salt. I strongly believe no one should ever consume white table salt. And why would we need to when sea salt is available to us?

Many people are still afraid of salt, fat, and carbohydrates because of all the crazy articles they read decades ago. The problem is not with salt, per se; we just need the right salts. People who are deprived of salts can suffer many health issues. You can include sea salts in your cooking, smoothies, or even just mix some in water and it will give you those trace minerals you need. Salt helps the human body function at its best.

Although sea salt may contain trace iodine, it is not the best source of iodine. Iodine-rich foods include seaweed, cod fish, shrimp, tuna, eggs, organic dairy, and prunes. Iodine is an essential mineral, needed for proper thyroid functioning. With too little, our metabolism slows down. In children, a deficiency can affect brain and bone development. Dr. Christiane Northrup recommends dried dulse flakes (a sea vegetable) as a source of iodine.

EVEN *MORE* CANCER-HEALING FOODS

This concludes our tour of the top 15 anticancer foods. But I feel encouraged to carry on because there are so many wonderful ingredients to choose from that have healing properties. So here, in a nutshell, are the next 15 cancer-healing foods to incorporate into your dietary plan as often as possible:

- Walnuts
- Wheatgrass
- Beets
- Green tea
- Cauliflower
- Berries (strawberries, raspberries, cherries, and blackberries)
- Celery
- Olive oil
- Artichokes
- Onion
- Cabbage
- Brussels sprouts
- Carrots
- Kakadu plum

OTHER FOODS THAT ARE VERY HEALTHFUL

Based on their high nutrient levels and antioxidant power, here are other top anticancer ingredients—some you may never have heard of before! The herbs are often used in healing teas.

- Acai
- Alfalfa sprouts
- Apples
- Apple cider vinegar
- Apricots—dried, raw, and seeds
- Artichokes
- Asparagus
- Avocado
- Baking soda
- Banana
- Basil
- Bee pollen
- Black beans
- Black pepper
- Black seeds (nigella)
- Blue-green algae
- Boswella
- Burdock root
- Butternut squash
- Camu camu berries
- Cat's claw
- Cauliflower
- Cayenne pepper
- Chamomile
- Chia seeds
- Chickpeas/ garbanzo beans
- Chili pepper
- Chlorella
- Cinnamon
- Cloves
- Coconut
- Coconut oil, including MCT oil (MCT stands for medium-chain triglyerides, fatty acids that are easily absorbed and digested as an energy source for the brain and digestive system)
- Coffee
- Cucumber
- Cumin
- Dates
- Dulse
- Eggs (only organic/ pasture raised)
- Fenugreek
- Figs
- Ginseng
- Goji berries
- Goldenberries
- Grapefruit
- Green beans
- Hemp seeds
- Jackfruit
- Jalapeño peppers
- Kidney beans
- Lavender
- Leeks
- Lentils
- Lettuce
- Lime
- Lucuma

- Maca
- Mango
- Mangosteen
- Manuka honey
- Mint
- Mulberries
- Mung beans
- Mustard
- Navy beans
- Nectarines
- Noni
- Nuts (almonds, Brazil nuts, cashews, hazelnuts, macadamia nuts, pecans, walnuts)
- Oats
- Olives
- Onions (including yellow, green, and red onions)
- Orange
- Papaya
- Passion fruit
- Parsnip
- Peach
- Peas
- Peppers
- Pineapple
- Plum
- Pomegranate
- Potatoes
- Psyllium seed husks
- Pumpkin and pumpkin seeds
- Raisins
- Radish
- Red Pepper Flakes
- Rice (organic, including brown rice)
- Saffron
- Sea salt
- Sesame seeds
- Samphire
- Spices (including basil, thyme, oregano, sage, paprika, rosemary, nutmeg, fennel, marjoram, coriander, dill)
- Spirulina
- Squash
- Sunflower seeds
- Sunflower sprouts
- Sweet potato
- Teff
- Valerian root
- Vanilla bean
- Willow Bark
- Yucca
- Zucchini

INDIGENOUS HEALING FOODS FROM AROUND THE WORLD

Every region of the globe offers us natural healing. When people ate food provided by Earth without tampering with it, there were fewer cases of cancer. Many globally oriented organizations are concerned about the nature of the food supply, salvaging its positive elements, and sustaining Earth's original genetic resources—both for the sake of biodiversity and for the chemistry of different crop variations.

Organized by region, the following fruits and vegetables offer record levels of vitamins and high-potency, cancer-healing compounds. Many of the foods on this list were researched and recommended by Ellen Gustafson, founder of Food Tank, a think tank on food issues.[104] In addition to the Food Tank blog, my research led me to a list of indigenous plants compiled by Kathryn Gorman-Lovelady, an Aboriginal medicine woman who resides in Canada.[105]

In my opinion, it's most powerful to eat cancer-healing foods farmed in your local area. One of the reasons why is that their nutrients are intact because they haven't been shipped halfway across the world to reach you, been refrigerated or frozen, gone through a high-altitude flight, radiation from security screening, and so on. Seek out the cancer-fighting foods that are grown locally to you because they do strengthen the immune system.

Foods from Australia and Oceania

- Kakadu plum, which contains the highest vitamin C of any fruit in the entire world
- Quandong, which contains twice the vitamin C of an orange
- Boab leaves
- Desert limes

- Lemon myrtle. While healing my tumor, I drank lemon myrtle tea from leaves I plucked off a tree outside my home and steeped in boiling water.
- Blushwood berry
- Lifou Island yam
- Bunya nut

- Kumara
- Perry pear

- Rourou
(taro leaves)

Foods from Africa

- Amaranth
- Cowpea
- Spider plant, also known as African cabbage

- African eggplant
- Argan

Foods from the Americas

- Yacón (Peruvian ground apple)
- Papalo
- Hinkelhatz pepper
- Gravenstein apple
- Guayabo
- Indian pink
- Chicory/cornflower
- Ironwood
- Pipsissewa
- Fleabane
- Common thistle
- Wild sarsaparilla

- Ground ivy
- Bittersweet
- Bloodroot
- Celandine
- Yellow dock
- Witch hazel
- Violets
- White cedar
- Red clover
- Wild indigo
- Goldenseal
- Comfrey
- Guanabana

Foods from Asia

- Bitter melon
- Pamir mulberry
- Okra

- Mung bean
- Lemongrass
- Tamarind

Foods from Europe

- Perinaldo artichokes
- Formby asparagus
- Filder pointed cabbage
- Målselvnepe turnip
- Ermelo orange

CHAPTER 3

TOP ANTICANCER SUPPLEMENTS

A supplement is a pill, capsule, tablet, or liquid that is designed to complement the diet by providing missing nutrients or higher doses of certain nutrients. Supplements can be incredibly useful for rapidly putting sufficient amounts of a nutrient into your body—especially if your gut is not absorbing nutrients properly due to illness or cancer treatments. Supplements are a multibillion-dollar industry, and many companies are motivated by profits rather than ethics, so we need to be careful of what we buy.

It is important to always read the ingredient label, as some contain fillers, additives, colors, and synthetics. Watch out for the following unnecessary and toxic ingredients.

- Silicon dioxide (this makes vitamin tablets heavier)
- Titanium dioxide (gives clear supplements opacity)
- Methylsynephrine or oxilofrine (a stimulant substance)
- *Natural flavors*, a term that is often code for monosodium glutamate (MSG)

A plant-based vegetarian outer capsule is best when a supplement comes in powdered form. We have to be careful with the supplement industry because they can be sneaky with their ingredients, and often will manufacture a product that costs very little to make while charging a huge price for it.

I was shocked one day to find a supplement bottle at an organic store whose ingredient list read "vitamin E." When I called the company to ask them the source of the vitamin E in their product, they told me it was corn. I was outraged that they did not list the proper ingredient! This just goes to show that unscrupulous companies will put whatever they want in their supplements and mislabel them if they think it will make them money. The supplement that was meant to provide the body with vitamin E was instead filling up the guts of those who took it with, no doubt, genetically modified corn. If they had a need of that vitamin, their deficiency would be ongoing. If they had a corn allergy, they could be in danger. You must get to know the supplement brands you can trust and then stick to them.

Now let's jump right in to a brief A-to-Z guide of the most recommended anticancer supplements!

ACAI

Acai berries are a superfood for their potency as an antioxidant. This comes from being high in polyphenols, which are anti-inflammatory and soothe intestinal inflammation.[1] In Part II, you'll find several smoothie recipes that include acai berries as an ingredient. To supplement with acai, take them in powdered form in capsules.

Suggested dosage: Follow packaging instructions.

ALOE VERA/ALOE JUICE

Aloe vera is a gelatinous substance obtained from a succulent plant that grows in tropical climates. You can either harvest it directly from an aloe plant yourself and blend it to make it a drinkable liquid or buy fresh aloe juice from a store.

Ideally, aloe juice should be used fresh. To the best of my knowledge, at present there is only one fresh aloe company in the United States, Aloe 1 (see Resources). You want pure aloe with no preservatives and absolutely nothing else added. Aloe juice sold in supermarkets and organic stores typically contains some preservative to make it shelf stable.

Aloe juice is antiviral and can aid in healing Crohn's disease, irritable bowel disorder, GERD, diabetes, immune system disorders, eczema, psoriasis, dermatitis, and vaginal yeast overgrowths (which can be a side effect of chemotherapy). Many cancer patients incorporate aloe juice into their daily diets to assist with immune boosting, hydration, and cleansing the gut of cancer cells. In combination with colloidal silver (see entry), aloe does intensive healing and repairs.

Suggested dosage: Drink 1 ounce of aloe vera daily to prevent cancer. If you have cancer, you can drink up to a cup or more. (Also see the Aloe and Colloidal Silver Protocol in the colloidal silver entry.)

Amygdalin

Amygdalin is a naturally occurring chemical compound found in many plants. (The synthetic equivalent is laetrile.) The best sources are fruit pits from apricots, almonds, apples, peaches, and plums. It's also found in lima beans, clover, sorghum, berries (including blueberries, raspberries, elderberries, strawberries, and blackberries), grains and millets, and sprouts—but to a lesser degree. You can eat whole or powdered apricot seeds or receive amygdalin injections. If you are interested in the latter, search for an alternative doctor (for example, a naturopath) in your area who can administer amygdalin shots.

Amygdalin breaks down in the body to hydrogen cyanide, which many natural healers believe is a potent cancer-killing compound.[2] Amygdalin is being researched as a treatment for malignant tumors, especially lung tumors, which have a tremendously high mortality rate.[3] According to one report, amygdalin is a "promising" antitumor drug, "if combined with conditional chemotherapy drugs, which can produce synergistic effect."[4] Studies have indicated that amygdalin may be helpful for prostate cancer.[5]

APRICOT SEEDS, POWDER, AND/OR SUPPLEMENTS (SEE AMYGDALIN)

ASHWAGANDHA

Ashwagandha (aka *Withania somnifera,* or Indian ginseng) is a shrub. In Latin, the species name, *somnifera,* means "sleep-inducing." Most ashwagandha is cultivated in India, Nepal, and China, where it is made into a root powder. This has been used for centuries to alleviate fatigue and improve general well-being.

Ashwagandha is known as an herb with powerful anticancer, antistress, antioxidant, anti-inflammatory, and adaptogenic properties. A study of 100 breast cancer patients in different stages of chemotherapy suggested to researchers that ashwagandha is a potential remedy for cancer-related fatigue and to improve the quality of life—though further study with a larger population is needed.[6] Another study proved that ashwagandha has the ability to selectively arrest the growth of cancer cells.[7]

You can buy ashwagandha in the form of a powder or as a tea, capsule, leaf, and/or leaf extract. I take the capsules, but also have the powder in my cupboard, which I add to smoothies, shakes, soups, and hot water—to make a tea. Some people boil it in water with milk and butter or honey. You could also use almond milk, macadamia nut milk, ghee, or coconut oil and manuka honey.

Suggested dosage: If taking capsules, use the serving size recommended on the bottle. Or take 1 to 2 teaspoons (600 to 1,200 milligrams) of the leaf extract twice daily.

ASTRAGALUS

Astragalus is famously known for boosting immunity! Everyone with cancer should be taking an astragalus supplement (if doctor's orders permit). A plant that belongs to the legume family, in traditional Chinese medicine there is a history of its use as an herbal remedy; it is known to reinforce chi (life-force energy), help discharge pus, and aid in the growth of new tissue. Astragalus helps the body build new cells. You can buy dried astragalus root and make tea by boiling it in hot water. Or you can purchase it in the form of a powder, liquid extract, or capsule. The powder or liquid can be added to smoothies, teas, and soups.

Research at the UCLA AIDS Institute focused on the function of cycloastragenol (a compound extracted from astragalus) in the aging process of immune cells. Their interest was its positive effects on the cell's response to viral infections. It appeared to increase the production of telomerase, an enzyme that plays a key role in cell replication and protects cells from DNA damage.[8]

Suggested dosage: Integrative physician Andrew Weil, M.D., says there are no known interactions between astragalus and other herbs and supplements. He recommends taking the extract (250 to 500 milligrams), three to four times a day. When making tea, boil three to six grams (0.21 ounces) of dried root per 12 ounces of water three times a day.[9]

BAKING SODA

Baking soda—sodium bicarbonate—is a natural substance found in mineral springs around the globe. You likely have some in your kitchen cabinet. It is commonly used in baking and also has therapeutic benefits, due to its high pH value of 9 to 9.5, which is extremely alkaline. You may, for instance, have sipped some dissolved in a glass of water when you had indigestion—to counteract an "acid stomach." It bubbles in water, so when you drank it, it might have made you burp. This is an inexpensive, quick home remedy to change the pH of your body and make it less hospitable to cancer cells.

Always be sure to read the label carefully. Do not confuse baking soda with baking powder. Your package should contain only one ingredient: sodium bicarbonate.

BAKING SODA BEVERAGE

Ingredients:

12 ounces purified water

1 teaspoon baking soda

1 tablespoon fresh lemon juice

1 teaspoon apple cider vinegar

Actions:

Add all the ingredients to a cup and stir well. Once the mixture stops bubbling, drink.

Caution: Only one alkalizing strategy should be used per day, so do not drink more than one Baking Soda Beverage a day and do not drink it in combination with other alkalizing strategies.[10] Do not drink Baking Soda Beverage 30 minutes before or after consuming food to avoid reducing stomach acid that is necessary for digestion of food to occur.

Suggested dosage: If you have cancer, you could drink this once per day. I wouldn't recommend drinking baking soda as a sole treatment, but rather as a complement to other treatments.

To prevent cancer, you could drink this once per week.

BENTONITE CLAY

Bentonite Clay was a huge part of my healing and the number-one supplement I used. See the Bentonite Clay Drink on page 193.

BLACK SEED OIL

Black seed oil comes from the seeds of *Nigella sativa*, which is also known as black caraway, black cumin, and kalonji. A flowering plant native to Asia, well-known for its antioxidant, anti-inflammatory, and antibacterial properties, nigella has been used in traditional medicine to treat many diseases. And now there are many contemporary studies showing it has anticancer properties as well, particularly one animal study that proved it can stop the growth of tumor cells.[11] Gary Null, Ph.D., says:

"Black cumin oil is probably the single most important oil you can put in your system."[12]

What kinds of cancers does it hold promise for healing? Black seed oil significantly reduces viability of human lung cancer cells.[13] It is also said to be a potential therapeutic agent for human cervical cancer.[14] An active ingredient in black seed, thymoquinone, is now being looked at as a potential cure for inflammatory disorders and cancer.[15] Black cumin seed oil increases the activity of immune cells that target cancer cells.[16] There is also speculation that black cumin seed (via injections) may be useful in protecting against the side effects of radiation therapy.

So, spread the word. I recommend every household get its hands on some black seeds and/or black seed oil and start using these in your kitchen at least once a week. If you have cancer, you can consume black seed oil daily.

Suggested dosage: Health experts recommend taking 1 teaspoon of the oil on an empty stomach two times per day for anticancer effects. It's also best to consume the oil raw. You can also:

- Incorporate black seeds into your recipes for salads, soups, and smoothies.
- Dry-roast black seeds to flavor curries, vegetables, pulses, beans, and lentils.
- Add the oil or seeds to spreads and dips like tahini, hummus, and guacamole.
- Add the seeds to homemade organic baked breads or Gluten Free Tortillas.
- Add them to potatoes or Cauliflower Popcorn.
- Add black seed oil to teas.
- Apply black seed oil topically.

Caution: Do not consume black seeds or oil if you are taking cytochrome P450 substrate drugs: *Nigella sativa* may increase the risk of side effects of these drugs.[17]

Blue-green Algae (E₃ Live, Spirulina, Chlorella, Blue majik, Cyanobacteria)

Blue-green algae is one of the most nutrient-dense foods on the planet. It is found in almost every terrestrial and aquatic habitat: oceans and freshwater ponds and lakes, damp soil, moistened rocks in the deserts, and bare rocks and soil—even Antarctic rocks! This pervasive life-form owes its superfood status to high concentrations of proteins, vitamins, and nutrients. Blue-green algae produces oxygen in the body, something that most cancer patients need more of!

WebMD reports that people use blue-green algae for treating precancerous growths inside the mouth, boosting the immune system, improving memory, increasing energy and metabolism, lowering cholesterol, healing wounds, and improving digestion and bowel health.[18]

The studies are intriguing. One study on blue-green algae revealed that it selectively induced cancer cells to die and to stop reproducing—meaning, healthy cells were spared.[19] Another study showed that blue-green algae substantially decreased the proliferation of pancreatic cancer cells.[20]

You can buy blue-green algae in loose powdered form or capsules. The powder is the most magical, sparkly blue I have ever seen, so I sometimes use it in raw vegan desserts to make them a vibrant blue color. You can also sprinkle it on your oats and cereal or mix it into your smoothies.

There may be side effects when taking blue-green algae, so check with your doctor.

Suggested dosage: The recommended daily dose is 2,000 to 3,000 milligrams, taken in divided doses throughout the day.

Burdock Root Powder (Happy Major, *Arctium lappa*)

Burdock root is used in some countries as a vegetable. You can buy burdock tea, supplements, liquid extract, or even the whole root. The active ingredients it possesses have been found to detoxify the blood and promote circulation.

After review of the literature, researchers said: "Antioxidants and antidiabetic compounds have also been found in the root. In the seeds, some active compounds possess anti-inflammatory effects and potent inhibitory effects on the growth of tumors such as pancreatic carcinoma."[21] An animal study of its effects when used in combination with various regimens of chemotherapy to treat lung cancer and melanoma revealed promising avenues for additional research.[22]

In Chinese medicine, burdock root is used for skin conditions such as eczema, and to treat colds and flu. It may be helpful in treating skin inflammation and/or other issues that crop up when receiving chemotherapy and radiation; however, I caution you to work with a health-care provider trained with Chinese herbs.

Suggested dosage: If you have cancer, add 1 to 2 teaspoons dried powder mixed in water, tea, or smoothies. If you have cancer, prepare 1 to 2 cups of burdock root tea daily by boiling the root in water for 15 minutes, then allowing it to steep and cool before drinking.

CHLOROPHYLL

Chlorophyll is a light-absorbing green pigment present in plants that helps them feed on the energy of sunlight. Chlorophyll is nontoxic to humans and contains magnesium. The molecule is similar to the hemoglobin in our bloodstreams that carries oxygen to our cells. As far as cancer goes, a study showed that the growth of melanoma cells in mouse tumors were effectively inhibited after being treated with chlorophyll. This is an indication there may be promise for using chlorophyll as an anticancer supplement.[23]

You consume chlorophyll every time you eat a green vegetable, have a leafy salad, or drink a green juice. If you are not consuming these foods, a supplement could effectively provide your body with chlorophyll. Because of its dark-green tint, I use chlorophyll as a food dye, and so do many other natural-food chefs, for making things green like a green frosting.

Suggested dosage: You can buy it in liquid or capsule form. Follow the package instructions; a small amount goes a long way.

COLLOIDAL SILVER

Colloidal silver is naturally found in soil, mushrooms, and breast milk. And yes, it's the same metal we wear as jewelry. (In chemistry, a *colloid* is any insoluble substance that is suspended in another, usually a liquid. This is a description of how it is delivered.) As a dietary supplement, we are able to consume it in small quantities safely. The liquid contains only nanoparticles.

Poor-quality preparations of colloidal silver can cause a condition known as argyria, which causes the skin to turn ashy blue. Good-quality colloidal silver preparations do not turn the skin blue. *Do not make your own at home.*

Avoid impure products with additives, protein, and salt.[24] My recommendation for purity is Sovereign Silver (see Resources).

Did you know that if you went to the hospital for burn treatment, the first thing they would do is put a form of silver on your wounds? "Silver repairs the skin faster than anything else on the planet," says Robert Scott Bell, author of *Unlock the Power to Heal.*[25] Colloidal silver has been used for centuries by natural healers to treat infections due to yeast, bacteria (tuberculosis, Lyme disease, bubonic plague, pneumonia, leprosy, gonorrhea, stomach ulcers, cholera), parasites (ringworm, malaria), and viruses (HIV and herpes). Modern research studies are beginning to assess colloidal silver with positive results.[26]

I find two cancer studies most intriguing. In one, colloidal silver was shown to elicit antitumor activity on human breast cancer cells.[27] Another showed that silver nanoparticles (AgNPs) displayed antileukemic activity. Researchers reported: "These results reveal that silver combined with ROS-generating drugs could potentially enhance therapeutic efficacy against leukemia cells." Ask your doctor about this study if you are currently undergoing treatment for leukemia.[28]

Suggested dosage: To prevent cancer, you could take a teaspoonful a day.

Aloe and Colloidal Silver Protocol

The aloe and silver protocol is used to cleanse the digestive tract, reduce inflammation, boost immunity, and promote healthy gut microflora. I have found this to be the most successful cleanse protocol for my digestive system to date, and I do it annually. The protocol is as follows:

- Combine 1 ounce of colloidal silver and 1 ounce of aloe juice, and drink three times a day on an empty stomach (morning, noon, and night). Also take one dose of probiotics (see entry) before sleeping.

- Wait to eat until 45 minutes have passed from drinking the mixture.

- Do the protocol for two to eight weeks. (If you absolutely cannot drink aloe juice, substitute coconut water or a green juice.)

DIGESTIVE ENZYMES

It can be helpful to take digestive enzymes to assist in routine digestion or in cases of stomach inflammation. The body has enzymes to digest and metabolize every type of food substance we are likely to eat—protein, fat, carbohydrates, fiber, and so on. The older we get, the more likely we are to have insufficiencies of certain ones. You can identify which ones because you won't feel good after eating those foods! And, some of us are born unable to properly metabolize certain foods, such as beans or onions.

Digestive enzymes have names like amylase, protease, lipase, cellulase, and alpha-D-galactosidase (my favorite, as it helps to digest beans). Without enough enzymes, we can get clogged up or flatulent. Fortunately, we can source them from foods too—from ginger root, pineapple, and papaya, to name a few.

Digestive enzymes will boost your immunity and reduce the metabolic burden on your liver.

Suggested dosage: Check with your doctor if you need to supplement with enzymes.

ESSENTIAL OILS

Plants evolve in harmony with their environments. The chemistry that is embodied in them has properties that will sustain their lives, such as the ability to withstand molds, fungi, insects, bacteria, viruses, and UV rays from harsh sunlight. When distilled, those chemical properties are amplified in the concentrated essence which can then be bottled for our use.

Essential oils are volatile liquids distilled from plants either by steam extraction or cold-pressing. This means that you do not need to put heat under them for their active properties to be unleashed. All you need to do is open the bottle and the scent of the oil molecules will begin to waft around the room.

Regulated by the government as food supplements, some essential oils are not appropriate for internal use, as they would be toxic. But many are edible: essential oils made from the peels of citrus fruits like lemons, oranges, limes, grapefruits, and bergamots, for instance. Ones that are edible have food supplement labels on the bottle.

There are edible essential oils made from herbs and spices, like rosemary, thyme, basil, marjoram, oregano, black pepper, cardamom, cilantro, coriander, dill, peppermint, and spearmint. Some essential oils come from bark, such as cinnamon bark. Others come from roots, such as ginger, or berries, such as juniper berry. Still others come from flower petals, like lavender.

Although essential oils are called "oils," they are not greasy in the slightest. They have no calories and no macronutrients. In general, edible oils are used in tiny quantities, such as 1 to 3 drops per 4 ounces of a liquid that they are mixed into, such as water or almond milk.

Essential oils have been used for millennia as therapy for every kind of condition you can imagine. Some have aromas that are healing simply when they are inhaled. Others can be applied topically (directly to the skin) along with a carrier oil, such as coconut oil or almond oil, which helps them to stay put without evaporating and to penetrate the layers of the skin.

Essential oils have been used by the food industry for decades as a flavoring. In recent years, scientists have begun conducting research on essential oils for therapeutic purposes. Lavender essential oil and clove bud essential oil are high in antioxidants. Frankincense has been shown to be potentially useful in healing from brain cancer,[29] colon cancer,[30] pancreatic cancer, prostate cancer, stomach cancer, and breast cancer.

Surgeon and doctor of natural medicine David Steuer, D.M.D., D.N.M., Ph.D., had a tumor on a pancreatic duct that ruptured and was operated on successfully. Shortly afterward, he started getting tremors. He went back to the hospital where doctors discovered he had a brain tumor the size of a gumball. They gave him a surgical option, but he chose not to risk losing functions. Since then he has shrunk the tumor to the size of a tiny pea through emphasizing nutritional strategies, which include daily use of essential oils. His daily regimen includes frankincense, grapefruit, clove, and copaiba essential oils.[31]

Suggested dosage:

- For nausea or constipation, try smelling peppermint essential oil or drink a few drops in a glass of water.

- For an antioxidant boost, put a few drops of a citrus essential oil, like lemon, in a glass of water.

- To rev up your metabolism, try adding a drop of ginger essential oil to your smoothie or tea.

Here are a few ways to use frankincense:

- Put it in a water diffuser so it emanates into the air around you.

- Rub it on your neck four times daily mixed with a carrier oil.

- Drink 4 drops in a 12-ounce glass of water three times daily.

Magnesium

Magnesium is a naturally occurring mineral found in food, a silver-white metal of the alkaline earth series that are known to relax the brain and body. Magnesium is beneficial in the treatment of migraines, insomnia, depression, and coronary artery disease. It may also help reduce your risk of getting cancer. Cancer patients may take magnesium supplements to assist their bodies in killing cancer cells and inhibiting tumor growth.

Studies have shown that magnesium intake may be beneficial in terms of primary prevention of pancreatic cancer and colorectal cancer.[32,33] Epidemiological studies identify magnesium deficiency as a risk factor for some types of human cancers.

One study showed that women consuming magnesium while undergoing chemotherapy for breast cancer improved treatment against breast metastasis (cell replication). Researchers concluded, "[Magnesium] is significant to enhance anti-tumor and anti-metastasis efficacy simultaneously."[34]

You should regularly consume magnesium-rich foods: sunflower seeds, pumpkin seeds, cashews, mung beans, wild rice, almonds, cacao, walnuts, Brazil nuts, chickpeas, lentils, salmon, bananas, avocados, and spinach. But I would also recommend taking a magnesium supplement. After I started taking them, feelings of depression I was experiencing were reduced and my sleep improved. Drinking magnesium can also be helpful for severe constipation.

Many people are deficient in magnesium, the main reason being low dietary intake. Low plasma magnesium (hypomagnesemia) is found in 2.5 to 15 percent of the general population. Check with your doctor if you are deficient and then you can supplement if you are. Intravenous magnesium is available to patients who are deficient.

Suggested dosage: The recommended dietary allowance (RDA) for magnesium is 400 milligrams for men ages 19 to 30 and 420 milligrams for older men. For women ages 19 to 30, it's 310 milligrams and 320 milligrams for older women. For therapeutic doses, consult with your doctor.

Pancreatic Enzymes (also see Digestive Enzymes)

Pancreatic enzymes typically contain a combination of lipase, amylase, and protease to assist in the digestion of fat, carbohydrates, and protein, respectively. If your pancreas is not functioning well enough to secrete about eight cups of pancreatic juice into the duodenum (the first part of the small intestine, located in the digestive tract right after the stomach) every day, then pancreatic enzymes may be clinically necessary or helpful.

Many causes of a pancreatic insufficiency, such as cystic fibrosis, pancreatic cancer, acute and chronic pancreatitis, and pancreatic surgery, require the initiation of pancreatic enzyme replacement therapy (PERT).[35] PERT involves taking digestive enzymes in the form of a capsule or an IV.

You may also choose to take a comprehensive digestive enzyme supplement to help your body out while you are healing or undergoing a cleanse.

In 1906, Scottish embryologist John Beard, D.Sc., proposed that pancreatic proteolytic enzymes represent the body's main defense against cancer.[36] In 1981, Nicholas J. Gonzalez, M.D., evaluated the concept at Cornell University Medical College. Then other researchers started to seriously reconsider the pancreatic and proteolytic enzyme approach to cancer therapy.

Suggested dosage: Take 5 grams of proteolytic enzymes three times daily on an empty stomach between meals to reduce inflammation.[37]

Proteolytic Enzymes (also see Digestive Enzymes)

Like pancreatic enzymes, proteolytic enzymes aid in digestion— in this case, in the digestion of protein. Proteolytic enzymes can be found in pineapple, asparagus, buckwheat, ginger, kiwi, sauerkraut, miso soup, figs, and papaya. They can also be taken as supplements.

One study showed the impact of proteolytic enzymes in colorectal cancer development and progression and revealed how four different proteolytic enzymes play a major role not only in colorectal cancer invasion and metastasis, but also in the transformation of precancerous lesions into malignant cancer.[38] Other studies have shown that enzyme therapy with bromelain, papain, and other proteolytic enzymes significantly decreased tumor-induced fatigue, weight loss, and restlessness, and obviously stabilized the quality of life. The enzymes helped with chemotherapy- and radiation-therapy-induced side effects, such as nausea and gastrointestinal distress.[39]

You can take proteolytic enzymes in supplement form, drink pineapple juice, or eat other foods containing the enzyme. See the Paradise Smoothie on page 175, which contains both pineapple and papaya, making it high in proteolytic enzymes.

Suggested dosage: Follow package instructions.

PREBIOTICS

Prebiotics are food ingredients that encourage the growth and activity of beneficial microorganisms (aka probiotics) so we can establish a healthy microbiome in our digestive tracts. This is what probiotic microbes themselves "like" to eat! You can get prebiotics naturally from tigernuts, asparagus, bananas, and garlic. Or you can buy prebiotics in powder or capsule form.

Suggested dosage: Follow package instructions.

PROBIOTICS

Probiotics are the "good bacteria" in the human gut that help us get our vitamins—microorganisms. You naturally get probiotics when you eat foods such as raw milk and raw milk products, including cheese, kefir, and yogurt. You can also take probiotic supplements: for people like me who eat little to no dairy, or lactose-intolerant people, that's the best way to get them into our system.

Bio means "life." *Pro* means "for." Thus, the aptly named probiotics promote life. Imbalance of gut microbes has been implicated in many disorders—everything from inflammatory bowel disease to obesity, asthma, psychiatric illnesses, and different cancers. By helping the gut function properly, probiotics play a role in protecting us against cancer.

Clinical application of probiotics may also diminish the incidence of postoperative inflammation in cancer patients. Chemotherapy- or radiotherapy-related diarrhea was relieved in patients who were administered oral probiotics.[40] At present, it is commonly accepted that most commercial probiotic products are generally safe and can improve health. That said, modulating intestinal microbiota with a variety of strains is likely to boost the immune response the most.

Some strains can be used as an adjunct to cancer treatment. Probiotics have been shown to suppress tumor growth in breast cancer.[41] And a lot of studies say that further investigations are required to reveal the effectiveness of probiotics in clinical settings.

In Chinese medicine, gut health is considered paramount to optimal wellness. It makes sense to have good gut balance, and if probiotics help with this, then it is something we all should explore. If you try them for a month and feel better, then you'll have your answer.

Suggested dosage: Follow package instructions.

Spirulina (see Blue-Green Algae)

Vitamin C

Interest in vitamin C began in the 1970s as an understanding of the relationship between oxidation and inflammation emerged. One of the world's great antioxidants, it can be taken by mouth as a supplement or given intravenously, as a drip. It also can be consumed from fresh produce like oranges, lemons, limes, and grapefruits. As an antioxidant, it plays a key role in the growth of collagen—a structural protein found in skin and connective tissue throughout the body.

Even now we don't have definitive information about vitamin C and its effect on cancer. However, as far back as the 1990s, the epidemiologic evidence of a protective effect of vitamin C for nonhormone-dependent cancers has been strong. For cancers of the esophagus, stomach, rectum, breast, cervix, larynx, oral cavity, and pancreas, evidence for a protective effect is consistent. Several lung cancer studies also found significant protective effects of vitamin C.[42]

A 2018 *Frontiers in Physiology* review of numerous studies looking at high-dose vitamin C concludes: "Recently, biological and preclinical studies suggest that high-dose intravenous vitamin C combined with conventional chemotherapy agent synergistically increase the effectiveness of cancer therapy."[43]

Suggested dosage: The RDA for adults is 75 to 120 milligrams. However, the therapeutic dose is much higher. Consult with your doctor for ingesting vitamin C in megadosages.

Vitamin D/Sunshine

Vitamin D is a necessary vitamin, as it helps us to absorb minerals, like magnesium and calcium, in our intestines. We get vitamin D from sunshine and from some foods. Vitamin D_3 and D_2 are compounds from food. D_2 is found in fungi (mushrooms). Vitamin D_3 is found in fish and grass-fed beef or calf liver. Some foods in the supermarket are fortified with vitamin D.

Foods that contain vitamin D:

- Mushrooms (button, cremini, portobello, shiitake)
- Fish liver oils, such as cod liver oil
- Wild fish (salmon, tuna, sardines, mackerel)
- Shell fish (shrimp, oysters)
- Egg yolks (another reason we should be eating the entire egg and not just the whites!)
- Beef liver
- Cheese

Vitamin D supplements are promoted to offer anticancer properties.[44] Observational studies have shown that low vitamin D levels raise the risk of developing certain cancers including colon cancer.[45] But getting sufficient sunshine may be key, rather than elevating blood serum levels. One study shows that breast cancer death rates tend to be higher in areas with low winter sunlight levels and lower in sunny areas.[46]

If you live in a place with little sunshine, chances are good that you are vitamin D deficient. I have heard from many people that said when they took vitamin D supplements (based on blood work showing they were deficient), a lot of their health issues improved. Maybe this is why we typically feel better in spring and summer?

Suggested dosage: Have your doctor check your vitamin D levels through a blood test and prescribe a proper amount of supplemental vitamin D. Get 10 to 15 minutes of sun on bare skin daily.

———————

Often a blood test can show you what vitamins and minerals you are deficient in. Then you can plan to eat more of the foods that provide the vitamins you need, or you can take supplements. Oftentimes supplements are a helpful means to put nutrients into the body quickly!

CHAPTER 4

AVOID THE 15 MOST TOXIC FOODS ON THE PLANET

Researchers have known about the dangers associated with unhealthy habits and cancer-causing foods for decades. A wide range of extensive research agrees that the substances listed in this chapter increase the risk of cancer. They wreak havoc on the body, creating stress, inflammation, acidity, brain fog, and hormonal imbalances. Our own common sense tells us that overloading our bodies with poisonous substances in either a small or an excessive quantity would produce some kind of negative health effect. I contend that if we eat too much of these things, cancer is the result.

I hope this information can be taught in schools someday, so children can get a great head start in knowing what foods to avoid, both as their bodies and minds are developing and for the rest of their lives. Even if we are not able to eliminate all of these items from our diet completely, every human being should at least cut down on their intake of these substances.

THE CUT-IT-OUT FOOD LIST:
WHAT YOU DON'T KNOW MAY KILL YOU

The following are the types of foods and ingredients I'd strongly recommend avoiding. When you cut these things out of your life, you will lower the toxic load going into your body and significantly reduce your risk of cancer.

I personally don't even call this list "food." The items below really are chemicals and toxins. Food is what grows and is harvested in nature—fruits and vegetables, free-range meat, and wild-caught fish.

1. Refined sugar: white sugar, brown sugar, and corn syrup

2. Food additives: artificial sweeteners (e.g., aspartame), stabilizers, and preservatives (e.g., benzoate)

3. Soda

4. Food from cans and plastics made with BPA

5. Genetically modified organisms (GMOs)

6. Conventional white flour (GMO), which contains gluten

7. Excessive alcohol

8. Meat from animals treated with hormones or fed nonorganic food

9. Meats that are charred or processed

10. Nonorganic fruits and vegetables

11. Nonorganic dairy products

12. Farmed seafood

13. Pasteurized food

14. Foods containing trans fats and partially hydrogenated oils (for example, margarine and processed cakes, cookies, and potato chips)

15. Microwaved food

Now, let's look at each of these cut-it-out foods in turn.

REASONS TO CUT OUT REFINED SUGARS

Cancer cells are basically "addicted" to refined sugar. In fact, when they can't consume enough, they begin to die. The sugar molecules feed the cancer, creating an environment in the body in which it can thrive. For these reasons, highly processed sugar (which has no nutritional value) should be banned, especially in hospitals and schools.

Sugar creates problems for the body, the mind, and the emotions. The average American consumes way too much sugar—152 pounds a year. Every time sugar is consumed, it triggers the release of the hormone insulin, which causes blood sugar to drop. Then there are cravings for more glucose (the molecule in table sugar), and the cycle is perpetuated. It leads to crazy swings in energy and mood—real highs and lows.

The bottom line is: If you cut white sugar out of your diet, you will reduce your risk of cancer. Cancer is ravenous for sugar.

However, all sugar is not created equal. The body can metabolize some forms of sugar more successfully than others, including the sugar in fruit (fructose). The beauty of eating a piece of fruit is that it contains phytonutrients and fiber as well as carbohydrates. By contrast, refined sugars wreak havoc in the body. These are processed until they are far removed from their natural state—oh boy, cane sugar goes through quite a lot to become white and crystalized. Ditto for corn and high-fructose corn syrup. It's tempting to eat sugary foods, but the temporary pleasure of the intense sweetness is not worth it.

Dr. Otto Warburg won the Nobel Prize in Physiology or Medicine in 1931 for his discovery that cancer cells are primarily fueled by the burning of sugar anaerobically (meaning, without oxygen). Sugar gives these abnormal cells the energy to grow, whereas healthy human cells get their energy from oxygen. Without sugar, most cancer cells simply lack the metabolic flexibility to survive. This discovery has become an important diagnostic tool. As noted in *New York Times Magazine*: "[The Warburg effect] is estimated to occur in up to 80 percent of cancers. It is so fundamental to most cancers that a positron emission tomography (PET) scan, which has emerged as an important tool in the staging and diagnosis of cancer, works simply by revealing the places in the body where cells are consuming extra glucose. In many cases, the more glucose a tumor consumes, the worse a patient's prognosis."[1]

In addition to feeding cancer cells, sugar feeds toxic microbes in the gut that we don't want to proliferate, like yeasts. If the microbiome becomes imbalanced, problems can result. Candida is a yeast that feeds on sugar and craves it; as it grows, the more sugar we feel driven to feed it. So, if we know we have excess candida, it's important to do a very-low-sugar cleanse to deprive it of this food so that it dies. (Foods high in chlorophyll—like dark leafy greens—also kill candida.)

Another thing sugar does is acidify the blood. It's been said that cancer cells cannot grow and thrive in an alkaline body. If you cut out sugar and consume vegetables, you'll be helping to create conditions in your body for optimal wellness.

REASONS TO CUT OUT ARTIFICIAL FOOD ADDITIVES

The most significant reason to avoid artificial food additives of all kinds is that when we metabolize them they release free radicals into the body that damage our cells. This process, known as oxidative stress, is a key factor in disease and aging. Antioxidants protect us from free radicals.

Fruits and vegetables are great sources of all kinds of antioxidants. The most abundant water-soluble antioxidant in the body is vitamin C. The most abundant fat-soluble antioxidant in the body is vitamin E.[2]

Preservatives like nitrates and sulfites; food colorings; and flavor enhancers like monosodium glutamate (MSG) have all been linked to free-radical damage in the body, which increases the risk of developing cancer. The best way to avoid these are to stay away from products that contain unknown and unpronounceable ingredients.

One of the most common—and toxic—preservatives in processed foods is benzoic acid. Sodium benzoate (the salt form of benzoic acid) is used in foods like processed fruit juice, syrup, jams, jelly, preserves, sauerkraut, pickles, and so on. Its purpose is to keep them from spoiling by limiting the growth of microbes. Sometimes, when benzoic acid comes into contact with citric acid, it is converted into benzene, a chemical that has been linked to leukemia and other blood cancers.[3] Journalist Deborah Mitchell writes: "In a laboratory study, scientists evaluated the genotoxic impact of sodium benzoate in cultured human cells. They found that the chemical significantly increased damage to DNA (which triggers cell mutation and cancer) when it was added to the cells in various concentrations."[4]

Sodium benzoate and potassium benzoate were investigated and discovered to be toxic to living cells and an agent of mutation. Both damage chromosomes.[5] Sodium nitrate and sodium nitrite were classified by the International Agency for Research on Cancer as probably carcinogenic to humans, particularly in the colon.[6]

BHA and BHT (E320) are stabilizers for foods containing oils and fats whose purpose as additives is to keep those foods from becoming rancid too soon or under high heat. They are actually considered antioxidants. Found in potato chips, gum, cereal, frozen sausages, enriched rice, lard, shortening, candy, and gelatin, supposedly they're safe for human consumption, but we know they cause cancer in lab rats—and, oh yeah, they're used to manufacture rubber.[7] Ick!

Artificial sweeteners such as aspartame, saccharine, and sucralose generate damaging free radicals in the body when we digest them. Preliminary research suggests they may contribute to the development of urinary or bladder cancers.[8] After digestion, they also can remain present in the liver, kidneys, and the brain for a while. Mental side effects can include headaches, migraines, dizziness, and mood swings.

Food dye is carcinogenic partly because the body cannot digest it properly. The Center for Science in the Public Interest published a report titled "Food Dyes: A Rainbow of Risks," laying out the evidence on nine common blue, red, green, orange, and yellow dyes that have been derived from petroleum products and coal tar—things we would never eat wittingly. And now you know, so you can avoid them![9]

REASONS TO CUT OUT SODA

There are several reasons why soda is terrible for us—even diet soda. For starters, soda is pumped full of carcinogenic additives like colorings and preservatives. Caramel-colored soda may expose you to a carcinogen, 4-methylimidazole (4-MEI), linked to pancreatic cancer.[10] Keep in mind that it's only there for so-called aesthetic purposes!

Regular soda is filled with sugar, which we know is bad for us, and its calories are "empty," with no nutritional value—so why ingest them?

Diet soda has artificial sweeteners, a food additive that we know is bad for us, and although it has no calories, it still has no nutritive value. And oddly, people who drink diet soda typically are more overweight than those who don't. According to MD Anderson Cancer Center: "Being obese increases your risk for breast cancer (after menopause) and colon, endometrial, kidney, and pancreatic cancers.[11]

There is apparently no cause for concern with carbonated seltzer. But you should steer clear of tonic water, which is full of salt.

REASONS TO CUT OUT FOODS PACKAGED IN PACKAGING LINED WITH BPA

Canned food lined with bisphenol A (BPA) has been linked to cancer. BPA is used in the production of plastics used to package or coat items that come in direct contact with food and liquids—everything from bottle caps and plastic packaging to kitchenware and the inside of aluminum cans.

BPA is metabolized by the liver. From there you pee most of it out, but over time it accumulates in your tissues. It is an endocrine disruptor, which means it messes with our hormones. Among other diseases and conditions, including high blood pressure, BPA has been directly linked to breast cancer, prostate cancer, and polycystic ovary syndrome.[12]

It is safest to not apply heat to any plastic containers, because they may leach BPA. Try not to drink water from plastic bottles either. Buy food in pouches or BPA-free packaging.

REASONS TO CUT OUT GENETICALLY MODIFIED ORGANISMS (GMO FOODS)

In the food industry, gene splicing has become a common technology for altering the characteristics of the produce sold—in some instances to make it more appealing to customers, or less vulnerable on the farm to insects or fungi, or hardier and less likely to be damaged in transit to the store. Agribusiness wants to own patented food, so how and in what ways they have modified the genetic code of a plant or animal is a closely guarded secret. It is not in their financial interest for the public to complain about it.

Well, it is in our interest not to let them experiment with our bodies! The science may not yet be in on whether or not GMOs are okay to eat, but common sense dictates we do not find out the hard way—if we can avoid it.

I believe that we should not eat GMO foods, including packaged foods made from GMO ingredients, because we don't know if we can digest them or what they will do to us. The human body evolved in harmony with nature, and we are not adapted to these ingredients.

Furthermore, science has proven that certain GMO products are carcinogenic—and the food industry doesn't care! Case in point, the company Monsanto makes an herbicide, Roundup, that contains a GMO ingredient, glyphosate. When this herbicide is sprayed on crops, it makes farmworkers and people living close to farms sick—doubling the incidences of non-Hodgkins lymphoma and multiple myeloma.[13,14]

Recently, a jury in the Superior Court of San Francisco ordered Monsanto to pay $289.2 million to Dewayne Johnson, who got terminal cancer as a result of overexposure to Roundup.

His attorneys proudly announced: "We were finally able to show the jury the secret, internal Monsanto documents proving that Monsanto has known for decades that glyphosate and specifically Roundup could cause cancer."[15] In May 2017, CNN reported that more than 800 other patients with cancer were suing Monsanto, claiming Roundup caused their illness.[16]

Be cautious of the most common GMO crops:

- Corn
- Soybeans
- Cotton
- Canola (for oil)
- Squash and zucchini
- Papaya

What can you do to protect yourself? According to MD Anderson Cancer Center:[17]

- Buy organic, as the designation precludes the use of GMO herbicides.
- Shop at local farmers markets—most GMO is used at industrial, not small, farms.
- Read the labels—look for products marked "non-GMO" and "GMO-free."
- Buy grass-fed meats—since the pigs, cattle, and chickens are grazing, they're not being fed GMO corn or alfalfa.
- Avoid products that contain corn syrup and soy lecithin.

REASONS TO CUT OUT WHEAT AND WHITE FLOUR

If you want to prevent cancer, I recommend eating foods containing gluten-containing flours and grains only on special occasions—and be sure that they're organic. For example, if you come across a baker making beautiful, fresh loaves of organic bread baked with high-quality non-GMO wheat, it might be an occasion to have some gluten. But even organic gluten is likely to be inflaming to the gut. A little may be okay to eat because the body can recover from its presence, but you don't want to make it a habit. In general, it's best to avoid foods made from wheat and white flour, including bread and other refined carbohydrates.

If you have a family heritage of celiac disease, avoid gluten at all times, as for you, gluten is truly a poison. One in 100 Americans—roughly three million people—have celiac disease, though many don't know it.

A 40-year study of 30,000 people in Sweden, reported in the *Journal of the American Medical Association*, compared mortality rates of people with celiac, people with inflamed guts and no celiac disease, and people with gluten sensitivity (which can come from overexposure). The researchers discovered that even for individuals with no genetic predisposition to celiac disease, inflammation and gluten sensitivity were high risk factors for heart disease and cancer.[18]

Gluten occurs naturally in grains such as wheat and rye. Rye is in a lot of fillers and additives, which is why gluten is present in nearly all highly processed foods. But it wasn't until wheat began to be modified for industrial breadmaking in the 1960s that it became triggering to people without the gene for celiac intolerance. In *Wise Traditions in Food, Farming and the Healing Arts*, the Weston A. Price Foundation published a fascinating article by Katherine Czapp on the history of wheat, explaining that common people rarely ate wheat until the 19th century. In 1777, George Washington was one of the first wheat farmers in America, and he was merely a hobbyist.[19]

These days we have so much food at our disposal that the amount of gluten in our diets has become excessive. Gluten, just like white sugar, is everywhere. You can find it in white bread, pastries, cakes, cookies, bagels, muffins, gummy bears, candy, and even in shampoo. After repeated exposures, many people develop a sensitivity to it of which they are unaware. Babies are even being born gluten intolerant.

When we are intolerant to a food we have eaten, it creates inflammation in the body that weakens our immune system. Remember, cancer cells thrive when conditions are right. If you are an emotional eater and battling overeating, I recommend cutting glutinous foods—like white flour—from your diet, as those foods are a trigger for the mind to go into a negative space. Refined carbs have sugars in them that light up the reward centers in the brain, which keeps us binge eating more foods containing gluten.

During their cancer treatments, people report that they sometimes urgently crave sugary or glutinous foods. If you stay nourished with smoothies and juices, you will be less likely to respond to a craving by grabbing something not conducive to healing. You can continue the momentum of healing your body by sticking with nutrient-dense foods.

Reasons to Cut Out Alcohol

In a metanalysis of the data from more than 200 studies on alcohol, researchers at the National Institute on Alcohol Abuse and Alcoholism report: "Alcohol most strongly increased the risks for cancers of the oral cavity, pharynx, esophagus, and larynx. Statistically significant increases in risk also existed for cancers of the stomach, colon, rectum, liver, female breast, and ovaries. Excessive alcohol can put major stress on the liver."[20]

The Centers for Disease Control and Prevention recommends a maximum of one drink per day for women and two drinks per day for men. Oncologist and hematologist Thomas Froehlich, M.D., who works at the Harold C. Simmons Comprehensive Cancer Center at the University of Texas Southwestern Medical Center, says: "Although many people believe that daily consumption of red wine (which contains the plant antioxidant resveratrol) prevents cancer, no clinical evidence suggests this to be true. Limit alcohol consumption to lower your risk for cancer."[21]

Furthermore, alcohol contains a lot of sugar, so it perpetuates sugar addiction and contributes to inflammation. Another reason to cut out alcohol is that it impairs judgment. When you're drinking at a social gathering, for example, you are much more likely to throw caution to the wind and reach for a toxic food choice.

Reasons to Cut Out Meat from Nonorganic, Hormone-Treated Animals

Conventionally produced meats are often produced using antibiotics and hormones to treat the animals and make them grow bigger. Effects in the human body, such as estrogen disruption, occur when this meat is consumed. A better choice is to buy local pasture-raised, grass-fed meats that are labeled "hormone-free" and "antibiotic-free."

Organic meat is better for you than nonorganic, as it is sourced from animals that are not fed GMO grains or foods treated with toxic pesticides and herbicides. To prevent and heal cancer, it is important to keep your level of exposure to environmental toxins low.

Reasons to Cut Out Processed and Charred Meats

Processed meats are prime sources of preservative salts, like nitrates and nitrites, which have been linked to gastrointestinal cancers for years.[22] Think hot dogs, bacon, ham, lunch meat, cured meat, corned beef, smoked fish, and so on—skip those.

Smoking, charcoal-broiling, and pan-frying meat can result in the formation of cancer-causing compounds, like polycyclic aromatic hydrocarbons (PAHs) and heterocyclic amines. There is reasonable evidence that this can increase your risk for developing kidney cancer.[23] It is best to limit the amount of meat you consume that is cooked at excessively high temperatures.

Reasons to Cut Out Nonorganic Fruits
and Vegetables

Avoid nonorganic fruits and vegetables as if your life depends on it. It does! Nonorganic produce is laden with the residues of toxic herbicides and pesticides used during farming.

Industrial farming practices have loaded our produce, air, water, soil, and animals at the bottom of the food chain (which we feed with our produce) with deadly chemicals. Always try to buy organic—ideally, locally grown foods. It is a must to buy some fruits and vegetables organic, like strawberries, as these absorb more of the pesticides and herbicides sprayed on them. By contrast, there are some you can get away with buying conventionally, like avocados, for example, as they have a harder shell and are less absorbent. The consumer watchdog organization the Environmental Working Group (EWG) keeps track of pesticides in 80,000 items sold in the marketplace (see Resources). You can also find a list of safe and unsafe fruits and vegetables on my website: CancerFreewithFood.com.

REASONS TO CUT OUT CONVENTIONAL DAIRY PRODUCTS

Like wheat, dairy is a hidden source of food sensitivity. It contributes to inflammation and chronic health problems. Fortunately, we don't need it. We can get calcium in dark leafy greens, like kale, spinach, and watercress. We can enjoy drinking organic nut and seed milk.

Here are the top three reasons to cut out conventional dairy, and remember if you do choose to include dairy in your diet the rule is it must be organic and come from healthy grass-fed cows.

- Dairy and calcium have been linked to prostate cancer in men.[24]

- Most of the population (75 percent) is genetically unable to digest lactose, the sugar in milk, beyond the age of two to five. Research shows that 79 percent of Native Americans, 75 percent of blacks, 51 percent of Hispanics, and 21 percent of whites lack the ability to produce the enzyme lactase.[25] Thus, dairy causes inflammation and weakens their immunity, increasing their risk of cancer.

- Nonorganic milk could be laden with hormones, antibiotics, and growth factors given to cows on dairy farms. Also, those cows may be fed GMO corn or grains grown with pesticides and herbicides. All these chemicals get passed along to us, increasing our risk of getting cancer and making it harder to heal from cancer.

Modern milk is different than milk of past millennia. Cows on factory farms are kept pregnant and lactating year-round, and as a result their bodies are flooded with estrogen. One study found that countries with the highest consumption of dairy products had the highest incidence of prostate and testicular cancer. In 2005, the same was found true for breast, ovarian, and uterine cancer.[26]

A final reason to avoid dairy is that it is high in fat, which is a carrier for aflatoxin B_1 and polychlorinated biphenyls (commonly referred to as PCBs). Although these toxic chemicals are now banned, they nonetheless have contaminated the food chain. They are in the soil and the riverbeds, which means they get into the fatty tissues of the fish and the animals we consume. Because they are stable under heat, for a long time these chemicals were used to coat electrical wiring, and now they are ubiquitous. Avoiding fatty foods lessens the risk of consumption.[27]

REASONS TO CUT OUT FARMED SEAFOOD

Farm-raised salmon is nutritionally different than wild-caught salmon in a few ways. First, it has considerably more calories. It is also much higher in fats, especially omega-6s, which can contribute to inflammation. Further, it is lower in minerals like potassium, zinc, and iron. Finally, and this is the main reason to avoid it, it is much higher in contaminants.[28]

Fish pick up chemicals, such as dioxins and PCBs, from the water they swim in. And they pick them up from the feed they are given, which in salmon farming often means grains grown with pesticides. Fisheries also raise animals in crowded conditions, so they give the fish antibiotics to reduce the chance of infection. Everything is in their flesh.

REASONS TO CUT OUT PASTEURIZED FOOD

Pasteurization is a technology of high heating that was invented to make milk from sick cows and cows living in unsanitary conditions safe to drink. It is also used to kill bacteria in other foods and beverages. High heat can change the molecules in the food and lead to the creation of free radicals, which may damage our DNA and lead to cancer.

In addition to destroying "bad" bacteria, pasteurization destroys "good" bacteria—the probiotics—and enzymes that can help us digest a variety of foods. Ty Bollinger of the Truth about Cancer likens pasteurization to dropping an atomic weapon on our food.[29]

REASONS TO CUT OUT TRANS FATS AND PARTIALLY HYDROGENATED OILS

For decades, we were told by the "experts" that we had to avoid eating fat. But this was poor advice. As we discussed, we need "good" fat in our diets. What we need to avoid is "bad" fat—trans fats and hydrogenated oils, to be specific.

Understanding the chemistry of fat molecules can make your eyes cross. There are saturated and unsaturated fats. And subcategories of each type—for example, mono- or polyunsaturated fats. On a food label, you will also see the category trans fats. Trans fats are the worst of the worst, and are officially banned in the United States.

There are a few naturally occurring trans fats, but most are byproducts of industrial food-preparation processes. This is why they are found in margarine, chips, crackers, baked goods, and fast foods. They are such a threat to public health that in May 2018 the World Health Organization released a six-point plan, known by the acronym RELEASE, to remove them from the global food supply.[30]

According to Dr. Mark Hyman, eating foods that are sources of omega-3 (good) fats, like flaxseeds, chia seeds, egg yolks, walnuts, and salmon, is imperative because, among other benefits, they heal inflammation. He says: "Inflammation is the common thread connecting most chronic disease including cancer. In fact, out-of-control inflammation causes insulin resistance, which, as we now know, is the main factor in all these diseases apart from autoimmunity and allergy. The insulin resistance then creates even more inflammation, and the whole biological house burns down."[31]

Partially hydrogenated oils should be cut out of your diet without hesitation. Hydrogenation is the process of adding hydrogen to a liquid fat to turn it into a solid. Partial—not full—hydrogenation is where trans fats come from. (Full hydrogenation may have other risks you would wish to avoid, like eating too much saturated fat or consuming oil made from chemically contaminated produce.)

Do not try to avoid fats altogether; God designed healthy fats for a purpose. We need them to metabolize fat-soluble nutrients and for our brains to function properly. When you avoid fats, you ruin your health. You can experience burnout—complete exhaustion—and this leads to craving fast food and fried food. Stay nourished by healthy fats and you will find the other stuff less appealing. Healthy fats will also reduce your inflammation.

Replace bad fats with healthy fats like the following.

- Olives and olive oil
- Coconuts and coconut oil
- Raw nuts, such as macadamias and pecans
- Seeds, such as sesame, pumpkin, hemp, and chia
- Organic egg yolks from pastured poultry
- Meat from grass-fed, pasture-raised animals
- Butter or ghee made from raw, grass-fed, organic milk
- Animal-based omega-3 fat, such as krill oil
- Wild-caught salmon
- Cacao butter

Reasons to Cut Out Microwaved Foods

As convenient as they may be for the rapid heating and thawing of foods and beverages, microwave ovens are carcinogenic for several reasons. First, a microwave oven emits radio frequency radiation that is vibrating incredibly fast; the water molecules in the food resonate with this frequency and begin to move faster, heating them. Outside radiation, our food and beverages are chemically transformed by this heating process.

Do you typically make your morning oatmeal in the microwave? Have you ever popped in a bag of spinach to steam-cook it? Do you use the microwave to thaw meat from your freezer? Or to reheat day-old slices of pizza? Here are just a few changes in food molecules that may be evoked by using one of these time-saving devices, according to Lloyd Burrell, an expert on electromagnetic fields.[32]

- Amino acids in milk and cereal grains may be converted into carcinogens.

- Sugars in thawed frozen fruits may be converted into carcinogens.

- Alkaloids in vegetables may be converted into carcinogens.

- Meat may form chemical compounds that are known carcinogens.

- Chemicals from plastic packaging, wraps, and bowls—in which many foods are heated—leach into the food. Benzene is one, among several.

The World Health Organization classifies microwave radiation as a class 2B possible carcinogen.[33] Burrell tested the electromagnetic fields (EMFs) around microwave ovens and found them to be more significant than manufacturers would lead us to believe. Even if the oven is in brand-new, pristine condition, as it came from the manufacturer, microwaves will be escaping it. And over time, most oven doors get a little wobbly, so the seals are not as good as they're supposed to be. Do not stand near your microwave when it is on because it *will* be leaking radiation.[34]

In addition, the electrical cords for ovens emit radiation—as do all our household appliances. Some people reject this as a problem, but the science is clear.[35] If you have many plugged-in electrical appliances in your home or office, you can rent an EMF detector from a hardware store and read their fields to ascertain your exposure.

———◆———

Sorry to scare you by describing so many toxic foods and substances, but it is certainly better to know than to poison your body through ignorance. Now that you know, you get to make the powerful choice to demonstrate that you value your body by only putting good-quality, wholesome foods into it. The reward for treating your body well is good health, high energy, strong immunity, mental clarity, and happiness. It's everything.

Given that we now know what's toxic, where do we start? How do we achieve the changes in our eating habits every day that make the most difference and still get to eat and drink what we love—foods with sweet, salty, crunchy, savory deliciousness? In the next chapter, I'll teach you my Upgrade Mind-Set. You'll see how the Cancer-Free with Food plan is doable.

CHAPTER 5

LIVING THE FOOD UPGRADE MIND-SET

After my diagnosis of precancer, I still felt the urge to eat junk food. This troubled me very much, because I *knew* that eating like this would not help me heal and would only worsen my condition, yet there was a part of me that wanted to go out and eat food that was terrible for me. This is one of those confusing human moments that at the end of the day we can laugh at, although it may seem overwhelming while it's occurring.

Someone once told me—and I believe it—that the greatest spiritual teachers on earth don't take themselves or events too seriously; they are lighthearted and can laugh at the craziness of life. But I wasn't there yet. Assessing the seriousness of my condition, I saw I had to figure out a way not to eat junk foods or else I was going to make the cancer grow and spread.

THE UPGRADE APPROACH

One approach I tried and quickly failed at was fasting. This approach lasted just one day for me because I noticed that I felt worse when I tried to fast. I felt so tired and so weak, so deprived and so starved, that I could tell that my blood sugar level had dropped dramatically. At first, I liked the idea of fasting. I had spent so many years overeating that the idea of being light and empty appealed to me. But as soon as I tried it, I realized that I needed to *strengthen* my body with nutrients; fasting was weakening for me.

Failing at fasting is what led me to develop the approach that I now call upgrading.

Once I left the hospital, I fully surrendered to the idea that I needed something bigger than myself to transform my eating habits. Something I could use to confront the problem of my cravings head on. That's when I got the idea to adopt the thought process, *Every time I am craving something to eat, I will find a way to eat it in the most natural way possible—in a way that nourishes my body at the same time as tastes really good.*

I was excited to try to find or invent new, healthier versions of the foods I loved. And the very first item I craved was chocolate. So, I set out to find how to make it in a healthier way.

This was a decade ago and there weren't as many organic choices available to us then. Although I did locate some organic chocolate in a health-food store, which was an upgrade from conventional chocolate, it was sweetened with white sugar, an ingredient I wanted to avoid.

When I am doing nutritional coaching, I always say: Start with your greatest obstacle first. Replace that food and the rest of the changes you want to make will be easier. It will also give you a lot of relief to move a huge rock from your path to wellness. For some people, the food blocking the path might be pizza, or pasta, or bread, or cheese, or candy. What is yours?

For five years, chocolate was always my biggest weakness and greatest obstacle to healthy eating. I had recently read a study about how in ancient Egypt they'd made chocolate from cacao beans, so I purchased some cacao powder, some almond flour, and some honey, and I made a raw chocolate brownie mixture with just those three ingredients.

Then I made variations of this dessert with almond butter and peanut butter to give it some additional flavor. And wow, I was blown away! The result was like a moist, buttery, delicious chocolate brownie, although it contained no gluten, no dairy, no soy, no preservatives, no GMO ingredients, and no refined sugar. It tasted absolutely delicious, all the while providing my body with protein, fiber, antioxidants, and other nutrients. It was a dream come true.

Upgrading is how we can have our cake and eat it too!

I used the upgrade approach to replicate all my favorite foods. I made chicken tenders with organic chicken and a coating of turmeric, almond flour, and sea salt. I made cheesecake with cashews. I made ice cream with almond milk. I used coconut oil instead of butter. I made cookie dough from almond flour and maple syrup. And I discovered that there is a healthier alternative for absolutely everything that we want to eat.

This means we can continue to eat the foods we love for the rest of our lives guilt-free! We can eat them and achieve optimal wellness.

Truly, it's not realistic for any of us to think, *I will start a new diet on Monday—after which I will never, ever eat cookies again.* We are not biologically programmed for deprivation. That's why millions of people are stuck in an *I'll start tomorrow* pattern and are still eating junk food.

But when we adopt the approach of asking "How can I eat cookies *in a healthy way?*" and then find a way to do so, we fulfill our cravings and have a pleasurable experience. Because this food tastes good and nourishes the body, it also leaves us with a sense of real satiety.

That's the key. Flood the body with nutrients at the same time as you are indulging in happy-tasting flavors. I was mind-blown to discover this and wished I had learned it before I had first tried processed foods with refined sugars and become hooked on the sugar.

If you get stuck and can't find an alternative to something you would like to eat, please let me know. So far, there hasn't been one food that I haven't been able to find an upgrade for that hasn't worked for someone. Tweet me @theearthdieter or send me a message via another social network such as Facebook or Instagram. I would love to hear from you and help you upgrade your diet.

The Upgrade Thought Process

When you have a craving think, How can I satisfy this in the best way possible?

> *Worst-case scenario:* Low-quality fast food and conventional options; GMO and nonorganic ingredients; high-sugar, high-fat foods; anything with artificial colorings, flavors, and preservatives
>
> *Better upgrade:* The organic option with clean ingredients
>
> *Best upgrade:* Make your own with the highest-quality ingredients you can buy.

Let's say, for example, you want some French fries. The worst-case scenario is buying fries at a fast-food franchise made from GMO potatoes cooked in low-quality oil and seasoned with preservative-ridden salt. What is the upgrade in this situation?

The *better* version is to get them at an organic restaurant where the cook uses non-GMO potatoes and high-quality oil.

The *best* version is to cook them at home yourself, using the Coconut Basil Sweet Potato Fries recipe (page 233), with extra-virgin coconut oil and sea salt with a high mineral content, prepared in a nontoxic stainless-steel pan.

If you do opt for the worst-case scenario—perhaps because you're traveling and nowhere near an organic cafe or a kitchen—then, rather than berate yourself for choosing that option, you can *upgrade the experience* by following the fries with Lemon Water (page 191) or a freshly squeezed vegetable juice to assist with digestion and elimination of toxins.

Living this way reduces guilt. When you know you're moving toward health, even by a small, incremental step, you feel better and have more peace of mind. Plus, you feel way less deprived if you do the right thing. It's empowering!

Deprivation diets will only drive you crazy, leaving you feeling worse than when you started. It's important to be kind to yourself. Health is the goal—and feeling good and being at ease with yourself are indicators of good health. This is why upgrading is such a great tool.

When you want chocolate, eat chocolate. Just try to make sure it's organic. Organic cacao, which is an ingredient in chocolate, is featured in different recipes in this book. You can also have cheesecake, cupcakes, ice cream, mousse, burgers, burritos, fries—just upgrade them from the old familiar junk-food versions. There are recipes for all these foods here as well.

When you upgrade, you're making a better choice. You're not sacrificing anything—except things that are harmful, like preservatives. The result is that you're eating food that tastes amazing and provides your body with the nutrition it needs.

In case you haven't noticed, I *love* eating dessert, and I ate a lot of dessert, which contributed to my recovery from cancer. If you do too, you'll be pleased to know that you can find almost anything to cure your sweet and creamy cravings in the dessert recipe section. Just follow the rule: Upgrade it. Make sure it is as natural as possible. The quickest upgrade decision is to choose organic ingredients.

EXAMPLES OF UPGRADES

The following upgrades will come up again and again. If you commit these to memory, you'll save yourself some time.

The Bread Upgrade: When you crave bread, go get the highest-quality freshly baked organic bread you can. If you're worried about the price difference, remind yourself that you are a high-quality person and you deserve high-quality foods that don't make you sick! Upgrade further by baking your own bread using organic, non-GMO ingredients.

The Salad Dressing Upgrade: When you're having your salad, instead of using a premade, store-bought salad dressing filled with sugar and preservatives, choose an organic salad dressing. Upgrade further by making your own salad dressing from simple ingredients like extra-virgin olive oil and lemon, or sesame oil and vinegar. (See "Sensational Sauces and Life-Changing Condiments" on pp. 311–322.)

The Burger Upgrade: When you crave a burger, get it from an organic restaurant that uses free-range meat. Upgrade again by making your own burger at home. (Try the Grass-Fed Beef Burger on page 286, the Bean Burger on page 219, and the Chickpea Burger on page 220, with the Ketchup on page 318.)

The Pizza Upgrade: When you're having a pizza, upgrade by buying it fresh from a pizza parlor that makes it with high-quality flour and cheese. Upgrade further by making it yourself with organic cheese and dough, topped with your favorite vegetables. (Try the Cauliflower Crust Mini Pizza on page 214.)

The Pasta Upgrade: You can upgrade pasta by using brown rice pasta, quinoa pasta, or black bean pasta, which taste amazing. All three of these types of pasta are good sources of protein and fiber, and they're also gluten-free, meaning you can eat them without getting bloated. (Try the Mac 'n' Cheese on page 227, the Zucchini Pasta with Broccoli Sprouts Pesto on page 212, and the Cajun Spice Pasta with Oat Cream on page 225.)

The Salt Upgrade: Any salt that has fillers and preservatives is toxic for the body. Upgrade your salt by using pure sea salt.

The Oil Upgrade: Instead of using GMO vegetable oil (including plain "vegetable oil" and canola oil), use non-GMO oils from the following list: extra-virgin olive oil, extra-virgin coconut oil, avocado oil, hempseed oil, flaxseed oil, tigernut oil, sesame oil, almond oil, and chia seed oil.

The Dairy Upgrade: Make sure to upgrade your milk, yogurt, and cheese products to organic, non-GMO, hormone-free, antibiotic-free, growth hormone–free (BGH-free) dairy from the milk of grass-fed, free-range cows—and sourced as locally as possible.

The Cheese Upgrade: Make sure if you are eating dairy cheese that it is organic and high quality. For a vegan upgrade, make your own recipes with nutritional yeast. Nutritional yeast is a vegan's best friend!

The Flour Upgrade: If you want to make a recipe that calls for flour, you must absolutely go for organic flour; flour is often genetically modified, and you don't not want those chemicals going into your body. For a gluten-free flour mix, these work really well: arrowroot, tapioca, brown rice flour, potato starch, and buckwheat.

The Egg Upgrade: Upgrade your eggs to organic, non-GMO, hormone-free, antibiotic-free, growth hormone–free eggs from pasture-raised, free-range chickens. Buy local, if possible.

The Fries Upgrade: When you crave French fries, get a batch from a café that uses high-quality oil. Upgrade further by making them at home using organic potatoes and extra-virgin coconut oil. (See Coconut Basil Sweet Potato Fries on page 233 and Chickpea Fries on page 302.)

The Chocolate Upgrade: When you crave chocolate, buy organic chocolate made from pure ingredients: no dairy, soy, preservatives, or refined sugar. Upgrade further by making your own raw chocolate at home. (See Chocolate Almond Buttercups on page 332, Chocolate Avocado Mousse on page 328, and the Classic Three-Ingredient Chocolate Ball on page 324.)

The Potato Chip Upgrade: When you feel like eating chips or crisps, go for non-GMO, organic potato products. There are some excellent brands out there. Upgrade further by making Baked Kale Chips (page 305).

The Candy Upgrade: When you crave candy, get organic candy that is also free of corn syrup, gluten, gelatin, and preservatives. Upgrade further by dehydrating a fruit puree at home, which is squished into different shapes. (Try Fruit Leathers on page 347).

The Cookie Upgrade: Buy organic, non-GMO cookies with few, simple ingredients. Upgrade further by making your own. Even more of an upgrade is eating the nutrient-dense Raw Cookie Dough, which is eggless and therefore safe to eat raw (page 326), and its baked variation, Melt in Your Mouth Baked Chocolate Chip Cookies. You can actually get vitamins and minerals from this!

The Soda Upgrade: Conventional soda is dangerous because it contains ridiculous amounts of GMO sugar, caffeine, preservatives, colorings, flavorings, additives, and aspartame. Upgrade with organic sodas made from honey and fruit or kombucha, which is a probiotic and aids digestion.

The Energy Shot Upgrade: Excessive reliance on caffeine can cause adrenal burnout. Furthermore, many of the most popular brands of energy shots contain damaging chemicals. Upgrade with the Lemon Ginger Shot (page 156). Also seek out one of the new, more enlightened fruit-based energy shots made with yerba mate, stevia, and containing high levels of B vitamins (often these do also contain caffeine, so you may wish to read the labels).

Organic vegetables and fruits don't need upgrades. Eat plenty every day.

———◆———

It's time to release any guilt you feel about your past food choices. Now that you know that there are healthier alternatives, you can choose those instead! Remember what Maya Angelou said: "Do the best you can until you know better. Then when you know better, do better."

When cravings hit, take a moment to remember the Upgrade Mind-Set. There is a healthy upgrade for every kind of craving imaginable—crunchy, sweet, creamy, savory, and salty.

CHAPTER 6

HEALING GUIDES FOR COMMON CANCERS

More than 100 different cancers can affect humans. According to the National Cancer Institute, the following are the 30 most commonly diagnosed types listed in order of prevalence.[1]

1. Skin cancer
2. Lung cancer
3. Breast cancer
4. Prostate cancer
5. Colorectal cancer
6. Bladder cancer
7. Non-Hodgkins lymphoma
8. Kidney cancer
9. Leukemia
10. Thyroid cancer
11. Pancreatic cancer
12. Uterine cancer
13. Liver cancer
14. Stomach cancer
15. Brain and spinal cord cancers
16. Esophageal cancer
17. Cervical cancer
18. Hodgkins disease
19. Endometrial cancer
20. Heart cancer
21. Extrahepatic bile duct cancer
22. Gallbladder cancer
23. Bladder cancer
24. Ovarian cancer

25. Salivary gland cancer

26. Urethral cancer

27. Bronchial cancer

28. AIDS-related cancers

29. Lip and oral
    cavity cancer

30. Larynx cancer

In this chapter, we'll look at several of the top cancers from the list above, exploring what foods to eat to get and stay well. Specific recipes will be recommended from Part II of this book. And as my aim is to empower you with knowledge about all-natural approaches to upgrade your self-care—here and there you'll also find a smattering of quick tips and home remedies, if those are relevant.

SKIN CANCER

There are three main categories of skin cancer: squamous cell carcinoma, basal cell carcinoma, and melanoma. Rarer types are Merkel cell tumors and dermatofibrosarcoma protuberans.

Best Foods to Eat

Registered dietician and skin cancer survivor Anne Cundiff recommends increasing your consumption of lycopene-rich foods. She explains: "This powerful antioxidant found in reddish-colored fruits tends to act as a natural sunscreen, providing an SPF of 3 or 4 from the inside out. In addition, lycopene helps your skin act as a natural filter, allowing enough sunlight through for your body to produce vitamin D."[2]

To prevent or heal skin cancer, try preparing meals that contain:

- Beta-carotene (carrots, kale, mango, spinach, squash, and sweet potato)
- Curcumin (turmeric and curry)
- Epigallocatechin gallate (EGCG) and polyphenols (cacao, garlic, green and black tea, oregano, rosemary, and thyme)
- Lutein (collard greens, kale, and spinach)

- Lycopene (apricot, guava, ruby red grapefruit, tomato, and watermelon)
- Selenium (Brazil nuts and some meats)
- Sulforaphane and a variety of other phytochemicals, minerals, and fiber (cruciferous veggies like broccoli, brussels sprouts, cabbage, cauliflower, and kale)
- Vitamin A (sweet potatoes and eggs)

Try These Cancer-Free with Food Recipes

- Anita Moorjani's Coconut Curry (page 222)
- Cauliflower Rice (page 224)
- Superpowerful Green Juice (page 148)

- Chocolate Smoothie (page 171)
- Walnut "Meatballs" (page 210)
- Superfood Kale Salad (page 245)

Mama Z's Serum

In *The Healing Power of Essential Oils*, Eric Zielinski, D.C., tells the story of his wife, Sabrina Ann Zielinski aka Mama Z, and her dad, who battled melanoma and had precancerous lesions on his arms and hands. As Mama Z described it: "I ended up making my dad two varieties of my antiaging cream for him to try: one with lavender oil only and another with a blend of lavender, tea tree, and frankincense. He used both my cream and the prescription stuff for a short time and ended up using my concoctions alone. From what we can tell, the precancerous lesions were not a sign of a candida infection and they simply disappeared and didn't progress to melanoma. Within six weeks, his hands and arms were completely clear, and now he's a believer in the power of DIY with essential oils!"[3]

Mama Z's supereasy serum is very good for the skin on its own, but even better with the essential oils. Use it as a carrier oil for a blend of any of your favorite essential oils!

Ingredients:

4 ounces aloe vera gel

4 ounces organic, unrefined coconut oil, melted

32 drops lavender essential oil

16 drops frankincense essential oil (any species will do)

16 drops tea tree (melaleuca) essential oil

8 drops sandalwood essential oil

Actions:

1. Blend the aloe gel, coconut oil, and essential oils in a food processor or blender until smooth.

2. Once well mixed, store in a glass jar or salve container in a cool place (like the fridge) so the coconut oil remains hardened.

3. Apply over any problem areas on your skin at least once per day.

Quick Tips

- For diagnostic purposes, get regular skin checks by your doctor or a dermatologist.

- Stay out of tanning beds, and always wear sunblock with an SPF of at least 30, even when it's not sunny. Buy natural skincare products or make your own. Stay away from any sunscreen or lip product that has these ingredients: avobenzone, homosalate, oxybenzone, octisalate, octocrylene, octinoxate, retinol, retinyl palmitate, or vitamin A.

- Oxybenzone alone is a synthetic estrogen that penetrates the skin and can disrupt your endocrine system. More than half of the beach and sport sunscreens in the marketplace contain oxybenzone. Its primary function is to absorb ultraviolet light, but some research shows it can be absorbed through the skin. Staff at the Environmental Working Group and other toxicology experts believe that oxybenzone is linked to hormone disruption and potentially to cell damage that could lead to skin cancer.[4]

- According to the EWG, we should look for mineral products that include zinc oxide, titanium dioxide, 3 percent avobenzone, or Mexoryl SX. These ingredients protect skin from harmful UVA and UVB light rays.[5]

For more ideas, visit CancerFreewithFood.com/SkinCancer

2. LUNG CANCER

There are three types of lung cancer: non-small cell lung cancer, small cell lung cancer, and lung carcinoid tumors.[6] Fewer than 5 percent of lung cancer falls into the latter category, which are also sometimes referred to as lung neuroendocrine tumors.[7]

Best Foods to Eat

Ever heard the expression "An apple a day keeps the doctor away"? Well, there's truth in those words. Flavonoids found in apples, like quercetin, can destroy cancer-causing free radicals in the lungs. According to a 1999 study published in the *Journal of the National Cancer Institute*, people who eat apples on a regular basis can lower their risk of lung cancer by up to 60 percent.[8]

To prevent or heal lung cancer, try preparing meals that contain:

- Anthocyanosides (acai, blueberries, chokeberries, black and red currants, eggplant, purple cauliflower, concord grapes, and dried red cabbage)
- Beta-carotene (whole fruits and veggies—usually orange in color—like carrots, cantaloupe, squash, mangoes, and sweet potatoes). But stick to whole foods; supplements that isolate beta-carotene seem to have the opposite effect—especially in smokers—though researchers don't know why.[9]
- Curcumin (turmeric and curry)
- Ellagic acid (blackberries, raspberries, strawberries, and walnuts)

- EGCG and polyphenols (green and black tea, oregano, rosemary, and thyme)
- Isoflavones (non-GMO soy foods, like tofu, tempeh, and soymilk[10])
- Quercetin (apples, capers, dill, cilantro, cranberries, grapes, kale, radicchio, red onions, watercress, and white grapefruit)
- Selenium and sulfur (garlic)

Try These Cancer-Free with Food Recipes

- Blueberry Chia Seed Jam (page 316)
- Cauliflower Popcorn (page 223)
- Chocolate Cauliflower Smoothie (page 177)
- Cauliflower Rice (page 224)
- Mashed Cauliflower (page 241)

Quick Tips

- The late Louise Hay, renowned mind, body, soul expert and author of *You Can Heal Your Life*, believed that all physical illness was linked to an emotional and mental state. According to Hay, lung issues may be caused by depression, grief, or feeling unworthy of living a full life. To counteract the energy of those types of feelings, you could practice sitting upright and taking big breaths while using the following affirmations, *I am safe, I am supported, and I am loved. I have the capacity to take in the fullness of life. I lovingly live life to the fullest.* Every time you feel fear or sadness say these affirmations, even if you don't believe them yet. This can help the subconscious mind and help to override a negative emotion.

- The Dana-Farber Cancer Institute recommends exercise for people with lung cancer. Even if you have shortness of breath, exercise can help you to decrease fatigue and the risk of secondary illnesses related to the cancer. Definitely consult with your care team before you begin. Light walking or physical therapy is the safest option. Listen to your body. Try not to get frustrated if you cannot do as much as you used to do right away; just start low and slow, doing 5–10 minutes at a time several times per day. Easy cycling or swimming are good too.

- Improve your posture to take in more oxygen. Keep your shoulders and chin back and open your chest to encourage deeper breathing.

For more ideas, visit CancerFreewithFood.com/LungCancer

3. BREAST CANCER

Breast cancer cells can begin in different areas of the breast such as the ducts, the lobules, or the tissue in between.[11] It may be invasive, noninvasive, or metastatic, among a number of subtypes.

Best Foods to Eat

Women who eat a diet supplemented with extra-virgin olive oil and mixed nuts may have a reduced risk of breast cancer.[12] If you follow the *Cancer-Free with Food* recipes, you'll naturally choose sources of healthy fats such as these oversaturated fats like butter. Also, flaxseeds may play a role in slowing breast cancer cell growth and may even improve the effectiveness of some cancer treatments.[13] They are rich in omega-3 fatty acids, minerals, vitamins, and fiber. You can add flaxseed oil or flaxseeds to smoothies, soups, and salad dressings. For breakfast, add them to your eggs or cereal. You can add flaxseed meal to desserts and snacks like the Chocolate Balls (page 324).

In addition to healthy fats, focus on your intake of antioxidants and phytochemicals. When my mum was diagnosed with breast cancer a couple of years ago, she made fresh juice at home multiple times a day with lots of orange and lemon for vitamin

C, to which she would add a whole clove of garlic. Johns Hopkins Breast Center recommends five or more servings a day of fruits and vegetables, especially those high in fiber, as fiber may protect against the hormonal actions of breast cancer. Aim for 25 to 30 grams of soluble and insoluble fiber per day.[14]

To prevent or heal cancer, try preparing meals that contain:

- Coumarins, flavones, and carotenoids (umbelliferous herbs and vegetables like carrots, celery, cilantro, dill, fennel, parsley, and parsnips[15])

- Indoles and sulforaphane (cruciferous vegetables like broccoli, broccoli sprouts, brussels sprouts, cabbage, collard greens, kale, kohlrabi, mustard greens, turnips, turnip greens, and watercress[16])

- Isoflavones (non-GMO soy, legumes, and flaxseeds[17])

- Lentinan (mushrooms, especially Asian varieties like shiitake and maitake)

- Lycopene (carrots, mangoes, tomatoes, and watermelon)

- Potassium, magnesium, iron, and various other nutrients (cucurbitaceous vegetables like cucumber, pumpkin, squash, zucchini, and watermelon)

- Protein (vegetarian options like legumes and lentils; poultry; and fish)

- Solanaceous vegetables (capsicum, chili peppers, eggplant, and potatoes)

- Sulfur (allium vegetables like garlic, chives, leeks, onions, and shallots[18])

- Green leafy vegetables (beet greens; endives, romaine, and other lettuces; spinach; and Swiss chard)

- Non-GMO whole grains (barley, bulgur, oats, quinoa, and rye)

Try These Cancer-Free with Food Recipes

- Vitamin C Blaster Juice (page 151)
- A Splash of Sunshine Smoothie (page 173)
- Vibrant Orange Carrot Ginger Juice (page 154)
- Sick-Kick Smoothie (page 169)
- Orange Arugula Avocado Sesame Seed Salad (page 249)

Mama Axe's Cancer Story

Josh Axe, D.N.M., D.C., C.N.S., is a doctor of natural medicine, a chiropractor, and a certified nutrition specialist. His mother has had two bouts with breast cancer. The second time she followed an all-natural plan with his support and got significant results—after a year she was declared "disease-free." Although when he shared this story with me, Dr. Axe was careful to stipulate that the plan might not lead to the same results for everyone, he believes that whether in conjunction with conventional treatments or on its own, it may support the body in its healing process.[19]

Here are some elements drawn from his mom's protocol.

- Eating turmeric and coriolus mushrooms
- Chlorella, blue-green algae, and spirulina, because they bind with heavy metals, thus helping eliminate them
- Dietary supplementation with digestive enzymes, probiotics, vitamin D_3, and frankincense essential oil
- Conjugated linoleic acid (CLA), which is helpful in preventing colon, rectal, and breast cancers
- Folate, which is helpful for breast, colorectal, and pancreatic cancers
- Melatonin, for better sleep
- Vitamin C chelation
- Oxygen therapy in a hyperbaric chamber

- Gerson Therapy, which consisted of consuming organic, plant-based foods, raw juices, beef liver, and natural supplements, as well as doing coffee enemas (see Resources)

- Sunshine

- Praying and building peace

Quick Tips

If you've been diagnosed with cancer, take your time deciding what course of treatment you want to do. In a podcast on managing breast cancer, surgical oncologist Alexander Miller, M.D., says: "Breast cancer is not something that develops overnight, and so you should feel very comfortable taking a week or more to make a decision."[20]

Avoid nonfermented soy products like tofu and edamame, which can raise estrogen levels. Fermented soy products like miso, natto, and tempeh, are acceptable—and good sources of vitamin K_2.

Women's health expert Christiane Northup, M.D., wisely insists: "All women can create healthy breasts."[21] In an article on creating optimal breast health, she explains that bolstering our immunity is critical. I love that her focus is on wellness, not fear! She offers several tips for creating healthy breasts.

- Cultivate a practice of self-care and self-love. She says the most important factor in creating health is carving out time to care for and love yourself unconditionally.

- Get enough sleep. Sleep restores the body, and it's during sleep that our bodies metabolize stress hormones. Aim for eight hours per night.

- Optimize your vitamin D intake. The best way to get your vitamin D is from safe exposure to sunlight, but many people need to take a supplement.

- Exercise regularly and eat a healthy diet.

- Get social. Get off your cell phone, computer, tablet, or whatever, and get out with friends. Volunteer in your community or at your church. Take up a new activity, such as dancing or yoga. Having a fulfilling social life improves your immune system. When your immune system is healthy it naturally kills off pathogens and rogue cells that can lead to disease.[22]

For more ideas, visit CancerFreewithFood.com/BreastCancer

4. PROSTATE CANCER

Prostate cancer may begin in different areas—the gland, the ducts, the urethra, or tissues around the gland. The most common type is acinar adenocarcinoma.[23]

Best Foods to Eat

Dean Ornish, M.D., is president and founder of the nonprofit Preventive Medicine Research Institute in Sausalito, California, and a clinical professor of medicine at the University of California, San Francisco. He is perhaps best known for his lifestyle-based approach to fighting heart disease, showing that it can be treated and even reversed through modification of the diet and exercise. In the past decade, he has applied a similar approach to research on cancer.

In July 2007, *Harvard Men's Health Watch* published a report of a study he and four other researchers conducted to examine the impact of lifestyle therapy on mild to moderate prostate cancer. Ninety-three men participated. None was abusing alcohol, tobacco, or drugs. Half were in a control group and half adopted a program that included an ultra-low-fat diet, nutritional supplements, brisk walking, and stress reduction. After a year, results showed that 70 percent in the lifestyle-modification group had blood that inhibited cancer growth as compared to 9 percent of the control group. In other words, a healthy lifestyle sets up your body for health rather than cancer.[24]

Ornish advises limiting calories from fat to 10 percent of your diet. Eat a menu that consists mainly of fruits, vegetables, whole grain products, legumes, and organic soy products.

Physicians measure the presence of prostate specific antigens (PSAs) as one factor that can help them determine the presence of prostate tumors and the speed at which these may be growing. The slower a tumor grows, the better.[25] Research done at the Sidney Kimmel Comprehensive Cancer Center in Baltimore, Maryland, along with several private clinics, has shown that the phytonutrient-rich pomegranate can reduce the rate of PSA doubling in men with prostate cancer. Similarly, at the University of California, Los Angeles, researchers found that pomegranate juice significantly slowed progression and recurrence in men who had already undergone surgery or radiation for prostate cancer. Researchers say: "Overall, the doubling time increased from 11.9 months at baseline to 18.5 months after treatment with pomegranate extract."[26]

In my opinion, it's best to eat pomegranate whole; however, you could instead take a pomegranate powder or supplement if you were determined to avoid the fruit's sugars.

Another measure that prostate doctors pay attention to is the level of dihydrotestosterone (DHT). DHT is a hormone that can create abnormal cell growth and cancer production. Testing is done for the biomarker insulin-like growth factor 1 (IGF-1). If you needed another reason to eat plant-based foods, here it is! A study in *Cancer Epidemiology, Biomarkers & Prevention* reported that IGF-1 levels were elevated among eaters of animal protein but not among eaters of plant proteins (beans, legumes, lentils).[27]

To prevent or heal cancer, try preparing meals that contain:

- Bromelain (pineapple)
- Capsaicin (cayenne pepper)
- Curcumin (turmeric and curry)
- Ellagitannin (pomegranate seeds or juice)
- EGCG and polyphenols (green and black tea, oregano, rosemary, and thyme)

- Lentinan and l-ergothioneine (mushrooms like king oyster, oyster, reishi, maitake, and shiitake)
- Lycopene (carrots, mangoes, tomatoes, and watermelon)
- Lysine (almonds, peanuts, pecans, and walnuts)
- Omega-3 fatty acids (astaxanthin [algae], flaxseeds, sardines, trout, walnuts, and wild-caught salmon)
- Quercetin (apples, capers, dill, cilantro, cranberries, grapes, kale, radicchio, red onions, watercress, and white grapefruit)
- Selenium (Brazil nuts)
- Sulforaphane and indoles (cruciferous vegetables like broccoli, broccoli sprouts, brussels sprouts, cabbage, collard greens, kale, kohlrabi, mustard greens, turnips, turnip greens, and watercress[28])
- Vitamin D_3 (beef liver, cheese, egg yolks, and oily fish such as albacore tuna, cod, cod liver oil, herring, mackerel, mussels, salmon, sardines, and trout)
- Zinc (cashews, kale, pumpkin seeds, spinach, wheat germ, and white mushrooms)

Try These Cancer-Free with Food Recipes

- Anticancer Omelet (page 205)
- Baked Walnut-Crusted Salmon (page 291)
- Black Bean Bowl with Sweet Potatoes and Roasted Chickpeas (page 216)
- Chocolate-Covered Pomegranates (page 340)
- Vanilla Pudding (page 335)[29]

Quick Tips

- Drink a glass of fresh tomato juice or vegetable juice at breakfast daily.

- Avoid nonfermented soy products like tofu and edamame, which can raise estrogen levels (men have a small quantity of this hormone). Fermented soy products like miso, natto, and tempeh are acceptable—and good sources of vitamin K_2.

- Foods that raise PSA levels most are those that contain acrylamide, such as processed French fries, potato chips, cakes, and doughnuts.[30] Acrylamides come from heating oil to a high heat in the presence of certain sugars. Make these foods at home so you can control both the cooking process and the quality of your ingredients.

For more ideas, visit CancerFreewithFood.com/ProstateCancer

5. COLON CANCER

Colon cancer is cancer of the large intestine, the last segment of your gastrointestinal tract. It usually starts with the development of benign polyps. Over time, some of these become cancerous.[31] This kind of cancer is also sometimes referred to as colorectal cancer or bowel cancer.

Best Foods to Eat

To prevent or heal cancer, try preparing meals that contain:

- Calcium (almonds and almond milk); figs, currants, rhubarb; dark green leafy vegetables like collard greens, bok choy, kale, broccoli, watercress, and mustard greens; salmon, shrimp, sardines; and white beans) [32]

- Iron, fiber, magnesium, and folate (whole grains like steel-cut oats, quinoa, and brown rice)

- Omega-3 fatty acids (avocados; chia seeds; flaxseeds; oily fish such as albacore tuna, salmon, cod, cod liver oil, herring, mackerel, mussels, salmon, sardines, and trout; olive oil; and walnuts)

- Nitric oxide and betaine (beets and beet juice)

Try These Cancer-Free with Food Recipes

- Beet Juice (page 147)
- Chocolate Tigernut Milk (page 162)
- Five-Ingredient Green Salad (page 244)
- Super Detox Broccoli Sprout Green Salad (page 250)
- Superfood Kale Salad (page 245)

Chris Wark's Cancer Story

Chris Wark, author of *Chris Beat Cancer*, was diagnosed with stage IIIC colon cancer in December 2003. He explained to me how it was a panicked time, as doctors quickly rushed him into surgery. After he underwent surgery to remove part of his colon, the hospital fed him a sloppy joe. Something clicked for Chris then. He had been eating the standard American diet, meals containing a lot of meat and processed foods. He made a connection that perhaps his diet had contributed to his cancer. What if he did something different?

Chris decided to opt out of chemotherapy and began eating a plant-based diet that incorporated juices and raw foods. Cancer-free to this day, Chris is now an advocate for a plant-based protocol when it comes to healing and preventing colon cancer.

Quick Tips

Colorectal cancer can interfere with digestion and elimination. The Dana-Farber Cancer Center advises that eating small, frequent meals may ease digestion and absorption, and help you manage all kinds of symptoms, including fatigue, acid reflux, and diarrhea.[33]

For more ideas, visit CancerFreewithFood.com/ColonCancer

6. BLADDER CANCER

The main types of bladder cancer are transitional cell bladder cancer, squamous cell bladder cancer, and adenocarcinoma, which is also known as bladder carcinoma. Transitional cell cancer is noninvasive and accounts for 90 percent of cases. Inflammation, exposure to irritants, and infections are factors leading to the development of the other two types. [34]

Best Foods to Eat

To prevent or heal bladder cancer, try preparing meals that contain:

- Carotenoids (apricot, chlorella, egg yolks, kale, and sweet potato)
- Catechins (green tea and green tea extract[35])
- Chlorophyll (spinach and wheatgrass juice)
- Flavonoids, polyacetylenes, and monoterpenes (parsley)
- Iron (spinach)
- Isothiocyanates (cruciferous vegetables like broccoli, cabbage, and cauliflower, especially eaten raw[36])
- Limonene (citrus fruits like grapefruit, lemon, lime, and orange; and citrus essential oils made from the peels of these same fruits)
- Lycopene (asparagus, papaya, tomato, and watermelon)
- Selenium (Brazil nuts, brown rice, eggs, spinach, and sunflower seeds)
- Sulfur (garlic)

Try These Cancer-Free with Food Recipes

- Energy Soup (page 268)
- Super Detox Broccoli Sprout Green Salad (page 250)
- Heal from Within Green Juice (page 151)

Bill Stewart's Cancer Story

Back in 1998, Bill Stewart began urinating large amounts of blood. His general practitioner scheduled an appointment with a kidney specialist for testing the next day. On returning to the kidney specialist, he confirmed that there was kidney cancer and it was urgent that one of his kidneys be removed. The doctor scheduled the surgery for the following week.

Not keen on having surgery, Bill chose to go home and contemplate the options. His wife, Linda, read the pathology report over the weekend, and through research began to question the accuracy of the diagnosis. The Stewarts went back to the doctor on Monday and asked if there was an error in his interpretation of the findings. He didn't like being challenged and said, "Absolutely not, and if you persist in getting a second opinion, don't come back."

Something didn't sit right with the Stewarts, despite the doctor's persistence about his diagnosis. Bill declared, "Have you ever seen a miracle? Well, you are going to see one." The doctor, who said "no," was shocked when they left the room and canceled their future appointment.

(In my opinion, if a medical doctor says this kind of thing to you or is aggressive in your treatment and doesn't seem supportive of your concerns, then I suggest that you get a new doctor or at the very least get a second, and possibly a third, opinion. There is nothing wrong with getting another professional opinion or in exploring all your options.)

Linda began an aggressive search for any-and-all modalities that might be able to heal his cancer. These included biofeedback, massage therapy, energy healing, wheatgrass therapy, meditation, and a purely vegan diet. Bill decided he would do anything that promised hope to treat his cancer. Doing more research, Linda came across the Creative Health Institute in Michigan where they could learn about juicing, colonics, coffee enemas, wheatgrass enemas, and a plant-based diet under a model that was established in the 1960s by the late Ann Wigmore, an early proponent of raw-food diets. They offered a two-week detox program where Bill and Linda would learn how to work in the kitchen. They would learn about fermenting and blending foods, growing sprouts, how to grow wheatgrass and juice it, and how to soak seeds. Everything Bill ate was made by hand. He enjoyed an energy soup daily (see Energy Soup on page 268) along with many microgreens, such as broccoli sprouts (see Five-Ingredient Green Salad on page 244). The instructors even taught him how to make immunity-building pies and desserts! (See Chapter 19 for recipes for comparable nutrient-rich desserts that are absolutely delicious.)

Back at home, Bill and his family continued to implement everything they learned. They bought organic soil with earthworms for their gardening efforts. They continued to detoxify his body and strengthen their immune system with wholesome food choices, and by pursuing other elements of a natural lifestyle, such as removing all chemicals from their home. They purchased a rebounder trampoline, and he jumped on it daily to stimulate his circulation and assist in draining his lymphatic systems.

However, Bill wasn't out of the woods yet, so the Stewarts sought further medical advice. They found a progressive kidney specialist at the University of Michigan who offered a second opinion and diagnosed Bill with bladder cancer. At that time, Bill felt confident in what he and Linda were doing with their diet and chose to move forward with holistic treatments at least for a short period of time. Surprisingly, the doctor agreed. Bill was relieved to hear he did not need to go into surgery immediately.

The Stewarts were happy with this plan. "It gave us time to apply everything we had learned and for Bill's body to respond," Linda said. Additionally, upon being referred to another specialist who had had success with treating cancer with mistletoe injections (Iscador) as a healing modality, the Stewarts decided to begin treatment.

When I asked what they did during the time before the next biopsy, Linda told me: "We continued using the protocols we researched, and we also began the injections. We put our lives on hold. Bill supplemented his diet with enzymes and took shark cartilage. We worked with dozens of different therapeutic-grade essential oils, in our water, our food, topically and with a diffuser. We ran the diffuser at night with oil blends to improve sleep quality, and throughout our home during the day to decrease stress. We also used essential oils to clean our home without exposing ourselves to chemicals.

"We drank filtered water. We would go to the local health store and fill up our water bins with reverse-osmosis filtered water, which is alkaline. We would then add drops of trace minerals to the water before drinking it. We followed a Mediterranean-style diet when we weren't eating raw foods, consuming lots of good, healthy fats, like olive oil, and ate green salads. All sugar was off the table. We only ate natural sugars from fruits. And no matter what we ate, we made everything by hand. For instance, we made salad dressing by hand. Because when it's made with your hands it is made with love, which transfers the energy of love to help you heal."

After seven months from beginning his journey, Bill had lost 75 pounds and was at a healthy weight. His health continued to improve and upon them further testing and follow-up, there was no evidence of any cancer.

This was 20 years ago, and Bill has been cancer-free ever since. The Stewarts have done their best to stay consistent with the dietary changes they made. Their daughter, Sarah, who was 14 at the time of her father's ill health, is now a health and wellness advocate herself.

Bill reports, "We turned my cancer diagnosis into a positive experience, and my children were part of the dietary changes, so they got to implement them too, which I think laid a foundation for them to be healthy for the rest of their lives. They learned the power of nutrition and the power of positive thinking from a young age. One of the most important things we learned was that you have to work on the subconscious beliefs and be very careful about letting other people influence you away from your goals. Words and beliefs build your reality. A positive mind-set and faith that you can heal and lead a healthy life are important when your wellness is at stake.

"We were so excited to share our story with everyone. It can be scary to be given a cancer diagnosis [but] empowering yourself will completely change your view on beating it. Ask questions. Get multiple opinions. Your body has the innate tools and capabilities to heal anything."

Quick Tips

- The bladder stores urine until it can be excreted—holding up to two cups of liquid.[37] Therefore, exposure to carcinogens inside the bladder is relatively prolonged, so decreasing exposure any way you can is beneficial to your health.

- Use a deodorant or antiperspirant that is aluminum-free. There is a clear link between aluminum and bladder cancer.[38] And I don't want to hear that "natural deodorants don't work" —ha! You just have to find the one that works best for you without this ingredient. Alternatively, you can use lemon juice and baking soda as deodorant, or on some days you can even give your underarms a break from wearing anything. Anything we put under our arms goes straight into our lymphatic system through our pores, and then toxic substances are processed for elimination through the bladder. The last thing we want to do is clog things up with aluminum.

- Drink bentonite clay (see page 193 for recipe) to help you eliminate toxins you may have accumulated from long-term exposure to chemicals, heavy metals, or smoke in your workplace. Studies have found higher rates of bladder cancer among people in various occupations: hairdressers; textile workers; machinists and metal workers; housepainters; printers; truck drivers; dry cleaners; and workers in industries that process rubber, aluminum, and leather.[39] This technique is also recommended if you have been a cigarette smoker or drink alcohol.

- Get checked (and treated, if necessary) for parasitic infections, as there is a connection with certain parasites and bladder cancer.[40]

For more ideas, visit CancerFreewithFood.com/BladderCancer

7. Non-Hodgkins Lymphoma

There are two different kinds of lymphoma, or lymphatic cancer. Both types, Hodgkins disease and non-Hodgkins lymphoma (NHL), begin in the white blood cells known as lymphocytes. Lymphocytes are part of the body's immune system, so cancer that begins here shows up when the immune system is weakened, there has been a chronic infection (for example, the Epstein-Barr virus—aka mono—or HIV), or when someone is taking an immune suppressant medication on purpose—such as after an organ transplant. NHL is the more common type of lymphoma.[41]

Best Foods to Eat

An interesting nearly eight-year-long study at the Yale School of Public Health in New Haven, Connecticut, that compared more than 600 Connecticut women with non-Hodgkins lymphoma to more than 700 women without revealed: "If a person has a higher intake of animal protein, they will have a higher risk of non-Hodgkins lymphoma. And people who have a higher intake of saturated fat have an increased risk."[42] Researchers also determined that higher-than-average intake of dietary fiber—particularly from vegetables and fruits—reduces NHL risk. It's nice when the evidence is so definitive.

To prevent or heal non-Hodgkins lymphoma, try preparing meals that contain:

- Iron (beans)
- Flavonoids (elderberry)
- Lycopene (tomatoes)
- Magnesium (ginger)
- Pantothenic acid and other B vitamins (medicinal mushrooms like maitake and shiitake)
- Vitamin C (apples, broccoli, cauliflower, onions, and squash)
- Vitamin K (leeks)

Try These Cancer-Free with Food Recipes

- Superpowerful Green Juice (page 148)
- Beet Juice (page 147)
- Anticancer Omelet (page 205)
- Superfood Kale Salad (page 245)

Jimmy Lechmanski's Cancer Story

Jimmy Lechmanski was diagnosed with non-Hodgkins lymphoma and chronic lymphocytic leukemia in 2005. His doctors diagnosed his condition as stage IV and told James that he had a life expectancy of less than five years. Fortunately, the statistics were not borne out in his case. At the time we spoke, he was at 13 years and counting. He is still alive and enjoying his life with almost complete remission of the NHL and leukemia. His white blood cell count is close to normal.

Jimmy underwent chemotherapy to treat his cancer, but attributes his health turnaround and ultimate survival to his nutritional strategy. Once he learned about the healing power of plant-based food and the importance of alkalizing the body, he started drinking green juices and having salad for breakfast, and he cut out refined sugars (white sugar, brown sugar, and cane sugar). He allowed himself to eat some fruit.

I asked Jimmy what inspired his breakfast salad habit. He said it was to put as much oxygen into his body from the dark leafy greens in the bowl. He believes that cancer cannot survive in an oxygen-rich environment. If this sounds boring to you, I promise you it does not have to be. For protein, add eggs to your salad—fried, poached, scrambled, or hard-boiled eggs all contribute to the breakfasty vibe. Eggs can be a much easier protein to digest than meat for many people with cancer. (And, as we learned, there is a connection between animal protein and non-Hodgkins lymphoma.) Jimmy also loves having oatmeal for breakfast. He makes sure to drink greens powder mixed in water, an ounce or two of wheatgrass juice, and a pomegranate juice every day. He purchased a wheatgrass machine to support this positive habit.

Quick Tips

- Reduce your intake of animal protein and increase your fiber intake.

- People with blood disorders may find drinking wheatgrass supportive of their well-being, so consider purchasing a wheatgrass machine to have a steady source. Those dark leafy greens that James loves to eat also contain a hearty dose of chlorophyll. This molecule makes plants green and helps them synthesize sunlight into food. Remember, chlorophyll resembles the hemoglobin molecule in human blood that makes it red and helps us transport oxygen to our tissues, energizing us.

For more ideas, visit CancerDietBook.org/ NonHodgkinsLymphoma

8. KIDNEY CANCER

There are two main kinds of kidney cancer: renal cell carcinoma and urothelial cell carcinoma. Less-common types include Wilms' tumor, which young children are more likely to get.

Best Foods to Eat

Your two kidneys are part of your urinary tract system. Their functions are to filter waste from your blood and make urine with which to carry waste into the bladder and out of the body. Healthy kidneys also produce a hormone, aldosterone, that helps to regulate blood pressure. Anything that interferes with filtering waste is potentially cancer-causing if it leads to prolonged exposure to environmental toxins, like heavy metals (cadmium, for example), pesticides, or over-the-counter pain medications.[43] Keeping your toxic burden low is supportive of these organs.

To prevent or heal kidney cancer, try preparing meals that contain:

- Molybdenum (bell peppers)
- Sulfur (cabbage and cauliflower)
- Vitamin C (garlic and onion)
- B vitamins (cranberries)
- Quercetin (apples)
- Anthocyanosides (acai, blueberries, chokeberries, black and red currants, eggplant, purple cauliflower, concord grapes, and dried red cabbage)
- Resveratrol (grapes)
- Essiac tea
- Biotin (peanut butter made from organic, non-GMO peanuts—and nothing else)

Try These Cancer-Free with Food Recipes

- Bean Burgers (page 219)
- Crazy Sexy Bean Chili (page 215)
- Kidney Bean Soup with Watercress and Kale (page 273)
- Cauliflower Popcorn (page 223)
- Hummus-Stuffed Peppers (page 299)

Quick Tips

- Eat five or six small meals throughout the day instead of three bigger meals, so that your kidneys are never taxed by the need to filter massive amounts of waste at once.
- If you are undergoing treatment for kidney cancer, work closely with your health-care providers to ascertain the correct amount of protein to eat. Too much protein can overwhelm a diseased kidney.[44] Remember, everyone is different. Your needs may vary from another's.

- Thoroughly wash produce to ensure that all contaminants and chemical residue are gone. This will help reduce the toxic load on your kidneys.

For more ideas, visit CancerDietBook.org./KidneyCancer

9. LEUKEMIA

Leukemia is cancer of the blood that usually begins in the lymphatic system or bone marrow, and results in high numbers of abnormal white blood cells.

Best Foods to Eat

To prevent or heal leukemia, try preparing meals that contain:

- Antioxidants (blackberries, green tea, and raspberries)
- Betaine (beets)
- Chrysin (honey and passionflower)
- Citral purity (lemon myrtle tea)
- Curcumin (turmeric and curry)
- Fucoidan (brown algae and brown seaweeds such as mozuku, kombu, bladderwrack, wakame, and hijiki)
- Ginsenosides (ginseng)
- Glycyrrhizic acid (licorice root)
- Indoles (broccoli, broccoli sprouts, cabbage, and cauliflower)
- Oleuropein (olive leaf extract)
- Polyphenols (acai berry[45])

- Vitamin C (garlic, lemon, lime, onion, and orange)
- Xanthene (mangosteen)
- Vitamin B$_6$ (rosemary)

Try These Cancer-Free with Food Recipes

- Beet Juice (page 147)
- Ultimate Superfood Smoothie (page 178)
- Grape Juice (page 146)
- Acai Bowl (page 181)

David Lingle's Cancer Story[46]

On the blog Chris Beat Cancer, I was impressed by the story of a man named David Lingle, who refused chemotherapy when he was diagnosed with leukemia in 2011. From the outset, David knew he wanted to heal naturally. The first thing he did was pray and ask God to heal him, as he believed cancer did not belong in his body. Then he changed to a majority plant-based diet, eating 70 percent raw and 30 percent cooked foods.

Reviewing his daily plan, it is evidently alkalizing, and high in phytonutrients and simple proteins. David drank a Baking Soda Beverage (see Chapter 3) in the morning and took maitake supplements. For lunch, he followed a protocol of flax oil, cottage cheese, and blueberries. He also ate apricot seeds, hummus, and drank green tea, dandelion root tea, and smoothies that he supplemented with a greens powder and whey protein.

David says that one of the most important things is just to believe in yourself and that you *can* heal; otherwise, no matter what you do, you will not get the results you want. By 2013, his tests showed that the cancer was completely gone. To see his full testimonial visit ChrisBeatCancer.com.

Quick Tips

To support your blood health, give yourself a natural "blood transfusion" by mixing coconut water with green juice. Human blood is composed of about 55 percent plasma and 45 percent red blood cells. The coconut water has a similar molecular composition as plasma. The chlorophyll in the greens helps tired old blood to supply your bodily tissues with fresh oxygen because it mimics the hemoglobin molecules in the red blood cells in our bloodstream. Chlorophyll is the green pigment found in cyanobacteria and the chloroplasts of algae and plants. Remember, green plants = chlorophyll.

For more ideas, visit CancerDietBook.org/Leukemia

10. WOMEN'S REPRODUCTIVE CANCERS

The most common reproductive cancers in women are cervical cancer, ovarian cancer, uterine cancer, and endometrial cancer. Collectively these are also known as gynecological cancers. A major reason to group them together is that female hormones impact their progression.

Best Foods to Eat

To prevent or heal reproductive cancers nutritionally, plant-based foods are key. A major long-term study of more than 100,000 California schoolteachers concluded that women who ate a majority plant-based diet, versus dairy, meats, and vegetable oils had a lower risk of ovarian cancer.[47] Other protective factors included exercise (more than four hours a week is good), more than two pregnancies, low alcohol consumption (fewer than one drink per day), and nonuse of estrogen hormone therapy.

A remarkable finding was that eating one papaya per week reduces a woman's risk of contracting cervical cancer. Papaya is higher in vitamin C than oranges and it's loaded with pectin, which induces the death of cancer cells when the fruit is soft and ripe.[48] So eat up!

To prevent or heal reproductive cancers, try preparing meals that contain:

- Anthocyanins (blueberries)
- Antioxidants (green tea)
- Beta-cryptoxanthin and zeaxanthin (papaya)
- Curcumin (turmeric and curry)
- Ellagic acid (raspberries)
- Falcarinol (carrots)
- Flavonoids (apples, asparagus, black beans, broccoli, brussels sprouts, cabbage, cranberries, garlic, lettuce, lima beans, organic soy, spinach, and onions)
- Folate (avocado, chickpeas, lentils, oranges, romaine lettuce, and strawberries)
- Ginger root (especially good for ovarian cancer[49])
- Glutathione (asparagus)
- Lentinan and l-ergothioneine (mushrooms such as king oyster, oyster, reishi, maitake, and shiitake)
- Omega-3 fatty acids (astaxanthin [algae], flaxseeds, sardines, trout, walnuts, and wild-caught salmon)
- Pantothenic acid (cauliflower)
- Vitamin A (sweet potatoes, pumpkin, winter squash, spinach, kale and other dark leafy greens, sweet peppers, tomatoes, oranges, and papaya)

Try These Cancer-Free with Food Recipes

- Paradise Smoothie (page 175)
- Sick-Kick Smoothie (page 169)
- Superfood Kale Salad (page 245)
- Baked Walnut-Crusted Salmon (page 291)
- Chickpea Fries (page 302)

Quick Tips

- Maintaining a healthy weight is helpful for preventing women's reproductive cancers because estrogen is often stored in fatty tissue in women's bodies. Estrogen is a known risk factor for cancer. If a woman is obese, her exposure to estrogen is higher and more prolonged.[50]

- Avoid nonfermented soy products like tofu and edamame, which can raise your estrogen levels. Fermented soy products like miso, natto, and tempeh are acceptable—and good sources of vitamin K_2.

- Cervical cancer is considered a lifestyle disease as it is closely linked to the human papilloma virus (HPV). Go for routine pap smears at your gynecologist and follow up if one comes back abnormal. Also, practice safe sex by using a condom every single time!

For more ideas, visit CancerFreewithFood.com/
WomensReproductiveCancers

PART II

CANCER-FREE WITH FOOD RECIPES

CHAPTER 7

KITCHEN SUPPLIES AND CONVERSION CHARTS

Many of the recipes in this book are so simple that to make and eat most of them you just need a bowl and a spoon. This is how food should be—let's not complicate things! The Cancer-Free with Food plan is about getting back to basics and simplicity. When we are healing, we need to expend as much energy as possible on healing the body, and less on making unnecessary trips to the supermarket or standing in the kitchen and making complex recipes. In this book, I've got your back. You'll be able to make many of these recipes (and eat them) with your hands, like the Chocolate Balls and Protein Bars. The Cancer-Free with Food plan is quite like an ancestral diet.

Some recipes will require you to use a juice machine and some a blender. Some are made on the stovetop and a few are baked. But many of these recipes are for raw dishes. By nature, just mixing raw ingredients is quick and produces food that is ridiculously high in nutrients.

Kitchen Supplies

Here are the supplies you'll need to set up your anticancer kitchen. These would be the top three most important pieces of equipment to have if you must prioritize:

1. Juice machine
2. Blender
3. Teflon-free cookware

Juice Machine: If you asked me, "What is the number-one thing I need in my kitchen to prevent and or heal cancer?" I would say: "A juice machine to make juices!" If this is the only appliance you have, well at the very least you are getting a huge daily dose of vitamins and live enzymes by making your own homemade juices. Juicers come in different price ranges, so don't let the price stop you; you may find a perfectly good model being sold inexpensively on the Internet. Stainless-steel juice machines have proven to be the best quality. This is your greatest investment in your health and well-being. You can even purchase a hand juicer for a couple of dollars to juice citrus fruits; they literally work just as well as expensive machines to make orange juice, lemon juice, and grapefruit juice. They are also easier to clean. When purchasing a juice machine, look for one that is capable of juicing whole apples. This will save you time from having to cut up fruits and vegetables. Here are the different options:

- A regular juice machine: Prices of models start from around $40, and you can get a good one for $100 to $200. This is all you may need for a good five years. Juice should be drunk the day it is made.

- A "slow" juice machine, which is often considered a "healthier" machine, as it creates less heat and friction by exerting a pressing force on the produce you put into it instead of just giving you a lot of speed. This type of machine often costs more than a regular juice machine. Juice should be drunk the day it is made.

- A cold-pressed juice machine, which is normally only used commercially by juice shop businesses. These are expensive, costing at least $1,000. They press the juice from the produce by weight and leverage rather than using electricity, so they would help you save on your electric bills over time. Cold-pressed juices stay intact for up to five days.

- An entirely different machine is a wheatgrass juice machine, which you would only need if you decided you would be interested in juicing your own wheatgrass. Juice should be drunk the day it is made.

In addition to a juicer, you'll need some or all of the following equipment.

A **high-speed blender** to make smoothies, raw desserts, sauces, and more. A powerful blender with a reliable motor and sharp stainless-steel blades will work. If you have a strong enough blender, you probably won't even need a food processor. The exceptions are frozen desserts and mixing dry blends. Always take care not to burn out the motor. Blenders are better for wet mixtures. I use a Vitamix blender because this is how I achieve creamy and ridiculously delicious smooth desserts like Cashew Ice Cream, Cashew Cheesecake, Chocolate Avocado Mousse, and Chocolate Sauce.

A **food processor** is the best machine for mixing dry ingredients. You can get away with not having a food processor if your blender can also make these things.

Quality cookware that is nonreactive to the foods you cook in it, like stainless-steel, ceramic, glass, and lead-free cookware. My personal preference is stainless steel. The pots for cooking have thick bottoms. Ultimately slow heating, as you would use when cooking on a fire or over coals, is the most natural form of cooking. Stay away from flimsy pots or nonstick pots and pans coated with Teflon and other synthetic materials. According to experts I trust, once heated these can spoil the food and become toxic. Of particular concern is what damage these may do to the immune system.

Teflon nonstick coating may sound appealing and convenient, but it's really dangerous in the long run. Teflon is made from perfluorooctanoic acid (PFOA), which was shown to cause liver, testicular, and pancreatic cancers in rodents.[1] There is also suspicion that nonstick pans cause thyroid issues including thyroid cancer.[2]

PFOA was found in the blood of an estimated 98 percent of Americans.[3] Can you believe this? It's crazy!

PFOA is also found in carpet and microwave popcorn bags. Cancer-proofing your entire home can be helpful in preventing and healing cancer, which is why it's important to switch your foods and kitchen utensils to be as safe as possible. Throw out your Teflon-coated pots and pans if you can; they are not safe!

Make sure to have these kitchen essentials.

- A 12-inch-diameter stainless-steel skillet
- A large stainless-steel baking sheet
- A stainless-steel pot (six to eight cups)
- A stainless-steel or glass mixing bowl (six to eight cups)

Utensils. These will be helpful:

- A large spoon
- A sharp all-purpose knife for cutting and chopping
- A bamboo or wood cutting board
- A set of measuring cups
- A set of measuring spoons

You can get BPA-free and nontoxic utensils.

A food dehydrator to make dried fruit and fruit leathers for rollups and candy. You can even dry your own herbs! If you don't have a dehydrator you can use your oven; however, this isn't ideal as your oven would be on for 12 hours.

On my website, you can find coupon codes for discounts on equipment and kitchen supplies that I recommend as the healthiest and most effective: CancerFreewithFood.com/ resources. Come back and visit regularly, as the list of products and discounts is always evolving as I continue to search for new ways to make our lives easier, more time efficient, and healthier.

METRIC CONVERSION TABLE (MEASUREMENTS AND TEMPERATURES)

If you live in a country where people adhere to the metric system, then a metric conversion chart can help you convert the quantities of ingredients in the Cancer-Free with Food recipes from ounces and pounds to grams and kilos. Find one on page 373.

CHAPTER 8

IMMUNE-BOOSTING JUICES

The body is holographic; therefore, when you change one biomarker you influence them all.[1]

— DEEPAK CHOPRA AND DAVID SIMON

Juicing is a good solution that works for almost everyone. In terms of the nutrients you gain from it, it's roughly equivalent to taking 50 supplements. If you are concerned about the natural sugar in fruit juice, then don't juice fruits. Instead, exclusively juice vegetables. You could also drink soups and smoothies where fiber remains in the liquid. One a day does wonders.

Let's talk about the differences between juices and smoothies. Like juices, smoothies are great sources of nutrients! Because they are blended fruits and vegetables, you get more fiber in them than you do in juices. Juicing removes fiber.

I am a big advocate of juice because it saves us energy. When we are sick with cancer, the last thing we want to do is make the body use energy it doesn't need to. To digest fibrous foods and processed foods containing gluten, sugar, and dairy, the body must use a lot of energy. This expenditure makes us feel tired and channels energy away from the immune system where it could otherwise be used to heal. When we drink juices, the body needs very little energy to break them down, as juice is absorbed immediately into the bloodstream and cells. When we drink smoothies, which contain fiber, the body must use energy to break down the fibers.

If you want to include smoothies in your cancer healing plan I do recommend it, as they can be filling and delicious, but also be sure to include a juice a day. You can incorporate both in your dietary healing plan.

Juice has become a daily staple for me, a nonnegotiable. Basically, no matter how busy I am, or how stressed I am, or how healthy and happy I feel, I make sure to have one juice every single day. And I've done this now for the past eight years. On days that I am traveling and not able to make or buy juice, I will mix a dried green powder into water instead. That's my green drink for the day. Nothing makes me feel as alive and energetic as drinking fresh juice. And I hope that in your efforts to become cancer-free, you will also make juice a daily staple.

Either make your own juice or buy your juice from a local juice bar. The cost of a juice machine can run from as little as $40 to $100. Get one with a bigger mouth on it. You want to be sure you buy a juice machine that has the capacity to juice whole apples so that you don't need to spend time and energy chopping up all your ingredients into tiny pieces. When I was drinking six juices a day, I would juice every morning and then bottle it so I could drink it throughout the day. Each juice was 12 ounces. If you had to do chopping sufficient for 72 ounces of juice, you could be at it for quite a while—an unnecessary use of time and muscle.

Yes, it's always best to make a juice and drink it instantly to get the most nutrition out of it, and some people will insist it loses its nutritional value if it's left in a bottle for hours, but realistically we have to do the best we can, especially when the body is in a state of radical healing. Drinking juice five hours after it's been made is much better than drinking no juice at all. You still get nutrients from it, just not as much as if you drink it on the spot.

Please don't be worried about spending time making juices, because this is valuable time you get to spend healing yourself. While you are chopping produce and making the juice, you can stand there and visualize all the good you are doing for yourself; and you can revisit your intention to heal your body and become cancer-free. Get present in your body and say, *I am in control of the cancer. The cancer is not in control of me.* Practice affirmations as you are juicing. This is not a waste of time. It is an opportunity to do some healing!

You will need to adjust your schedule to accommodate your new healing diet and lifestyle. If you have cancer, you will have to be doing new things—trying new things, adjusting your behavior, shifting out of your old habits, and focusing on your new life. You will be spending more time making wholesome food, drinking juice, getting natural treatments, getting massages, taking baths, perhaps doing colonics, meditating, praying, reading, and so on. Be prepared to spend time in new, more healthful ways.

If you are concerned about wasting food when throwing away the pulp after you make juice, keep it and make brownies or muffins out of it. You can also add it to soups. The fiber from juicing is an excellent ingredient! You can also add it to your compost so that you are giving back to the earth by creating new soil.

If you are unable to make juice for yourself because of your illness, you could have a family member or friend do it for you. It is also helpful to your healing to ask as many of your loved ones as possible to help you through this time. The love, support, and prayers of others is so powerful for healing. We all need human connection to thrive—love and a sense of belonging. To be a member of a tribe or a community. To be touched. To know someone cares.

Another way to get a daily juice if you don't have the means to juice yourself is to buy juices from your local juice bar. It will cost more than making them yourself, of course, but at this point—when you're sick—the price really doesn't matter. No price should be put on good health. The most important thing is to get nutrients into your body to boost your immune system, so it can detox and flush out the cancer. Even if it seems costly, remember that juicing is much cheaper than chemo. Consider juicing the medicine you need to invest in right now.

I wish that health insurance covered juicing! Hopefully, one day it will.

Cold-pressed juices, like the ones sold in boutique juice shops and upscale supermarket chains, can last for a few days in your fridge, so feel free to stock up on them and be prepared for days ahead. Why is this possible? The process of cold-pressing fruits and vegetables prevents oxygen from getting into the juice, keeping it fresh for days with its original nutrients intact.

Without sufficient hydration, our cells simply won't function properly. And when our cells aren't functioning properly, things go wrong. Then cancer can emerge or flourish.

With juices, you can boost your antioxidant levels, immune function, and metabolic activity while regulating your blood sugar, body fat, cholesterol and lipid levels, and hormone levels. The health improvements that come from drinking juice every day are remarkable. This is one of the world's best cancer-fighting strategies.

ONE-INGREDIENT JUICES

You can juice literally anything you have on hand. You can juice vegetables, fruits, and herbs on their own or together. One reason why you would juice the ingredients rather than eat them is to get a highly concentrated dose of nutrition straight into your cells, feeling instant energy, supporting the immune system, and helping the body cleanse toxins. Juice becomes the building blocks for your new body. Often when I juice, I like to visualize and think, *Juice in, toxins out. Nutrition in, cancer out.*

At the Hippocrates Health Institute, the staff gives some patients juices rather smoothies as it is much easier for a cancerous body to digest juice. Smoothies have fiber, which takes energy to digest that some people are not able to spare. Juice without fiber penetrates into the cells with little effort.

Serving Size for One

Orange Juice: 4 oranges, peeled (pairs well with turmeric); for a Classic OJ Berry Smoothie, add 2 cups of berries (blueberries, strawberries, and raspberries)

Apple Juice: 4 green or red apples (pairs well with ginger)

Cherry Juice: 4 cups of pitted cherries

Pineapple Juice: ½ pineapple, skin off (pairs well with orange, ginger, and turmeric)

Carrot Juice: 10 carrots (pairs well with parsley, orange, and turmeric)

Celery: 1 whole bunch (pairs well with lemon and apple)

Tomato Juice: 5 tomatoes (pairs well with parsley and a dash of sea salt and pepper)

Wheatgrass: 2 big handfuls of wheatgrass make a 2-ounce shot

Broccoli Sprouts: You would need a lot of sprouts to make one juice, but this would be a powerful and potent concoction. You could mix this with cucumber.

Grape Juice: 3 cups of purple or red grapes

Kitchen Helper

Did you know that when you make a juice, such as carrot juice, you don't have to throw away the pulp? Feed your plants with it. Add the pulp to your compost heap and it will create nice, lush soil that grows a great garden. Or use the pulp in a muffin or cake recipe!

BEET JUICE

Beets are a great cancer cleanser. This juice not only detoxifies the blood and liver, it also helps lift compacted waste from the bowel wall. I drank this every single day during my healing and it cleaned out my body.

Total time: 10 minutes

Makes 1 serving

Ingredients:
1 small beet

2 red apples

4 carrots

Actions:
1. Put all the ingredients in a juicer.
2. Juice and drink.

Tips:
- Add 3 celery stalks for extra nutrients.
- Add 1 small lemon with rind for extra nutrients.
- Replace the apples with more carrots if you want to reduce your sugar intake.

Variation:
Add one 2-inch piece of ginger for Spicy Beet Juice.

Calories: 385.4 | Protein: 4.7g | Carbs: 90.8g | Dietary Fiber: 18.8g | Fat: 1.5g | Vitamin C: 18.4mg | Vitamin D: 0 IU | Vitamin E: 2.6mg | Calcium: 119mg | Iron: 1.8mg | Magnesium: 69.3mg | Potassium: 1,488mg

SUPERPOWERFUL GREEN JUICE

You can get all your essential greens in one drink with this recipe. The greens in this juice are so nutrient-rich and intense that the juice puts oxygen into your cells, which creates an alkaline environment where cancer cells are unwelcome. This is the green juice I drink most often.

Total time: 10 minutes

Makes 1 serving

Ingredients:

1 cucumber	½ cup dandelion greens
3 celery stalks	½ cup watercress
½ cup kale	1 cup broccoli sprouts
½ cup spinach	½ lemon (you can juice the rind)
¼ cup parsley	1 thumb-size piece of ginger
¼ cup cilantro	

Optional, for sweetness add 1 green apple or ¾ cup pineapple

Actions:

1. Put all the ingredients in a juicer.
2. Juice and drink.

Calories: 148.7 | Protein: 9.9g | Carbs: 23.7g | Dietary Fiber: 6.7g | Fat: 2.3g | Vitamin C: 197.5mg | Vitamin D: 0 IU | Vitamin E: 2mg | Calcium: 437mg | Iron: 5.8mg | Magnesium: 117.1mg | Potassium: 1,557mg

---

THE BIG 3: BLUEBERRY BROCCOLI SPROUTS TURMERIC JUICE

The top three anticancer foods are delivered all in one in this potent juice. Turmeric root is an ancient Indian spice containing the anti-inflammatory medicinal compound curcumin. 'Chiropractor Josh Axe, D.C., explains: "Curcumin modifies an internal process known as eicosanoid biosynthesis. Eicosanoids consist of four different molecules within the body that are involved in the natural inflammation process."[2]

Total time: 10 minutes

Makes 1 serving

Ingredients:

2-inch chunk of turmeric root (or 1 teaspoon dried turmeric powder)	1 cup broccoli sprouts
	3 celery stalks
2 cups blueberries (you can use strawberries and raspberries too)	1-inch chunk of ginger
	Dash of black pepper

Actions:

1. Put all the ingredients in a juicer, except for the black pepper.

2. Juice, sprinkle with black pepper, and drink.

Calories: 241 | Protein: 7.7g | Carbs: 49.1g | Dietary Fiber: 9.3g | Fat: 2.7g | Vitamin C: 157.5mg | Vitamin D: 0 IU | Vitamin E: 2mg | Calcium: 298.9mg | Iron: 3.6mg | Magnesium: 61.8mg | Potassium: 1,077mg

---

GREEN LEMONADE

This juice is highly alkalizing and also sweet and refreshing. This will be a great juice for you if you are new to juicing or want to enjoy a sweet but healthy juice and not feel like you are missing out on "lemonade."

Total time: 10 minutes

Makes 1 serving

Ingredients:

2 apples

1 large cucumber

1 large celery stalk

1 (roughly) thumb-size piece of ginger

½ large lemon, peeled

Actions:

1. Put all the ingredients in a juicer.

2. Juice and drink.

Tip:

Serve over ice cubes.

Calories: 262.7 | Protein: 3.9g | Carbs: 68.3g | Dietary Fiber: 12.5g | Fat: 1.2g | Vitamin C: 49.7mg | Vitamin D: 0 IU | Vitamin E: 1mg | Calcium: 107.7mg | Iron: 1.7mg | Magnesium: 70.9mg | Potassium: 1,086mg

VITAMIN C BLASTER JUICE

This juice is high in vitamin C to boost the immune system, but also tastes sweet. Vitamin C is crucial in fighting viruses and all forms of cancer. If you have gained weight during your cancer treatments, this is also a helpful juice to keep sugar cravings at bay. It evaporates fat cells because grapefruit contains 88 to 95 percent limonene.

Total time: 10 minutes

Makes 1 serving

Ingredients:

2 oranges, peeled

1 grapefruit, peeled

1 lemon (with rind optional)

1-inch piece of turmeric

Actions:

1. Put all the ingredients in a juicer.
2. Juice and drink.

Tips:

- You don't need a juice machine for this recipe; you can simply squeeze these fruits into a jug and add turmeric powder afterward. You can also use a hand squeezer.
- Add more oranges for a sweeter juice.
- Add cayenne pepper if you want an extra kick.

Calories: 225.2 | Protein: 4.8g | Carbs: 57.4g | Dietary Fiber: 10.7g | Fat: 0.8g | Vitamin C: 258mg | Vitamin D: 0 IU | Vitamin E: 0.8mg | Calcium: 152.5mg | Iron: 1mg | Magnesium: 51.3mg | Potassium: 946mg

HEAL FROM WITHIN GREEN JUICE

This recipe is from Linda Stewart, wife of Bill Stewart. After Bill's diagnosis of bladder cancer, the couple decided to change their diet before opting for surgery and chemotherapy. They were successful, and Bill was cancer-free within six months. They enjoy a healthy organic diet to this day and Linda shares with us the green juice they drank. Linda shares their story on page 121 and explains how sprouts were key in the healing process.

Total time: 10 minutes

Makes 1 serving

Ingredients:

2 celery stalks

2 kale leaves

1 small cucumber

1 cup spinach

1 garlic clove

½-inch piece of turmeric

½-inch piece of ginger

½ lemon

½ orange

½ apple

½ cup broccoli sprouts, sunflower sprouts, or other sprouts of choice

Actions:

1. Put all the ingredients in a juicer.
2. Juice and drink.

Calories: 196.9 | Protein: 8.5g | Carbs: 42.2g | Dietary Fiber: 9.4g | Fat: 1.9g | Vitamin C: 178mg | Vitamin D: 0 IU | Vitamin E: 1.7mg | Calcium: 320.5mg | Iron: 3.9mg | Magnesium: 116.9mg | Potassium: 1,501mg

RAINBOW VEGETABLE JUICE FOR DIABETICS

Epidemiologic evidence suggests that people with diabetes are at significantly higher risk for many forms of cancer.[3] The ingredients in this recipe are not starchy, so it is a great way to get the vitamins and minerals your body needs while preventing an excessive blood sugar response.

Total time: 10 minutes

Makes 1 serving

Ingredients:

1 head of lettuce (any kind works well, including iceberg or red leaf) or kale

2 medium-size tomatoes

3 carrots

1 red bell pepper

1 cucumber

Pinch of turmeric powder

Dash of black pepper

Actions:

1. Put all the ingredients in a juicer, except for the black pepper.

2. Juice, then sprinkle some black pepper on top and drink.

Tip:

Add one or all of the following ingredients to the juice:

- 2 parsnips
- 1 small purple onion
- ½ teaspoon sea salt
- ½ teaspoon cracked black pepper

Variation:

Add ¼ teaspoon cayenne pepper (more if you like it spicy) for Spicy Vegetable Juice.

Calories: 209.6 | Protein: 7.5g | Carbs: 46.8g | Dietary Fiber: 12.9g | Fat: 1.7g | Vitamin C: 206.5mg | Vitamin D: 0 IU | Vitamin E: 4.5mg | Calcium: 156.8mg | Iron: 3mg | Magnesium: 109mg | Potassium: 1,972mg

---

DIGESTION-HELPER JUICE

This delicious juice is helpful for people with issues such as constipation, bloating, and IBS, which are common side effects of chemotherapy treatment.

Total time: 10 minutes

Makes 1 serving

Ingredients:

1 small beet

1 cup pineapple

3 carrots

3 celery stalks

⅓ cup fresh parsley

1-inch piece of ginger

Pinch of turmeric

Actions:

1. Put all the ingredients in a juicer.

2. Juice and drink.

Calories: 225.6 | Protein: 5.4g | Carbs: 53g | Dietary Fiber: 12.5g | Fat: 1.2g | Vitamin C: 124.7mg | Vitamin D: 0 IU | Vitamin E: 1.7mg | Calcium: 172.3mg | Iron: 3.3mg | Magnesium: 87.4mg | Potassium: 1,489mg

VIBRANT ORANGE CARROT GINGER JUICE

The combination of orange, ginger, and carrot is elevating and will help lift your mood. On a gloomy day, this is a fun one to make because the colors are so vibrant that our eyes find it appealing. The more colorful fruits and vegetables we work with, the better to banish cancer.

Total time: 10 minutes

Makes 2 servings

Ingredients:

10 carrots

2 oranges, peeled

1 thumb-size piece of ginger

1 thumb-size piece of turmeric

Actions:

1. Put all the ingredients in a juicer.
2. Juice and drink.

Calories: 191.2 | Protein: 4.1g | Carbs: 45.5g | Dietary Fiber: 11.7g | Fat: 0.9g | Vitamin C: 87.8mg | Vitamin D: 0 IU | Vitamin E: 2.2mg | Calcium: 154.6mg | Iron: 1.1mg | Magnesium: 51.2mg | Potassium: 1,246mg

BERRY GREEN JUICE

This is one of my favorite combos because it mixes delicious anti-inflammatory berries with nutrient-rich, alkalizing greens. It's a great way to get your greens in without them being too bitter.

Total time: 10 minutes

Makes 1 serving

Ingredients:

1 cup blueberries

1 cup strawberries

1 small cucumber

1 large celery stalk

1 handful of kale

1 handful of fresh cilantro

¼ lemon, peeled

Actions:

1. Put all the ingredients in a juicer.

2. Juice and drink.

Variation:

Juice a 1-inch piece of turmeric with the other ingredients to boost the juice's anti-inflammatory properties.

Calories: 190 | Protein: 4.7g | Carbs: 46.6g | Dietary Fiber: 9.3g | Fat: 1.4g | Vitamin C: 124.2mg | Vitamin D: 0 IU | Vitamin E: 1.7mg | Calcium: 111.4mg | Iron: 2.1mg | Magnesium: 76.1mg | Potassium: 954.7mg

---

CELERY JUICE

Drinking celery juice is one of the healthiest things we can do. It can reduce your risk of getting cancer dramatically, as well as have beneficial roles in the treatment of cancer. Apigenin, a flavonoid found in celery, reduces oxidative stress and DNA damage, and suppresses inflammation and angiogenesis.[4]

Total time: 10 minutes

Makes 1 serving

Ingredients:

1 bunch celery

¼ lemon, peeled

Actions:

1. Put all the ingredients in a juicer.

2. Juice and drink.

Tips:

- Add 1 apple or more to make the juice sweeter.
- Add ½-inch piece of ginger for added health benefits.

Calories: 55.4 | Protein: 2.3g | Carbs: 10.8g | Dietary Fiber: 5.5g | Fat: 0.5g | Vitamin C: 17.6mg | Vitamin D: 0 IU | Vitamin E: 0.8mg | Calcium: 131.7mg | Iron: 0.7mg | Magnesium: 36.3mg | Potassium: 852mg

---

LEMON GINGER SHOT

An immune-boosting energizer that is perfect for whenever you feel like you're getting the sniffles or feeling sluggish, which is a common symptom if you are experiencing cancer.

Total time: 5 minutes

Makes 2 servings

Ingredients:

2 lemons, peeled

2-inch piece of ginger, peeled

Actions:

1. Put all the ingredients in a juicer.
2. Juice, then pour into shot glasses and drink.

Tip:

To amplify the heat even further, add a smidgen of cayenne pepper. Studies have shown that cayenne pepper, which contains capsaicin, can slow the growth of cancer cells.[5]

Variations:

Ginger Lemon Orange Turmeric Shot: add the juice of 1 orange and a 1-inch piece of turmeric. *Ginger Lemon Orange Juice*: add 7 oranges; it's absolutely so sweet and refreshing.

Calories: 22.7 | Protein: 0.7g | Carbs: 6.7g | Dietary Fiber: 1.7g | Fat: 0.2g | Vitamin C: 31.1mg | Vitamin D: 0 IU | Vitamin E: 0.1mg | Calcium: 16.2mg | Iron: 0.3mg | Magnesium: 7.8mg | Potassium: 110.6mg

CHAPTER 9

NUT MILKS, SEED MILKS, AND DAIRY-FREE SHAKES

Nuts and seeds are a great alternative to making dairy-free plant-based milks. It has even been said that dairy can be dangerous for your health. Dairy avoidance is wise for preventing and healing cancer. However, if you feel strongly that dairy will help you in your healing, I fully advise you to make sure it is organic, so it comes without the growth hormones. It would be ideal to find a local farmer who sells fresh milk. It's important to see the state of the farm, so you know where the milk is coming from.

HOMEMADE NUT MILK AND SEED MILK

This recipe makes a delicious and refreshing dairy-free milk base! It's way better than purchasing from the store because it is free of additives, such as sweeteners, preservatives, and thickeners.

When you make your own plant-based milk, you see everything that goes into it.

You can add other ingredients to make different flavors.

Total time: less than 5 minutes

Makes 4 servings

Ingredients:

1 cup of nuts or seeds or grains (almonds, cashews, macadamia nuts, Brazil nuts, hemp seeds, flaxseeds, sunflower seeds, pumpkin seeds, rice, oats, or tigernuts)

4 cups filtered water

¼ teaspoon vanilla extract

4 seedless dates, optional (or use figs, 1 tablespoon honey, or maple syrup)

Pinch of sea salt

Actions:

Put all the ingredients in a blender and mix together until a smooth, milky consistency is achieved. Drink.

Tips:

- For a creamier and smoother milk, soak your nuts or seeds for 4 hours. For example, when the almond skin becomes soft from soaking, you can pop the almonds right out of their skins before blending. Then you can drain the nut or seed milk with a cheesecloth to remove all the fiber.

- Make a batch of nut or seed milk every Saturday so you have your own homemade milk all week. This will save you from consuming the preservatives that are found in store-bought nut milks. And, it will save you a bunch of money!

Variations—add these ingredients to the above recipe:

- Add 3 tablespoons of cacao powder for Chocolate Milk.
- Add 1 cup strawberries for Strawberry Milk.
- Add 1 teaspoon cinnamon.
- Add 1 teaspoon turmeric.
- Add 2 cups of ice to make shakes.
- Add 8 cups of ice to make smoothies.
- Add 4 frozen bananas or any fruit to make smoothies.

ALMOND MILK

You can make delicious Almond Milk in less than five minutes. Drink as is or use it as a base for other recipes. If you have time, you can soak the almonds in water for 4 hours to make an even creamier milk.

Total time: 5 minutes

Makes 4 servings

Ingredients:

1 cup raw almonds, soaked for 4 hours

4 cups filtered water

¼ teaspoon vanilla extract

4 seedless dates, optional (or use figs, 1 tablespoon honey, or maple syrup)

Pinch of sea salt

Actions:

1. Pop the almonds out of their skins after soaking and add to a blender with all the other ingredients.

2. Mix until a smooth consistency is achieved.

3. Strain the Almond Milk with a cheesecloth to remove any lumps.

4. Drink or place in the fridge for up to 7 days.

Calories: 207.7 | Protein: 7.5g | Carbs: 7.7g | Dietary Fiber: 4.4g | Fat: 17.8g | Vitamin C: 0mg | Vitamin D: 0 IU | Vitamin E: 9.1mg | Calcium: 103.3mg | Iron: 1.3mg | Magnesium: 98.9mg | Potassium: 262.4mg

FLAX MILK

Flaxseeds are high in omega-3 fatty acids and have antioxidant and anti-inflammatory benefits that make them a superfood. A subtle smoky flavor makes Flax Milk a good base for Chocolate Milk and other milkshakes.

Total time: 5 minutes

Makes 4 servings

Ingredients:

4 cups filtered water

1 cup flaxseeds

4 seedless dates (or 1 tablespoon honey)

Dash of sea salt

¼ teaspoon vanilla extract

Actions:

1. Put all the ingredients in a blender and mix until a smooth consistency is achieved.

2. Drain with a cheesecloth or fine mesh strainer to remove any fiber.

Calories: 229.8 | Protein: 7.7g | Carbs: 13.4g | Dietary Fiber: 11.5g | Fat: 17.7g | Vitamin C: 0.3mg | Vitamin D: 0 IU | Vitamin E: 0.1mg | Calcium: 115.7mg | Iron: 2.4mg | Magnesium: 168.8mg | Potassium: 354.4mg

---

COCONUT MILK

Coconuts can be extremely helpful in healing cancer, especially reproductive cancers like breast cancer, ovarian cancer, and prostate cancer. Coconuts are one of the best sources of lauric acid, which has antibacterial and antiviral activities. Fifty percent of the fat in coconuts is lauric acid. Coconut Milk is also great for digestive health.

Total time: 10 minutes

Makes 1 serving

Ingredients:

1 fresh coconut, both the liquid and the meat

Actions:

1. Make a hole in the coconut (page 191).

2. Drain the liquid from the coconut into a blender.

3. Crack open the coconut with a hammer, then scrape out the white coconut flesh inside and add it to the blender.

4. Blend on high speed until a smooth, creamy coconut milk is achieved.

Tip:

Add a pinch of sea salt for added flavor.

Variations:

- Add ½ teaspoon of pure vanilla extract for Vanilla Coconut Milk.
- Add 1 teaspoon cacao powder for Chocolate Coconut Milk.
- Add ½ cup strawberries for Strawberry Coconut Milk.

Calories: 702.6 | Protein: 6.6 | Carbs: 30.2g | Dietary Fiber: 17.8g | Fat: 66.4g | Vitamin C: 6.5mg | Vitamin D: 0 IU | Vitamin E: 0.4mg | Calcium: 27.7mg | Iron: 4.8mg | Magnesium: 63.5mg | Potassium: 706.6mg

---

GOLDEN MILK

Golden Milk is a creamy, dairy-free, soothing milk made with ginger, turmeric, coconut oil, and naturally sweet coconut sugar. Its golden color can help you to imagine healing gold light going into your body as you drink it. This is great to have during the day or at night—just make it without the coconut sugar late in the day so it doesn't keep you up at bedtime.

Total time: 15 minutes

Makes 2 servings

Ingredients:

3 cups Coconut Milk (page 160) and/or Almond Milk (page 159)

1 ½ teaspoons turmeric powder

Pinch of black pepper

¼ teaspoon ginger powder

¼ teaspoon cinnamon

1 ½ teaspoons coconut sugar (more if desired)

1 tablespoon coconut oil (MCT is best)

Actions:

1. Add all the ingredients to a saucepan.
2. Whisk gently until the mixture is boiling. This will make it creamy.
3. Serve and enjoy. You can also add some beautiful edible flowers and a sprinkle of cinnamon powder on top before serving.

Tip:

You can make this with fresh turmeric and ginger instead of the powder; just grate it finely before adding to the saucepan.

Calories: 387.8 | Protein: 11.5g | Carbs: 15.3g | Dietary Fiber: 7.3g | Fat: 33.5g | Vitamin C: 0.03mg | Vitamin D: 0 IU | Vitamin E: 0.09mg | Calcium: 161.7mg | Iron: 3mg | Magnesium: 153.3mg | Potassium: 457mg

IRON-BOOSTING TIGERNUT MILK

Ancient civilizations in Africa knew about the health benefits of this incredible vegetable root. With a blender on hand, you can create a beverage that is filled with prebiotic starches, which nourish the good bacteria in our intestines that help us digest vitamins. When a body has cancer, it is important to make sure the digestive system can absorb as many vitamins as possible, so maintaining healthy gut flora is crucial. Tigernuts have the same amount of iron as a serving of red meat, so they are an ideal source of iron for vegans and vegetarians.

Total time: 5 minutes

Makes 4 servings

Ingredients:

1 cup tigernuts

4 cups filtered water

4 seedless dates or 1 teaspoon maple syrup

Pinch of sea salt

¼ teaspoon vanilla extract

Actions:

1. Put all the ingredients in a blender.
2. Mix together until a smooth, milky consistency is achieved.

Variation:

Add 2 tablespoons cacao powder for Chocolate Tigernut Milk.

Calories: 155.5 | Protein: 2.5g | Carbs: 25g | Dietary Fiber: 0.1g | Fat: 8.7g | Vitamin C: 2.3mg | Vitamin D: 0 IU | Vitamin E: 0mg | Calcium: 46.1mg | Iron: 2.3mg | Magnesium: 39.2mg | Potassium: 12.9mg

TURMERIC LATTE

This recipe comes from psychologist and author Dr. Mike Dow, as seen on *The Doctors*.

Ingredients:

1 cup coconut milk

½ teaspoon turmeric

½ teaspoon black pepper

½ teaspoon cinnamon

5 threads of saffron

Actions:

1. Heat the milk on medium heat on a stovetop until simmering.

2. Add the other ingredients and whisk well to make the mixture frothy.

Calories: 54.5 | Protein: 0.2g | Carbs: 4.5g | Dietary Fiber: 2.2g | Fat: 4.5g | Vitamin C: 0.07mg | Vitamin D: 120 IU | Vitamin E: 0.09mg | Calcium: 119.9mg | Iron: 1.1mg | Magnesium: 37mg | Potassium: 83.9mg

CHOCOLATE MILK

This milk will keep in the fridge for up to seven days.

Total time: 5 minutes

Makes 4 servings

Ingredients:

1 cup tigernuts (or almonds, macadamia nuts, cashews, or Brazil nuts)

4 cups filtered water

4 seedless dates or 1 teaspoon maple syrup

Pinch of sea salt

¼ teaspoon vanilla extract

Actions:

1. Put all the ingredients in a blender.

2. Mix together until a smooth, milky consistency is achieved.

Variation:

For a Chocolate Shake, add ½ cup ice to the blender.

Calories: 175.5 | Protein: 3.5g | Carbs: 28g | Dietary Fiber: 1.1g | Fat: 9.2g | Vitamin C: 2.3mg | Vitamin D: 0 IU | Vitamin E: 0mg | Calcium: 46.1mg | Iron: 3mg | Magnesium: 73.2mg | Potassium: 99.9mg

---

STRAWBERRY MILK

Total time: 5 minutes

Makes 4 servings

Ingredients:

1 cup cashew nuts (or almonds, macadamia nuts, or coconut)

4 cups filtered water

1 cup strawberries

12 seedless dates (or 3 tablespoons raw honey or maple syrup)

Pinch of sea salt

¼ teaspoon vanilla extract

Actions:

Put all the ingredients in a blender and mix until well combined.

Variation:

For a Strawberry Shake, add ½ cup ice to the blender.

Calories: 206.5 | Protein: 6.3g | Carbs: 16.3g | Dietary Fiber: 2.1g | Fat: 14.4g | Vitamin C: 21.5mg | Vitamin D: 0 IU | Vitamin E: 0.4mg | Calcium: 29.3mg | Iron: 2.4mg | Magnesium: 107.5mg | Potassium: 307.8mg

---

VANILLA SHAKE

Total time: 5 minutes

Makes 1 serving

Ingredients:

1 cup Almond Milk (page 159)

½ tablespoon pure vanilla extract

3 seedless dates (or 1 tablespoon raw honey or maple syrup)

½ cup ice

Actions:

Put all the ingredients in a blender and mix until well combined.

Tips:

- To be even closer to nature, substitute the seeds of 1 vanilla bean for the vanilla extract. Scrape the seeds out of the vanilla bean pod and discard the pod before using the seeds.

- Add a pinch of sea salt for enhanced flavor.

- You can swap out the Almond Milk for a milk of your choice, such as Sunflower Seed or Tigernut Milk.

Calories: 240.2 | Protein: 7.7g | Carbs: 12.2g | Dietary Fiber: 4.7g | Fat: 17.8g | Vitamin C: 0.2mg | Vitamin D: 0 IU | Vitamin E: 0.01mg | Calcium: 110.9mg | Iron: 1.5mg | Magnesium: 106mg | Potassium: 310.3mg

ICED COFFEE

Coffee beans are naturally provided by the earth and can give us a lot of positive health benefits when consumed in moderation. They have antidepressant properties to help elevate your mood. The more positive energy you have running through your body, the stronger your immune system will be to be able to fight off the cancer.

Total time: 5 minutes

Makes 1 serving

Ingredients:

1 cup brewed coffee

½ cup Almond Milk (page 159) or another nut milk or seed milk (page 158)

1 teaspoon honey or maple syrup to sweeten (more, if you would like it sweeter)

5 large ice cubes

Actions:

Mix all the ingredients together in a blender.

Tips:

Make Coffee Ice Cubes by freezing in an ice cube tray.

Calories: 127.5 | Protein: 4g | Carbs: 9.6g | Dietary Fiber: 2.2g | Fat: 8.9g | Vitamin C: 0.03mg | Vitamin D: 0 IU | Vitamin E: 0.02mg | Calcium: 60mg | Iron: 0.7mg | Magnesium: 57.7mg | Potassium: 251.9mg

---

CHERRY CHOCOLATE SHAKE

This is a delicious dessert treat, but it's also extremely high in magnesium (good for the brain and muscles) and antioxidants. Cherries contain Vitamin C, fiber, and carotenoids.

Total time: 10 minutes

Makes 2 servings

Ingredients:

2 cups pitted cherries

¼ cup cashews (or almonds or hazelnuts)

¼ cup seedless dates (or 1 tablespoon honey)

1 tablespoon cacao powder

1 ½ cups filtered water

2 tablespoons of hazelnut butter or almond butter

Actions:

Put all the ingredients in a blender and mix until well combined.

Tip:

If you want the shake to be sweeter, add more dates, honey, or maple syrup.

Calories: 273.1 | Protein: 6.8g | Carbs: 30.2g | Dietary Fiber: 5.5g | Fat: 15.7g | Vitamin C: 1,644mg | Vitamin D: 0 IU | Vitamin E: 0.1mg | Calcium: 30.2mg | Iron: 1.8mg | Magnesium: 91.8mg | Potassium: 414.4mg

HOT CHOCOLATE

Did you know cacao has more antioxidants than blueberries? Real chocolate is medicine!

Total time: 10 minutes

Makes 1 serving

Ingredients:

1 tablespoon cacao powder

1 cup boiling filtered water

1 tablespoon Almond Milk (page 159) or Coconut Milk (page 106)

2 teaspoons manuka honey, coconut sugar, or maple syrup

Actions:

Stir all the ingredients together in a mug and drink.

Variation:

Add a dash of turmeric and cayenne pepper for Spicy Hot Chocolate.

Calories: 75.5 | Protein: 1.5g | Carbs: 15g | Dietary Fiber: 1.3g | Fat: 1.6g | Vitamin C: 0.07mg | Vitamin D: 0 IU | Vitamin E: 0mg | Calcium: 14.4mg | Iron: 0.8mg | Magnesium: 42.8mg | Potassium: 110.6mg

CHAPTER 10

BRAIN-PROTECTING SMOOTHIES AND SMOOTHIE BOWLS

Some cancer patients lose their appetites, so a smoothie is an effective way to pack in calories and protein and superfood ingredients to ensure all their nutritional needs are being met. A smoothie can be a meal—breakfast, lunch, dinner—or a dessert or snack. And because smoothies are in liquid form, the nutrients can be easily absorbed in the digestive system, ensuring you get the most out of what is going into your body.

SICK-KICK SMOOTHIE

Here's a quick way to boost your body with vitamin C and support the immune system. This smoothie is packed with immune-boosting ingredients to help you feel better instantly.

Total time: 7 minutes

Makes 1 serving

Ingredients:

2 oranges, peeled

½ lemon, peeled

½-inch piece of ginger

½ cup filtered water

Dash of turmeric powder

Pinch of black pepper

Actions:

Put all the ingredients in a blender and mix together until a smooth consistency is achieved.

Tips:

- Add 1 small garlic clove, peeled, for an extra immunity boost.
- For spiciness, add a dash of cayenne pepper.

Calories: 149.7 | Protein: 2.9g | Carbs: 38.7g | Dietary Fiber: 7.1g | Fat: 0.5g | Vitamin C: 181mg | Vitamin D: 0 IU | Vitamin E: 0.4mg | Calcium: 133.1mg | Iron: 0.7mg | Magnesium: 36.7mg | Potassium: 527.7mg

---

SIMPLE VANILLA BANANA SMOOTHIE

This is the base to make a simple classic smoothie. Using frozen bananas (be sure to freeze them without the skin) makes a thick, smooth, and chilled smoothie. Then you can add any ingredients you like for other flavors such as a Chocolate Smoothie or Strawberry Smoothie.

Total time: 10 minutes

Makes 2 servings

Ingredients:

1 cup plant-based milk (any type)

2 frozen bananas

3 seedless dates

Pinch of sea salt

Dash of vanilla extract

Actions:

Put all the ingredients in a blender and blend on high speed until the mixture reaches a smooth consistency.

Variations:

- Add 1 ½ teaspoons cacao powder for a Chocolate Smoothie.
- Add 1 ½ teaspoons cacao powder and 2 tablespoons peanut butter for a Chocolate-Peanut Butter-Banana Smoothie.
- You can add a scoop of protein powder or almond butter to this smoothie too!
- Add ½ cup berries for a Banana Berry Smoothie.
- Freeze this smoothie for 2 hours for Banana Smoothie Ice Cream.

Tip:

To freeze a banana, peel it first, then wrap it in plastic wrap and place it in the freezer. This makes it easier when you are ready to make smoothies or instant ice cream: Just grab it out of the freezer, unwrap, and blend!

Calories: 216.8 | Protein: 5.1g | Carbs: 32.7g | Dietary Fiber: 5.4g | Fat: 9.3g | Vitamin C: 10.3mg | Vitamin D: 0 IU | Vitamin E: 0.1mg | Calcium: 59.8mg | Iron: 1mg | Magnesium: 84.1mg | Potassium: 572.8mg

THE SMOOTHIE CURE

Kelly Brogan, M.D., is an advocate for "healing your brain by changing your breakfast." She says, "People often ask me what I eat for breakfast. If you're looking for a quick and easy recipe to improve brain health and functioning, and give you energy to spare, try this smoothie. Loaded with healthy fats, lecithin, protein, and antioxidants, this smoothie packs a serious punch—and it tastes great!" Kelly is a Manhattan-based holistic women's health psychiatrist, author of the *New York Times* best-selling book, *A Mind of Your Own: The Truth About Depression and How Women Can Heal Their Bodies to Reclaim Their Lives*, and co-editor of the landmark textbook, *Integrative Therapies for Depression: Redefining Models for Assessment, Treatment and Prevention*.

She completed her psychiatric training and fellowship at New York University Medical Center after graduating from Cornell University Medical College, and has a B.S. from the Massachusetts Institute of Technology in systems neuroscience. In regard to cancer, Kelly says, "There is nothing to fight. There is no war to declare. In fact, it is the posture of aligning with the good to fight the bad that is keeping us stuck, tired, and losing precious ground. The sooner we recognize that what we are calling other is us, the sooner we heal. Cancer is a wise mechanism on the part of a body, mind, and spirit. It is a means of communicating a desperate message, a signal of danger, and a mandate for change. Change in relationships, in diet, in toxic exposures, and often, an indication that it is time to unearth old secrets, heal past trauma, and give voice to suppressed anger. It is, as all diagnoses, an invitation to be initiated to your more whole, healed self."

Total time: 5 minutes

Serves 1

Ingredients:

½ cup frozen organic cherries (or other berries)

1 cup fermented coconut water, coconut water, or filtered water

3 tablespoons collagen hydrolysate as a protein base

1 tablespoon sprouted nut butter or Sunbutter

3 pastured organic egg yolks

1 tablespoon coconut oil

1 to 2 tablespoons ghee

1 to 2 tablespoons raw cacao powder

Actions:

Blend all the ingredients.

Calories: 676.4 | Protein: 30.5g | Carbs: 25.2g | Dietary Fiber: 5.3g | Fat: 50.9g | Vitamin C: 7mg | Vitamin D: 111.1 IU | Vitamin E: 2.2mg | Calcium: 173.7mg | Iron: 3.7mg | Magnesium: 103.5mg | Potassium: 838.6mg

A SPLASH OF SUNSHINE SMOOTHIE

This recipe comes from holistic health practitioner Sarah Anne Stewart, AADP, who is the daughter of Bill and Linda Stewart (page 121). Sarah was 14 when her father was diagnosed with cancer and her family decided as a unit that they would change their eating habits. They were successful, and Bill became cancer-free. Sarah was positively affected and inspired for a lifetime to eat and drink nourishing, nutrient-rich foods. This is one of Sarah's favorite smoothies loaded with anticancer ingredients. It is both anti-inflammatory and high in protein.

Total time: 10 minutes

Makes 6 servings

Ingredients:

1 ½ cups ice

2 ½ cups Almond Milk (page 159) or coconut water

1 frozen banana

1 ½ cups chopped frozen pineapple

1 avocado

1 cup spinach

1 cup kale

1 tablespoon lemon juice

3 ½ medjool dates, pitted and soaked in filtered water for 4 hours

1 tablespoon flaxseeds

1 tablespoon chia seeds

1 tablespoon hemp seeds

1 tablespoon peeled ginger

¼ teaspoon cayenne

¼ teaspoon turmeric

Handful of coconut flakes

1 tablespoon pure maple syrup, to taste (if desired)

Actions:

Blend all the ingredients in a blender on high speed and serve with love.

Calories: 263.7 | Protein: 6.2g | Carbs: 28g | Dietary Fiber: 8g | Fat: 16.7g | Vitamin C: 30.5mg | Vitamin D: 0 IU | Vitamin E: 0.9mg | Calcium: 87.5mg | Iron: 1.7mg | Magnesium: 95mg | Potassium: 553.6mg

CLASSIC GREEN SMOOTHIE

This powerful concoction of greens will leave you feeling so vibrant! Packed with sulforaphane from the broccoli sprouts, vitamin A from the spinach, vitamin K from the cilantro and blueberries, and vitamin C from the kale, this smoothie will support your immune system immediately.

Total time: 5 minutes

Makes 2 servings

Ingredients:

1 ½ cups Almond Milk (page 159) or filtered water

2 cups kale

1 frozen banana

1 ½ cups blueberries

1 cup spinach

¼ cup fresh cilantro

1 cup broccoli sprouts

1 peeled cucumber

Actions:

Put all the ingredients in a blender and mix together until a smooth consistency is achieved.

Tips:

- If you want a smoother mixture, add more water.
- For more creaminess, add 1 peeled avocado.
- For more sweetness, add 3 seedless dates (or 1 tablespoon raw honey or maple syrup).
- For extra protein and vitamins, add 1 tablespoon spirulina.
- Reserve the cucumber skins and use them later as refreshing face wipes.

Calories: 315.2 | Protein: 11.1g | Carbs: 39g | Dietary Fiber: 9.2g | Fat: 14.9g | Vitamin C: 105.4mg |Vitamin D: 0 IU | Vitamin E: 1.3mg | Calcium: 254.7mg | Iron: 3.4mg | Magnesium: 142.3mg | Potassium: 1,018mg

PARADISE SMOOTHIE

Drink this smoothie and imagine you are in a tropical paradise. Visualize your body healthy and strong while you are sitting on a hammock looking at white sand and crystal-clear water.

Total time: 10 minutes

Makes 1 serving

Ingredients:

1 papaya, peeled and cut in chunks

1 pineapple, peeled and cut in chunks

2 passion fruit, scooped out

½ tablespoon flax oil

¾ cup ice

¼ cup noni juice (or coconut milk, almond milk, or filtered water)

Actions:

Put all the ingredients in a blender and mix together until a smooth consistency is achieved.

Calories: 884.6 | Protein: 9.3g | Carbs: 211g | Dietary Fiber: 29.6g | Fat: 10.1g | Vitamin C: 920.5mg | Vitamin D: 0 IU | Vitamin E: 2.5mg | Calcium: 282mg | Iron: 5.1mg | Magnesium: 288.3mg | Potassium: 2,534mg

CHOCO-MOCHA SMOOTHIE

If you love chocolate and coffee, this blend is for you!

Total time: 10 minutes

Makes 1 serving

Ingredients:

¾ cup Almond Milk (page 159) or Coconut Milk (page 160)

½ cup ice

1 frozen banana

1 tablespoon coconut oil or MCT oil

2 teaspoons cacao powder

1 teaspoon freshly ground coffee beans

4 seedless dates

1 teaspoon honey

½ teaspoon pure vanilla extract

Pinch of sea salt

1 tablespoon coconut flakes/ shavings

Actions:

1. Place the ingredients in a blender and mix until the liquid reaches a smooth consistency.

2. Sprinkle with extra ground coffee and cacao powder on top!

Calories: 483.5 | Protein: 8.5g | Carbs: 48.4g | Dietary Fiber: 8.8g | Fat: 30.7g | Vitamin C: 10.6mg | Vitamin D: 0 IU | Vitamin E: 0.2mg | Calcium: 96.8mg | Iron: 2.3mg | Magnesium: 147.8mg | Potassium: 812.7mg

CHOCOLATE NUT BERRY SMOOTHIE

This is my personal favorite because it tastes like a dessert smoothie. It's so delicious, smooth, thick, and chocolaty, and it's packed with health benefits including protein and antioxidants. You can add bee pollen for immune boosting and hemp for extra protein.

Total time: 10 minutes

Makes 1 serving

Ingredients:

1 cup berries of your choice (strawberries, raspberries, and/or blueberries—I like to use a mixture)

1 frozen banana

1 cup filtered water

2 tablespoons almond butter

1 tablespoon cacao powder or more, to taste

1 tablespoon raw local honey or maple syrup

1 teaspoon flax oil

Actions:

Put all the ingredients in a blender and mix together until a smooth consistency is achieved.

VARIATION:

For more protein, substitute Almond Milk (page 159) for the water.

Calories: 471.4 | Protein: 10g | Carbs: 64.3g | Dietary Fiber: 10.2g | Fat: 23.6g | Vitamin C: 95mg | Vitamin D: 0 IU | Vitamin E: 8.3mg | Calcium: 148.3mg | Iron: 2.8mg | Magnesium: 176.6mg | Potassium: 980mg

CHOCOLATE CAULIFLOWER SMOOTHIE

You can use frozen cauliflower in any smoothies to replace the frozen banana, which cuts down the sugar intake from the smoothie. I prefer it half and half—half frozen cauliflower and half frozen banana, so it's still got some sweetness. Surprisingly, you cannot taste the cauliflower!

Total time: 10 minutes

Makes 1 serving

Ingredients:

1 tablespoon cacao powder

1 ½ cups Almond Milk (page 159)

3 seedless dates or 1 tablespoon honey

1 cup frozen cauliflower

½ large frozen banana

Smidgen of sea salt

Dash of vanilla extract

Actions:

Put all the ingredients in a blender and mix together until a smooth consistency is achieved.

Tip:

You can add a scoop of protein powder to this smoothie too!

Calories: 439.6 | Protein: 15.9g | Carbs: 40.1g | Dietary Fiber: 12.8g | Fat: 27.8g | Vitamin C: 70.5mg | Vitamin D: 0 IU | Vitamin E: 0.1mg | Calcium: 191.8mg | Iron: 3.7mg | Magnesium: 222.1mg | Potassium: 1,017g

STRAWBERRIES AND CREAM SMOOTHIE

To fulfill those strawberry and cream cravings in a much healthier way, try this smoothie. While battling cancer it's empowering to think, *How can I fulfill my cravings in a healthier, more nourishing way?*

Total time: 10 minutes

Makes 1 serving

Ingredients:

½ cup Cashew Milk (page 158)

½ cup Coconut Milk (page 160), or macadamia nut milk

1 cup frozen strawberries

3 seedless dates

½ teaspoon honey or maple syrup

¼ teaspoon vanilla extract

Smidgen of sea salt

Actions:

Put all the ingredients in a blender and mix together until a smooth consistency is achieved.

Calories: 120.1 | Protein: 0.8g | Carbs: 21.8g | Dietary Fiber: 3.9g | Fat: 4.2g | Vitamin C: 61.6mg | Vitamin D: 130 IU | Vitamin E: 0.4mg | Calcium: 128.6mg | Iron: 1.4mg | Magnesium: 54.1mg | Potassium: 281.5mg

---

ULTIMATE SUPERFOOD SMOOTHIE

You can't beat the nutritional punch of 16 superfoods in one yummy beverage. These superfoods will give your body super-powers to give you a better chance of fighting cancer!

Total time: 10 minutes

Makes 2 servings

Ingredients:

2 cups Almond Milk (page 159) or Tigernut Milk (page 162)

1 ½ teaspoons pure vanilla extract

½ cup blueberries

½ cup kale

½ cup broccoli sprouts

1 tablespoon goji berries

3 seedless dates

3 figs

2 cups ice

½ teaspoon maca powder

½ teaspoon mangosteen powder

1 teaspoon pomegranate powder

½ teaspoon bee pollen

½ teaspoon spirulina

¼ teaspoon cacao powder

1 teaspoon coconut oil

1 teaspoon hemp seeds

1 teaspoon chia seeds

1 teaspoon flaxseeds

¼ teaspoon turmeric powder

Actions:

Place all the ingredients in a blender and mix until a smooth consistency is achieved.

Calories: 391.1 | Protein: 12.1g | Carbs: 36.4g | Dietary Fiber: 9.5g | Fat: 22.7g | Vitamin C: 56.5mg | Vitamin D: 0 IU | Vitamin E: 0.4mg | Calcium: 230mg | Iron: 3.2mg | Magnesium: 142.8mg | Potassium: 529.5mg

---

THE CHEMO BRAIN BUSTER

CC Webster, author of *So, That Happened,* drank this smoothie every morning to get through her courses of chemotherapy. *Chemo brain* is a term people use to describe difficulty concentrating, confusion, being unusually disoriented, struggling to find the right word, difficulty learning new skills or multitasking, fatigue from thinking, and any feeling of mental fogginess from mild to severe.[1] CC says this smoothie "brought my words back to me."

The secret of the smoothie is that it is rich in the highest-quality omega-3 and omega-6 fats. What's the science? The brain is one of the systems of the body that is MOST reliant on cell turnover. It needs to regenerate itself to continue making high-speed connections, to sift through memories for deductive reasoning, to dream and plan, and to facilitate word recall. Without fresh, new cells, neurotransmitter activity simply doesn't work. Chemo stops cell regeneration in its tracks, and with that your dreams, your memories, and your words are also affected. Healthy fats nourish your brain and coat it with literal brain food. CC still drinks this every morning! She is two years cancer-free.

Total time: 10 minutes

Makes 2 servings

Ingredients:

1 cup Coconut Milk (page 160)

½ frozen banana

1 cup frozen mixed berries

1 cup frozen wild blueberries

1 heaping handful of fresh spinach or kale

1 tablespoon coconut oil or MCT oil

2 tablespoons safflower oil

1 tablespoon PC oil (phosphatidyl choline), or break open PC gel capsules (optional)

2 tablespoons collagen powder (optional/nonvegan)

Actions:

Combine all the ingredients in a blender and mix until smooth.

Calories: 397.6 | Protein: 13.8g | Carbs: 25.1g | Dietary Fiber: 6.9g | Fat: 31.9g | Vitamin C: 9.6mg | Vitamin D: 60 IU | Vitamin E: 0.3mg | Calcium: 87.3mg | Iron: 0.9mg | Magnesium: 32.8mg | Potassium: 375.2mg

---

HIGH-PROTEIN SMOOTHIE

This smoothie is packed with protein: hemp seeds, chia seeds, pumpkin seeds, and almond butter. It's a great way to consume protein in liquid form if you are having trouble swallowing or digesting.

Total time: 5 minutes

Makes 2 servings

Ingredients:

1 cup plant-based milk (any nut or seed milk, page 158)

2 bananas

3 seedless dates

¼ cup pumpkin seeds

¼ cup hemp seeds

1 tablespoon chia seeds

1 teaspoon flax oil

2 tablespoons almond butter

Actions:

Place all the ingredients in a blender and mix until the liquid reaches a smooth consistency.

Calories: 584.6 | Protein: 22.9g | Carbs: 42g | Dietary Fiber: 10.8g | Fat: 40.2g | Vitamin C: 11.4mg | Vitamin D: 0 IU | Vitamin E: 4.1mg | Calcium: 167.8mg | Iron: 6mg | Magnesium: 393.7mg | Potassium: 1,110mg

BANANA BERRY SMOOTHIE BOWL

This smoothie bowl is packed with vitamin B6 and vitamin C, so it's bound to leave you feeling energized. Add some fun toppings.

Total time: 10 minutes

Makes 2 servings

Ingredients:

1 cup Almond Milk (page 159)

2 frozen bananas

¾ cup frozen berries, such as blackberries, cherries, blueberries, or strawberries

¼ cup fresh blueberries

¼ cup fresh strawberries, sliced

3 seedless dates

Actions:

1. Combine the Almond Milk, bananas, dates, and frozen berries in a blender. Mix until smooth.
2. Pour into 2 bowls and top with the fresh blueberries and strawberries.

Tip:

Serve with fun toppings such as Almond Butter Granola (page 200), chopped almonds, walnuts, or organic chocolate chips.

Calories: 255.7 | Protein: 5.8g | Carbs: 42.6g | Dietary Fiber: 8.1g | Fat: 9.4g | Vitamin C: 27.7mg | Vitamin D: 0 IU | Vitamin E: 0.2mg | Calcium: 71.7mg | Iron: 1.3mg | Magnesium: 87.8mg | Potassium: 618.4mg

ACAI BOWL

If you love smooth and crunchy textures together, you'll love the roasted almonds on top.

Total time: 8 minutes

Makes 1 serving

Ingredients:

Smoothie:
2 Açaí Superfruit Packs (Sambazon)

1 banana (fresh or frozen)

¼ cup liquid of your choice (filtered water, coconut water, almond milk, apple juice, noni juice, or pomegranate juice)

Topping options:

Roasted nuts, such as almonds

Raw nuts

Chopped fruit, such as banana, apple, strawberries, or peaches

Cacao nibs

Golden berries

Goji berries

Almond Butter Granola (page 200)

Oats

Coconut shavings

Actions:

1. Blend the acai, banana, and liquid until completely smooth.

2. Serve in a bowl and then add your toppings.

Calories: 245 | Protein: 1.2g | Carbs: 34.9g | Dietary Fiber: 3g | Fat: 10.3g | Vitamin C: 10.2mg | Vitamin D: 0 IU | Vitamin E: 0.1mg | Calcium: 87.6mg | Iron: 1mg | Magnesium: 32.4mg | Potassium: 542.4mg

---

LIANA'S FAVORITE SMOOTHIE BOWL

This is my favorite bowl because of the combination of berries with almond butter and cacao powder as a base. And then I love the crunchiness, textures, and flavor of the toppings.

Total time: 10 minutes

Makes 2 servings

Ingredients:

Smoothie:
2 cups frozen berries (strawberries, raspberries, and blueberries)

¾ cup filtered water

3 tablespoons almond butter

1 tablespoon cacao powder

1 tablespoon raw honey

Toppings:

1 teaspoon bee pollen

2 teaspoons hemp seeds

1 teaspoon flax meal or seeds

1 tablespoon roasted chopped almonds

½ tablespoon roasted chopped hazelnuts

1 tablespoon fresh blueberries

4 strawberries, sliced

Sprinkle of blue-green algae

Actions:

1. Add all smoothie ingredients to a blender and blend until completely smooth.

2. Add the toppings and enjoy.

Calories: 337.1 | Protein: 9.6g | Carbs: 37.1g | Dietary Fiber: 10.9g | Fat: 19.6g | Vitamin C: 60.3mg | Vitamin D: 0 IU | Vitamin E: 7mg | Calcium: 139.2mg | Iron: 3.1mg | Magnesium: 137.9mg | Potassium: 532.4mg

CHAPTER 11

DETOXING TEAS AND CLEANSING WATERS

During the cancer healing process, one easy way to ensure we are getting constant hydration, nourishment, and detox aid is to be drinking herbal teas and cleansing waters regularly. In between the juices and foods that I was consuming every day, I was also drinking a lot of herbal tea, mostly lemon myrtle with myrtle that came straight from a tree in my backyard. If you have a tree or plant that you can access from your own garden this is even better and more powerful for healing. If not, you can purchase teas.

Here are some easy cleansing waters that you can keep in your fridge, or even pour into ice cube trays and place in the freezer—then they are ready to pop out and add to filtered drinking water at any time.

IMMUNE-BOOSTING TURMERIC BLACK PEPPER TEA

This stimulating tea offers a great way to get your daily dose of the turmeric-and-black pepper remedy.

Total time: 10 minutes

Makes 1 serving

Ingredients:

2 cups filtered water

1-inch piece of ginger, diced

1 garlic clove, diced

Pinch of cayenne pepper (the beverage should be spicy but comfortable to drink)

¼ teaspoon turmeric powder

Dash of black pepper

1 lemon

1 tablespoon raw honey (optional)

Actions:

1. Bring the water, ginger, garlic, cayenne pepper, turmeric, and black pepper to boil in a saucepan. Reduce the heat to medium and simmer for 7 minutes.

2. Strain the liquid as you pour it into a teacup.

3. Squeeze in the juice of the lemon, add honey, if using, and stir well.

4. Drink warm.

Calories: 23.2 | Protein: 0.5g | Carbs: 6g | Dietary Fiber: 0.5g | Fat: 0.2g | Vitamin C: 19.1mg | Vitamin D: 0 IU | Vitamin E: 0.1mg | Calcium: 25.9mg | Iron: 0.4mg | Magnesium: 13.2mg | Potassium: 107.2mg

ANTI-INFLAMMATORY GINGER TEA

If you have cancer, or want to prevent cancer, always have some fresh ginger root in your home. You can cut it up and boil it to make a ginger tea. I recommend drinking a ginger tea every night before bed. Ginger is an incredibly powerful anti-inflammatory and assists in reducing pain, cramps, aches, and bloating. It also suppresses appetite, so it can help curb sugar cravings at nighttime.

Total time: 10 minutes

Makes 2 servings

Ingredients:

4 cups filtered water

2-inch piece of ginger, diced

Actions:

1. Boil the water and ginger in a saucepan for 7 minutes.

2. Strain the liquid as you pour it into teacups.

3. Drink warm.

Tip:

Make a huge batch, and then let it cool and later place in the fridge so the next day you have Ginger Water.

Calories: 5.9 | Protein: 0.1g | Carbs: 1.3g | Dietary Fiber: 0.1g | Fat: 0.06g | Vitamin C: 0.3mg | Vitamin D: 0 IU | Vitamin E: 0.02mg | Calcium: 15.3mg | Iron: 0.04mg | Magnesium: 7.9mg | Potassium: 30.5mg

---

PAIN-RELIEVING TEA

Before popping pain relievers, try this remedy for natural pain relief. No worries if you are missing one or two ingredients; make it with what you have on hand and it will help relieve your pain anyway. This recipe is also helpful for neuropathy, which can be a side effect of chemotherapy.

Total time: 10 minutes

Makes 2 servings

Ingredients:

4 cups filtered water

1-inch piece of ginger, diced

1-inch piece of turmeric, diced

¼ teaspoon chili powder

1 teaspoon dried valerian root powder

1 teaspoon white willow bark powder

1 teaspoon cat's claw powder

1 teaspoon Boswellia powder

2 teaspoons cloves

Actions:

1. Boil all the ingredients in a saucepan for 15 minutes or until well combined.

2. Strain the liquid as you pour it into teacups.

3. Drink warm.

Calories: 11.3 | Protein: 0.2g | Carbs: 2.4g | Dietary Fiber: 0.9g | Fat: 0.4g | Vitamin C: 0.1mg | Vitamin D: 0 IU | Vitamin E: 0.3mg | Calcium: 30.1mg | Iron: 0.4mg | Magnesium: 12.2mg | Potassium: 61.2mg

---

ENERGY TEA

This energizing combo of green tea, mint, and ginseng is bound to leave you pleasantly bouncing off the walls—heehee! Ginseng helps the body use oxygen more efficiently, which gives the body more energy. During and after cancer treatment, some patients reported to have had sexual issues. Ginseng has been proven as an effective alternative for treating male erectile dysfunction.[1] In Chinese medicine, ginseng is also used as an antidepressant quite effectively.[2]

Total time: 10 minutes

Makes 2 servings

Ingredients:

4 cups filtered water

1 teaspoon dried green tea leaves

1 small handful of fresh mint or
1 teaspoon dried mint

1 teaspoon ginseng root or powder

Actions:

1. Boil all the ingredients in a saucepan for 5 minutes.

2. Strain the liquid as you pour it into teacups.

3. Drink warm.

Calories: 5.9 | Protein: 0.4g | Carbs: 1g | Dietary Fiber: 0.3g | Fat: 0.09g | Vitamin C: 3.6mg | Vitamin D: 0 IU | Vitamin E: 0mg | Calcium: 27mg | Iron: 0.4mg | Magnesium: 8.1mg | Potassium: 24.2 mg

---

RELAXING BEDTIME TEA

All its ingredients make this a relaxation tonic. Even just chamomile is a relaxing bedtime tea in itself, if you aren't able to get the other ingredients. Chamomile is used to soothe muscles and has been proven to be effective in treating spasmodic gastrointestinal disorders.[3] And check this out—based on available data, chamomile has appeared useful in mitigating anxiety and depression. "Chamomile and other flowers including lavender can benefit cancer patients by minimizing medication load and accompanying side effects."[4]

Valerian root has been used in alternative medicine to aid in treating sleep problems including insomnia; it also may alleviate PMS symptoms.[5]

Total time: 10 minutes

Makes 2 servings

Ingredients:

4 cups filtered water

2 tablespoons chamomile flowers

1 tablespoon lavender leaves

1 teaspoon dried valerian root powder

1 teaspoon fenugreek powder or fresh leaves

Actions:

1. Boil all the ingredients in a saucepan for 5 minutes.
2. Strain the liquid as you pour it into mugs.
3. Drink warm.

Calories: 7.6 | Protein: 0.5g | Carbs: 1.1g | Dietary Fiber: 0.9g | Fat: 0.1g | Vitamin C: 0.2mg | Vitamin D: 0 IU | Vitamin E: 0mg | Calcium: 17.2mg | Iron: 0.1mg | Magnesium: 4.7mg | Potassium: 0mg

INFUSED WATERS

You can infuse water with literally any fruit, vegetable, herb, or spice you have on hand—even edible essential oils in moderation. You can infuse them on their own or together. One reason why you would infuse your water is to add nutrients, and the other—main reason—is for flavor. Staying hydrated is helpful to your elimination systems.

Some ideas:

Orange slices	Strawberries
Lemon slices	Blueberries
Lime slices	Pineapple slices
Apple slices	Cucumber slices
Halved cherries	Rosemary sprigs
Halved grapes	Mint leaves
Raspberries	Ginger slices

Apple cider vinegar (1 teaspoon or 1 capful per cup of water)

Essential oils, therapeutic grade only (1 to 2 drops per cup) such as cinnamon, clove, copaiba, frankincense, ginger, grapefruit, lemon, lemongrass, orange, peppermint, and spearmint

---

DETOX WATER

This is for people who find drinking plain water "boring." If you are used to drinking soda, this is the recipe for you—not that it is sweet in any way, but it adds an extra quick to your water, so you can feel good about doing some extreme cleansing for your body. Woo-hoo, kick it!

Total time: 5 minutes

Makes 1 serving

Ingredients:

2 cups filtered water	Pinch of sea salt
1 lemon	Sprinkle of turmeric
1 teaspoon apple cider vinegar	Sprinkle of black pepper
Pinch of cayenne pepper	

Actions:

1. Pour the water into a pitcher. Slice the lemon in half and squeeze its juice into the water by hand.
2. Add the remaining ingredients. Stir and drink.

Calories: 17.5 | Protein: 0.6g | Carbs: 5.5g | Dietary Fiber: 1.6g | Fat: 0.2g | Vitamin C: 30.8mg | Vitamin D: 0 IU | Vitamin E: 0.1mg | Calcium: 29.8mg | Iron: 0.4mg | Magnesium: 9.8mg | Potassium: 88.2mg

COCONUT WATER

Enjoying Coconut Water is as simple as poking a hole into a coconut and drinking straight from it. You can then eat the coconut meat or add it to a smoothie to make thick and creamy coconut milk.

Total time: 5 minutes

Makes 1 serving

Ingredients:

1 fresh whole coconut

Actions:

1. Make a hole in the coconut. Here is the easiest way: On one end of every coconut you'll see 3 darker circles together. One of the holes will be softer than the others. Poke through this hole with a screwdriver or a sharp kitchen utensil, like a thin knife or a metal chopstick.

2. Drain the coconut water into a cup or place a straw in the hole and drink directly from the coconut!

Calories: 34.2 | Protein: 1.3g | Carbs: 6.6g | Dietary Fiber: 1.9g | Fat: 0.3g | Vitamin C: 4.3mg | Vitamin D: 0 IU | Vitamin E: 0mg | Calcium: 43.2mg | Iron: 0.5mg | Magnesium: 45mg | Potassium: 450mg

---

LEMON WATER

A powerful way to start your day on the right healthy foot is to drink Lemon Water as soon as you rise (or after oil pulling). Lemon Water is highly alkalizing and helps to flush your digestive system, especially the stomach and liver. It is also beautifully hydrating.

Total time: 5 minutes

Makes 1 serving

Ingredients:

2 cups filtered water

1 lemon

Actions:

Hand squeeze the lemon into the water and drink.

Calories: 25 | Protein: 1g | Carbs: 6g | Dietary Fiber: 2g | Fat: 0g | Vitamin C: 30mg | Vitamin D: 0 IU | Vitamin E: 0mg | Calcium: 34.2mg | Iron: 0.3mg | Magnesium: 4.7mg | Potassium: 0mg

LEMON ICE CUBES

Keep these on hand so that whenever you want you can pop one into your water, juice, smoothie, or tea.

Total time: 5 minutes

Makes 1 serving

Ingredients:

1 lemon

2 cups water

Actions:

1. Hand squeeze the juice of the lemon into the water.
2. Pour the liquid into an ice cube tray and freeze for 2 hours.

Calories: 10 | Protein: 0.1g | Carbs: 3.1g | Dietary Fiber: 0.1g | Fat: 0.1g | Vitamin C: 17.7mg | Vitamin D: 0 IU | Vitamin E: 0.07mg | Calcium: 16.9mg | Iron: 0.04mg | Magnesium: 7.4mg | Potassium: 47.1mg

SEA SALT FLUSH

Sea salt is high in minerals. It's important to use the right kind of salt, which I would call "real" salt, not table salt with loads of preservatives. This is a great drink if your immune system feels down, or you want to gargle and clean your mouth.

Total time: 1 minute

Makes 1 serving

Ingredients:

½ teaspoon sea salt

2 cups water

Actions:

Mix the sea salt into the water until dissolved and drink.

Calories: 0 | Protein: 0g | Carbs: 0g | Dietary Fiber: 0g | Fat: 0g | Vitamin C: 0mg | Vitamin D: 0 IU | Vitamin E: 0mg | Calcium: 14.2mg | Iron: 0mg | Magnesium: 4.7mg | Potassium: 0mg

BENTONITE CLAY DRINK

Bentonite clay is ash that has accumulated from volcanoes over millions of years. This remarkable clay has magnetic properties that can assist us in expelling impurities, toxins, worms, parasites, and heavy metals from the blood, gut, and body. It is a natural chelator that absorbs toxins so they can be excreted safely. Bentonite clay contains an abundance of minerals, including magnesium, calcium, iron, potassium, and silica.

There are some great studies on bentonite clay and cancer, including one that talks about chickens with an accumulation of carcinogens in their tissue. After treatment, the chickens that received bentonite clay had reduced levels of aflatoxins in their livers and increased longevity.

This is one of the known benefits of drinking bentonite clay—it assists the liver in the natural detoxification process to ensure toxins are kept out. The clay absorbs toxins, which are then expelled with the remnants of the clay when we poop.

Based on different studies, here are two things the clay does.

- An in vitro study showed the clay inhibits the growth of spinal cord and brain tumors (glioblastomas).[6]

- Researchers tested the urine of people in an at-risk population and found that the clay reduces the bioavailability of carcinogens (aflatoxins and fumonisins). It reduces our risk of liver cancer (hepatocellular carcinoma) and esophageal cancer.[7]

Use a wooden spoon to mix the clay into the water, because a metal utensil will change the molecular structure. (See Resources for suppliers.)

Total time: 5 minutes

Makes 1 serving

Ingredients:

1 teaspoon bentonite clay

1 cup filtered water

Actions:

Use a wooden spoon to mix the clay into the water, stirring until there are no lumps.

Tip:

If you let this drink sit for 30 minutes before stirring, lumps often dissolve on their own, making it possible to achieve a smoother consistency.

Calories: 0 | Protein: 0g | Carbs: 0g | Dietary Fiber: 0g | Fat: 0g | Vitamin C: 0mg | Vitamin D: 0 IU | Vitamin E: 0mg | Calcium: 7.1mg | Iron: 0mg | Magnesium: 2.3mg | Potassium: 0mg

CHAPTER 12

EASY, BREEZY BREAKFASTS

Breakfast is your first meal of the day, so it can define your energy and the quality of your self-care. People can be too rigid in their definition of the ideal breakfast. It's okay to eat a salad for breakfast! You could add some eggs to your salad: fried, poached, scrambled, soft-boiled, or hard-boiled to add some more protein and breakfast vibes. Eggs can be a much easier protein to digest than meats for some cancer patients. You can also have a smoothie or smoothie bowl for breakfast. The following recipes include sweet and savory combinations. They are super easy and simple to prepare and great when you are low in energy—especially overnight oats.

CHIA SEED CEREAL

Chia seeds are a great way to start the day! You can make this cereal the night before so that in the morning the seeds are soft and swelled up like a pudding. Chia seeds are extremely comforting and can feel like a lighter "gluten" in the digestive system, helping you to crave less actual gluten like bread. There are also hundreds of articles on chia seeds detailing benefits such as decreased blood glucose; decreased waist, bloating, and weight in overweight adults; and improvements in pruritic skin and endurance in distance runners have been recorded.[1] This cereal can help fuel your body to be able to heal cancer!

Total time: 10 minutes

Makes 1 serving

Ingredients:

3 tablespoons chia seeds

½ cup filtered water, nut milk, or Sunflower Seed Milk (page 158)

Your choice of chopped fruit: 1 apple, banana, peach, pear, or nectarine, or ½ cup berries

Actions:

1. Place the chia seeds and liquid into a cereal bowl. Soak for 5 minutes.

2. Add the fruit and eat.

Tip:

Add 1 teaspoon of raw honey, maple syrup, or chopped dates for a sweeter cereal.

Variations:

Chia Hemp Seed Cereal: add 1 tablespoon hemp seeds.

Oatmeal Chia Seed Cereal: add 1 tablespoon oats.

Calories: 247.7 | Protein: 5.6g | Carbs: 38.4g | Dietary Fiber: 15.2g | Fat: 9.9g | Vitamin C: 8.8mg | Vitamin D: 0 IU | Vitamin E: 0.4mg | Calcium: 213.2mg | Iron: 2.6mg | Magnesium: 115.8mg | Potassium: 322.9mg

---

CHOCOLATE COCONUT MOUSSE

You can make this recipe, along with the Overnight Oats and Blueberry Chia Seed Jam, and stack it in a jar to make a beautiful breakfast parfait. This is my favorite combination because you have the savory overnight oats at the bottom, then a layer of decadent mousse, topped with another layer of oats or some fresh fruit like strawberries and blueberries, then finished with some jam, a sweet-tart fruity way to complete the jar. You can make up to three of these and take them with you to work—so sweet and so convenient!

Total time: 5 minutes

Makes 4 servings

Ingredients:

1 can 13.5 oz coconut cream

2 tablespoons cacao powder

6 seedless dates

¼ teaspoon vanilla

1 tablespoon MCT oil or coconut oil

Smidgen of sea salt

Actions:

Add all ingredients to a high-speed blender and whip until completely combined. It will be melted, so set in the fridge in jars or an airtight container for 2 hours until it's set and smooth like mousse.

Calories: 231.9 | Protein: 1.1g | Carbs: 30.7g | Dietary Fiber: 0.7g | Fat: 12g | Vitamin C: 0.1mg | Vitamin D: 0 IU | Vitamin E: 0.07mg | Calcium: 4.3mg | Iron: 0.5mg | Magnesium: 28.5mg | Potassium: 114.5mg

STEEL-CUT OVERNIGHT OATS

A five-minute recipe that you can leave in the fridge overnight and enjoy the next morning—woo-hoo! You can make these oats as many as three days ahead.

Total time: 5 minutes and setting overnight

Makes 1 serving

Ingredients:

½ cup steel-cut oats

¼ cup filtered water

¼ cup almond milk

⅛ teaspoon vanilla

1 tablespoon chia seeds (If you can't do chia seeds, add an extra tablespoon of steel-cut oats.)

Smidgen of sea salt

Actions:

1. Add all the ingredients to a jar and stir until well combined.

2. Place in the fridge and enjoy the next day with some toppings.

Tips:

- Add these as toppings: cinnamon, cardamom, nutmeg, cacao powder, cacao nibs, cashews, walnuts, pistachios, granola, shredded coconut, blueberries, strawberries, kiwi.

- You can use regular whole oats instead of steel-cut, but they expand more so use this recipe with ½ cup oats and do 1 cup of liquid.

Calories: 362 | Protein: 15.7g | Carbs: 54.9g | Dietary Fiber: 12.3g | Fat: 12.9g | Vitamin C: 0.1mg | Vitamin D: 0 IU | Vitamin E: 0.05mg | Calcium: 124.2mg | Iron: 4.4mg | Magnesium: 60.5mg | Potassium: 109.1mg

---

ANTICANCER MUFFINS

This is an epic muffin recipe that makes a great breakfast because it is delicious and filling and packed with loads of anticancer ingredients. These are truly mind-blowingly tasty and a must-try! They are also gluten-free, dairy-free, soy-free, and egg-free. To make them even more anticancer potent, add one apricot seed to each muffin—just poke one right in the middle after pouring the mix into the muffin tin!

Total time: 50 minutes

Makes 12

Ingredients:

2 tablespoons flax meal

2 tablespoons filtered water

½ cup almond milk

1 teaspoon apple cider vinegar

1 ½ teaspoons baking soda

2 organic apples or ½ cup applesauce

1 tablespoon MCT oil

¼ cup coconut oil

⅓ cup maple syrup

¼ cup coconut sugar

½ teaspoon sea salt

1 cup organic blueberries

2 tablespoons chia seeds

Gluten-free flour mix:

1 tablespoon potato starch

2 tablespoons tapioca starch

¼ cup tigernut flour

1 tablespoon brown rice flour

¾ cup plant-based protein powder, or more flour of any mentioned here

¼ cup almond flour

Actions:

1. Preheat the oven to 375°F and line a 12-cup muffin tray with paper baking cups.

2. Mix the flax and water together in a small cup until well combined. Let the mixture sit for 10 minutes until it becomes gummy like eggs. This is the egg replacement. Set aside.

3. In a separate bowl, mix the almond milk, apple cider vinegar, and baking soda until well combined. Set aside.

4. Peel and core the apples. Mix in a blender or food processor with the MCT oil until you have an applesauce.

5. In another, larger bowl, mix the coconut oil, maple syrup, coconut sugar, and applesauce. Add the egg replacement (see step 1) to this bowl and whisk.

6. Add the almond milk mixture and stir well.

7. Add the sea salt and gluten-free flour mix.

8. Add the blueberries and chia seeds.

9. Pour the batter evenly among 12 baking cups and bake for 24 minutes or until golden brown and you poke it with a toothpick and it comes out dry.

10. Let the muffins cool for 15 minutes.

Calories: 197.3 | Protein: 4.8g | Carbs: 23.9g | Dietary Fiber: 4.9g | Fat: 9.7g | Vitamin C: 2.6mg | Vitamin D: 0 IU | Vitamin E: 0.9mg | Calcium: 41.3mg | Iron: 2.2mg | Magnesium: 74.8mg | Potassium: 211.5mg

PROTEIN BARS

Total time: 10 minutes

Makes 5 bars

Ingredients:

7 tablespoons almond butter or peanut butter

½ cup almond meal or tigernut flour

5 tablespoons raw honey or maple syrup

3 tablespoons hemp seeds

3 tablespoons pumpkin seeds

Actions:

1. Mix all the ingredients together in a bowl until well combined. If the mixture is too dry to form together, add a bit of water.

2. Press the mixture into a baking tray. Sprinkle additional hemp seeds and pumpkin seeds on top and press them down. Set in the freezer for 5 minutes and then cut into 5 bars.

Calories: 325.6 | Protein: 10.5g | Carbs: 24.9g | Dietary Fiber: 4g | Fat: 23.3g | Vitamin C: 0.2mg | Vitamin D: 0 IU | Vitamin E: 8.4mg | Calcium: 109.4mg | Iron: 2.2mg | Magnesium: 165.5mg | Potassium: 289.6mg

ALMOND BUTTER GRANOLA

Making your own granola is always healthier and more rewarding than store-bought because you can control the ingredients that are going into it, and choose the sweetener you want to use. This recipe uses wholesome honey.

Total time: 10 minutes

Makes 6 servings

Ingredients:

¼ cup almond butter

1 tablespoon whole or sliced almonds

2 tablespoons honey or maple syrup

½ teaspoon cinnamon

½ teaspoon vanilla extract

½ tablespoon flaxseeds

½ tablespoon chia seeds

1 cup rolled oats

Actions:

1. Preheat the oven to 400°F.

2. Add all the ingredients to a bowl and mix until well combined.

3. Line a baking sheet with parchment paper or grease with coconut oil. Spread the oat mixture over the baking sheet.

4. Bake for 9 minutes. If you'd like a crunchier granola, bake for an additional 5 minutes.

Tip:

Eat as a snack on its own, in cereal, or as a topping on an Acai Bowl (page 181) or dish of Instant Ice Cream (page 330).

Variation:

Add this to almond milk or coconut milk for a granola cereal.

Calories: 168.1 | Protein: 4.7g | Carbs: 19.9g | Dietary Fiber: 3.7g | Fat: 8.4g | Vitamin C: 0.06mg | Vitamin D: 0 IU | Vitamin E: 2.5mg | Calcium: 55.3mg | Iron: 1.1mg | Magnesium: 57.7mg | Potassium: 152.8mg

FRESH MUESLI

Freshen up your morning by adding delicious wholesome ingredients to a bowl with some nut or seed milk and fresh fruit. The flax meal bumps up the chemopreventive effects.

Total time: 10 minutes

Makes 2 servings

Ingredients:

1 apple, diced

1 peach, diced

1 banana, sliced

1 tablespoon raisins

¼ cup whole or chopped walnuts

½ cup oats

1 teaspoon flax meal

1 tablespoon sunflower seeds

2 cups nut milk or seed milk

Actions:

Divide all the ingredients into 2 bowls, then pour milk over them and enjoy.

Tip:

If you want the muesli sweeter, drizzle with maple syrup or honey, or sprinkle coconut sugar on top.

Calories: 568 | Protein: 15.4g | Carbs: 64.2g | Dietary Fiber: 12.9g | Fat: 32g | Vitamin C: 14.5mg | Vitamin D: 0 IU | Vitamin E: 0.8mg | Calcium: 146.7mg | Iron: 3.6mg | Magnesium: 186.2mg | Potassium: 900.7mg

---

PERFECT PORRIDGE

Whole grains such as oats may protect against colorectal cancer and have benefits for people with inflammatory bowel disease.[1]

Total time: 10 minutes

Makes 4 servings

Ingredients:

Porridge:

1 cup gluten-free organic oats

2 cups filtered water

Choose your toppings:

Almond butter

Almond Milk (page 159)

Apples, diced

Bananas, sliced into rounds

Cacao nibs

Cacao powder

Chia seeds

Cinnamon

Coconut sugar

Flaxseeds

Flaxseed meal	Pomegranate seeds
Goji berries	Raisins
Honey	Sesame seeds
Maple syrup	Sunflower Seed Milk (page 158)
Nuts, including almonds, pecans, walnuts, and Brazil nuts	Tigernut Milk (page 162)
	Vanilla extract or powder

Actions:

1. Add the oats and water to a pot. Bring to a boil and allow the mixture to boil for 9 minutes.

2. Serve the oats in bowls, adding toppings to make it your style.

For recipe without toppings: Calories: 93.3 | Protein: 3g | Carbs: 16.6g | Dietary Fiber: 1.9g | Fat: 1.6g | Vitamin C: 0mg | Vitamin D: 0 IU | Vitamin E: 0mg | Calcium: 12.3mg | Iron: 1mg | Magnesium: 36.7mg | Potassium: 88.8mg

---

VEGAN YOGURT

Although this is ready to serve as soon as it is blended, it will keep in the fridge for up to four days. This is a great plant-based alternative, and it is very much cooling and comforting the same way traditional dairy yogurt is.

Total time: 6 minutes

Makes 4 servings

Ingredients:

½ cup almonds	½ cup coconut water
½ cup cashews	1 tablespoon lemon juice (from about ½ lemon)
½ cup filtered water	⅛ teaspoon vanilla extract

Actions:

1. Place all the ingredients in a blender.

2. Blend on high until the mixture reaches a smooth consistency.

Tip:

Add granola and your favorite fruit and nut toppings.

Calories: 200.3 | Protein: 6.9g | Carbs: 10.1g | Dietary Fiber: 3.1g | Fat: 16.1g | Vitamin C: 2.2mg | Vitamin D: 0 IU | Vitamin E: 4.7mg | Calcium: 62.4mg | Iron: 1.8mg | Magnesium: 103.8mg | Potassium: 317.5mg

SUPER SCRAMBLED EGGS

This is a great go-to for a quick breakfast, but also convenient for lunch, dinner, or a snack. All the cancer survivors I interviewed for this book confirmed how helpful it is to be able to make a quick meal in 10 minutes or less so they could reserve their energy for healing and absorbing nutrients and protein from the food. I add a handful of greens because I am always looking for more ways to add greens to my diet. You can add any spices or herbs that you like to this recipe. (I've included my favorite anticancer ingredients.) And don't be afraid of the egg yolks! They provide good, healthy fats that the brain and body need during healing.

Total time: 10 minutes

Makes 1 serving

Ingredients:

3 eggs

1 to 2 tablespoons extra-virgin coconut oil or olive oil

Pinch of turmeric

Pinch of black pepper

Pinch of cayenne pepper

Pinch of paprika

Pinch of thyme

Pinch of rosemary

Pinch of sea salt

Actions:

1. Crack the eggs into a bowl and whisk with a fork.

2. Heat the coconut oil in a frying pan over medium heat. Make sure that the oil covers the entire bottom of the pan—if not, add more oil. When the oil is hot, pour in the eggs and then add the spices.

3. Cook for a few minutes until the bottom begins to firm, then mash with a fork to scramble the eggs.

Tips:

- Serve with avocado slices.
- Add a handful of greens, like spinach or cilantro.

Variations:

Add 2 tablespoons nutritional yeast for Cheesy Scrambled Eggs.

Calories: 336.5 | Protein: 18.9g | Carbs: 1.5g | Dietary Fiber: 0.2g | Fat: 27.3g | Vitamin C: 0.1mg | Vitamin D: 123 IU | Vitamin E: 1.6mg | Calcium: 87.9mg | Iron: 2.8mg | Magnesium: 19.1mg | Potassium: 218.7mg

---

ANTICANCER OMELET

This omelet is packed with all the goods. It's a powerful serving on a plate with all kinds of anticancer spices and greens, including broccoli sprouts. I'd like to see cancer survive this healthy food bomb!

Total time: 15 minutes

Makes 2 servings

Ingredients:

5 eggs

¼ cup extra-virgin coconut oil

Black pepper and sea salt, to taste

1 small handful of spinach

1 small handful of fresh cilantro

1 small handful of fresh parsley

¼ cup diced broccoli

1 small handful of broccoli sprouts

1 small handful of leeks, diced (or diced yellow or green onions)

Optional spices that I usually include:

Pinch of turmeric

Pinch of paprika

Pinch of thyme

Pinch of rosemary

Smidgen of cayenne pepper

Actions:

1. Crack the eggs into a bowl and whisk with a fork.

2. Heat the coconut oil in a frying pan over medium heat. Make sure that the oil covers the entire bottom of the pan— if not, add more oil. When the oil is hot, pour in the eggs.

3. Cook for 1 minute, then add all the toppings. Continue to cook until the bottom is firm, then, using a spatula, fold it over in half so it's a half-moon shape.

4. Continue to cook the omelet until the desired doneness is achieved.

Tip:

Serve with avocado slices.

Variation:

Add 2 tablespoons nutritional yeast for Cheesy Omelet.

Calories: 440.4 | Protein: 17.1g | Carbs: 4.3g | Dietary Fiber: 0.9g | Fat: 38.2g | Vitamin C: 37.2mg | Vitamin D: 102.5 IU | Vitamin E: 1.7mg | Calcium: 127.2mg | Iron: 3.4mg | Magnesium: 32.5mg | Potassium: 362.8mg

---

MEDITERRANEAN OMELET

The eating habits of people from the Mediterranean region have been proven to reduce the risk of cancer, including breast cancer. Their meals incorporate plenty of good fats from eggs, olives, olive oil, and fish, as well as veggies and whole grains. They tend to snack on nuts, have fruit for dessert, and enjoy some red wine. The Cancer-Free with Food plan includes these ingredients.

Total time: 10 minutes

Makes 4 servings

Ingredients:

2 tablespoons extra-virgin olive oil

8 eggs

¼ cup olives, sliced

1 cup spinach

1 small tomato, sliced

1 small handful of fresh parsley

1 teaspoon minced garlic

Handful of organic cheese or nutritional yeast

Pinch of sea salt

Actions:

1. Heat the olive oil in a large pan.

2. Whisk the eggs in a bowl, then pour them into the pan.

3. As the egg mixture starts to firm up, top it with the olives, spinach, tomato, parsley, garlic, cheese (or nutritional yeast), and sea salt.

4. Using a spatula, fold the omelet over in half when the egg mixture is cooked and firm.

Calories: 263.1 | Protein: 15.4g | Carbs: 3.1g | Dietary Fiber: 0.5g | Fat: 20.8g | Vitamin C: 9.4mg | Vitamin D: 82 IU | Vitamin E: 2.2mg | Calcium: 137.7mg | Iron: 2.2mg | Magnesium: 22.1mg | Potassium: 253.1mg

COCONUT BACON

This is an extremely tasty plant-based bacon alternative! It's great served with eggs or as a topping on a salad. I also add it on top of Bean Burgers (page 219) and Grass-Fed Beef Burgers (page 286). Stored in an airtight container at room temperature, it will keep for seven days.

Total time: 30 minutes

Makes 3 ½ cups, serves 7

Ingredients:

¾ cup apple cider vinegar

¼ cup maple syrup

1 tablespoon sea salt

1 tablespoon paprika

2 teaspoons garlic powder

1 teaspoon onion salt

½ teaspoon dried cilantro

½ teaspoon dried parsley

3 cups coconut flakes

Actions:

1. Preheat the oven to 250°F.

2. Mix all the ingredients, except the coconut flakes, in a bowl with a spoon until well combined.

3. Add the coconut flakes to the bowl and stir until they are completely coated in the sauce. Let soak for 10 minutes.

4. Spread the coconut flakes out evenly on a baking sheet or other oven-proof dish, making sure they are not overlapping.

5. Bake for 5 to 12 minutes, or until the coconut flakes are crispy and golden brown.

Calories: 85.2 | Protein: 0.8g | Carbs: 6.4g | Dietary Fiber: 1.5g | Fat: 7.1g | Vitamin C: 0.1mg | Vitamin D: 0 IU | Vitamin E: 0.1mg | Calcium: 6.4mg | Iron: 0.3mg | Magnesium: 2.1mg | Potassium: 32.5mg

HASH BROWNS

Grate up a bunch of potatoes and keep hash browns in your freezer so you can have a fun, delicious, and vitamin C-rich snack, breakfast, lunch, or dinner.

Total time: 10 minutes

Makes 2 servings

INGREDIENTS:

1 tablespoon extra-virgin olive oil, coconut oil, or tigernut oil

1 large organic raw potato

⅛ teaspoon turmeric powder

Sea salt and pepper to taste

Actions:

1. Peel and grate the potato.

2. Heat the oil in a frying pan over medium heat.

3. Add the potato and turmeric to the pan and stir-fry for 9 minutes or until cooked to your liking.

Tip:

Garnish with some broccoli sprouts!

Calories: 205 | Protein: 3.7g | Carbs: 32.7g | Dietary Fiber: 3.8g | Fat: 7.1g | Vitamin C: 36.3mg | Vitamin D: 0 IU | Vitamin E: 0.8mg | Calcium: 22.1mg | Iron: 1.4mg | Magnesium: 42.4mg | Potassium: 784.1mg

CHAPTER 13

ENERGIZING LUNCHES AND HEALING DINNERS

If it's made in a garden, eat it. If it's made in a lab, then it takes a lab to digest.

— KRIS CARR

We can agree that a plant-rich diet is ideal for healing and pre-venting cancer. This chapter focuses on alkalizing raw vegan meals and cooked vegan meals that will amplify your energy. Our bodies were not designed to digest a lot of chemicals, tox-ins, preservatives, or additives. Sure, they are strong and resil-ient. But in the contemporary world, they simply have had to endure chemical exposure for years, both from our food supply and from the environment, and frankly, that toxic overload is making us sick. This is what the cancer statistics are showing!

The recipes here feature a mixture of easily digestible and nutrient-rich ingredients—lunch and dinner dishes that will nourish any body. There are a combination of soups and salads;

raw vegan, cooked vegan meals, and cooked vegetarian entrées; broths; and recipes for meat eaters here.

WALNUT "MEATBALLS"

For when you are craving meatballs but want to skip on the red meat, these are a tasty creative alternative that are surprisingly delicious and even appealing to meat eaters.

Total time: 10 minutes

Makes 4 servings

Ingredients:

1 ½ cups walnuts

1 cup sundried tomatoes

2 tablespoons extra-virgin olive oil

1 tablespoon fresh sage

1 teaspoon fennel seeds

1 teaspoon fresh thyme

1 teaspoon fresh rosemary

1 teaspoon fresh marjoram

Pinch of black pepper

Pinch of cayenne pepper

Pinch of sea salt

Actions:

Add all the ingredients to a blender and mix for 5 minutes or until well combined.

Tips:

- If you do not have a blender, you can make this recipe using a mortar and pestle. Crush the walnuts first, then dice the sundried tomatoes and add both to a bowl. Add in the remaining ingredients and stir until the mixture is moist enough to stick together.

- This recipe can be used as the meat to make a "raw burger," "raw tacos," Zucchini Spaghetti with Raw Tomato Sauce and Walnut "Meatballs" (page 213), or Raw Lasagna (page 211).

Calories: 423 | Protein: 8.8g | Carbs: 20.5g | Dietary Fiber: 5.2g | Fat: 35.7g | Vitamin C: 8.2mg | Vitamin D: 0 IU | Vitamin E: 1.1mg | Calcium: 54.5mg | Iron: 2.1mg | Magnesium: 72.7mg | Potassium: 208.4mg

RAW LASAGNA

Total time: 40 minutes

Makes 12 servings

Ingredients:

Walnut "Meatballs" (page 210)

Cashew Cheese (page 303)

2 large zucchinis

1 tablespoon dried oregano, divided (for sprinkling)

1 cup fresh spinach

1 cup fresh basil

2 tablespoons extra-virgin olive oil

Actions:

1. Prepare the Walnut "Meatballs" and the Cashew Cheese.

2. Peel and slice the zucchini into thin strips with a vegetable peeler. Place the first layer of zucchini in a deep lasagna dish (or 8 x 11 ½ x 2-inch baking dish) that holds 2 quarts. Layer the zucchini so that the strips are just overlapping each other. You could also build the lasagna directly on plates if you will be eating it immediately. Sprinkle ½ tablespoon of oregano over the zucchini strips.

3. Layer ½ of the Walnut "Meatballs" over the zucchini.

4. Spread ½ cup Cashew Cheese over the Walnut "Meatballs."

5. Place ½ cup each of spinach and basil leaves over the Cashew Cheese.

6. Add another layer of zucchini strips. (Keep in mind that you will need 1 more layer for the top of the lasagna.)

7. Repeat the layering of the Walnut "Meatballs," Cashew Cheese, spinach, and basil.

8. Add the last layer of zucchini strips and sprinkle the remaining ½ tablespoon of oregano on top. Finish with a drizzle of extra-virgin olive oil.

9. The lasagna is now ready to eat, but if you allow it to set in the refrigerator overnight it will be easier to slice.

Tips:

- If you want to add more layers, use the pesto sauce from the Pasta Pesto recipe (page 212) or the Raw Tomato Sauce (page 311).
- The lasagna keeps well in the fridge for 4 to 5 days.
- If you want a spicy lasagna, sprinkle cayenne pepper on one of the layers.

Calories: 296.4 | Protein: 8g | Carbs: 15.9g | Dietary Fiber: 3.3g | Fat: 24g | Vitamin C: 15.3mg | Vitamin D: 0 IU | Vitamin E: 1mg | Calcium: 48.3mg | Iron: 2.6mg | Magnesium: 103.4mg | Potassium: 395.5mg

ZUCCHINI PASTA WITH BROCCOLI SPROUTS PESTO

Total time: 20 minutes

Makes 4 servings

Ingredients:

4 zucchinis

1 cup fresh basil

½ cup broccoli sprouts

Juice of 1 lemon

4 garlic cloves

½ teaspoon sea salt

½ cup spinach

2 cups raw walnuts

½ cup extra-virgin olive oil (or more for smoother mixture)

Actions:

1. Make thin strips of zucchini using a vegetable peeler or pasta machine. Set aside.

2. Place the remaining ingredients in a blender and blend until the pesto mixture reaches desired consistency. Set aside.

3. Distribute the zucchini evenly among 4 plates.

4. Pour the pesto sauce over the zucchini pasta and serve.

Tip:

Top the dish with Cashew Cheese (page 303).

Calories: 683.1 | Protein: 12.5g | Carbs: 16.3g | Dietary Fiber: 6g | Fat: 67g | Vitamin C: 59.7mg | Vitamin D: 0 IU | Vitamin E: 4.3mg | Calcium: 145.6mg | Iron: 3.1mg | Magnesium: 142.2mg | Potassium: 899.4mg

ZUCCHINI SPAGHETTI WITH RAW TOMATO SAUCE AND WALNUT "MEATBALLS"

This is a raw, plant-based vegan dish—no cooking required. It is extremely nutrient-rich, leaving you feeling fulfilled, yet light so you can continue with your day without feeling sluggish.

Total time: 35 minutes

Makes 4 servings

Ingredients:

2 large zucchinis

1 cup Raw Tomato Sauce (page 311)

1 cup Walnut "Meatballs" (page 210)

Nutritional yeast, to taste upon serving (optional)

Actions:

1. Use a spiralizer or vegetable peeler to make spaghetti strips with the zucchini. Place in bowls.

2. Make the Raw Tomato Sauce and pour over the zucchini spaghetti.

3. Make the Walnut "Meatballs" and add to the bowls. Sprinkle some nutritional yeast on top, if desired, and serve.

Tips:

• To save some time, you can make this recipe without the Walnut "Meatballs" and just have the Zucchini Spaghetti and Raw Tomato Sauce.

• Make a batch of pasta each week and keep it in the fridge so you can pull it out and add sauces and toppings for a quick fresh meal!

Calories: 362.4 | Protein: 9.3g | Carbs: 34g | Dietary Fiber: 7.4g | Fat: 22.1g | Vitamin C: 53.8mg | Vitamin D: 0 IU | Vitamin E: 1.7mg | Calcium: 72.2mg | Iron: 2.9mg | Magnesium: 78mg | Potassium: 764.8mg

CAULIFLOWER CRUST MINI PIZZAS

This recipe is from my good friend chiropractor David Jockers, D.N.M, D.C., who says, "One of the most common complaints I get from people is that they can no longer eat pizza or must restrict their pizza intake when they begin a keto program. I always respond by saying that they just have to get more creative and innovative. Using a cauliflower crust makes this grain-free and anti-inflammatory for the body! This is a fantastic recipe for a true pizza flavor and texture without all the nasty inflammatory carbs and toxic fats. You get tons of incredible nutrients in this recipe, healthy fats and antioxidants. This is a whole-super-food-based meal that the family will love and enjoy for many meals to come!"

Total time: 40 minutes

Makes 8 servings (1 mini pizza each)

Ingredients:

2 cups fresh cauliflower, steamed and grated

2 large pasture-raised eggs

2 cups grass-fed cheddar cheese

1 teaspoon toasted and ground fennel

¼ teaspoon sea salt

1 teaspoon ground oregano

2 teaspoon dried parsley

2 teaspoons dried basil

1 teaspoon dried rosemary

2 garlic cloves, minced

Toppings of your choice:

Raw Tomato Sauce (page 311)

Cheese (organic dairy or vegan)

Pesto

Tomatoes

Olives

Actions:

1. For the mini pizza crusts, steam the cauliflower, then grate, rice, or chop it finely. (You can do this in a food processor a few pieces at a time.)

2. Beat the eggs in a bowl, then add the cauliflower and shredded cheese and mix together.

3. Press 8 large spoonfuls of the cauliflower mixture onto a cookie sheet covered with parchment paper.

4. Sprinkle with the spices and bake at 450°F for 8 to 10 minutes. Keep the oven on.

5. To complete the pizzas, add desired pizza sauce (or a slice of fresh tomato) or pesto, and then add toppings such as cheese, grass-fed meat, olives, chopped mushrooms, etc. Just put back in oven until the cheese is melted for completed mini pizzas!

Nutritonal facts are just for the pizza crust: Calories: 142.1 | Protein: 8.7g | Carbs: 3g | Dietary Fiber: 0.8g | Fat: 10.7g | Vitamin C: 13.4mg | Vitamin D: 17 IU | Vitamin E: 0.4mg | Calcium: 229.7mg | Iron: 0.8mg | Magnesium: 17.2mg | Potassium: 139.4mg

CRAZY SEXY BEAN CHILI

This recipe was created by Chad Sarno and Kris Carr, authors of *Crazy Sexy Kitchen*. Kris and I attended an event together where I told her about this book and asked what recipe of hers would be great to share with you. Straightaway, she said, "Beans! Something with beans. We need to bring beans back, and have people eat more beans!" Voilà! Here is their recipe. (Psst . . . for more delicious, plant-powered recipes, check out kriscarr.com/recipes.)

Total time: 45 minutes

Makes 8 servings

Ingredients:

1 ½ tablespoons cumin seeds

2 tablespoons olive oil

1 white onion, diced

3 garlic cloves, minced

1 jalapeño, finely diced (for less heat, remove the seeds and/or use ½ the pepper)

2 tablespoons chili powder

1 ½ cups ground seitan (alternatives: crumbled tempeh [wheat-free] or finely diced mushrooms [soy-free])

1 zucchini, diced

½ cup diced potato (any kind)

Two 15-ounce cans black beans, rinsed

One 15-ounce can kidney beans, rinsed

One 14-ounce can crushed tomatoes (San Marzano recommended)

2 cups filtered water

2 tablespoons maple syrup

1 teaspoon sea salt

½ bunch of fresh cilantro

1 cup kale, chopped

Diced avocado (optional)

Fresh cilantro (optional)

Actions:

1. Toast the cumin seeds in a dry soup pot on medium heat for 2 minutes, until you smell the robust aroma. (This process releases the full flavor of the spice.)

2. Add the olive oil, onion, garlic, and jalapeño. Stir constantly, until the onion is golden and translucent.

3. Add in the chili powder, seitan, zucchini, and potato and stir well. Sauté for 3 to 4 minutes, stirring to avoid sticking.

4. Add in the black beans, kidney beans, tomatoes, water, maple syrup, sea salt, and cilantro. Cover with a lid, reduce the heat to low, and allow the chili to cook for 20 to 25 minutes, or until the potatoes are tender.

5. Remove from the heat and stir in the kale.

6. Serve hot. Garnish with diced avocado and a handful of fresh cilantro, if desired.

Calories: 288.8 | Protein: 17.5g | Carbs: 40.2g | Dietary Fiber: 11.8g | Fat: 8g | Vitamin C: 16.3mg | Vitamin D: 0 IU | Vitamin E: 2mg | Calcium: 109.3mg | Iron: 3.4mg | Magnesium: 62.8mg | Potassium: 994.4mg

BLACK BEAN BOWL WITH SWEET POTATOES AND ROASTED CHICKPEAS

This recipe is by Chris Wark, author of *Chris Beat Cancer: A Comprehensive Plan for Healing Naturally.*

Total time: 40 minutes

Makes 4 servings

Ingredients:

Black Beans:

Two 15-ounce cans black beans, drained and rinsed

Sea salt and black pepper to taste

½ teaspoon cumin, divided

¼ teaspoon paprika

Roasted Sweet Potato and Chickpeas:

2 sweet potatoes, cubed

½ teaspoon cumin

¼ teaspoon chili powder, divided

¼ teaspoon turmeric

Sea salt and black pepper to taste

One 15-ounce can chickpeas, drained and rinsed

Serve over:

2 cups of cooked quinoa or 4 servings of Cauliflower Rice

Topping:

½ cup fresh cilantro

1 avocado, sliced

Handful of broccoli sprouts

1 lime

Actions:

1. Preheat the oven to 400°F.

2. Add the black beans to a pot with water so that the beans are just covered with a quarter-inch of water above, and bring to a rolling boil, then simmer for 4 minutes. Season with sea salt, black pepper, cumin, and paprika, adding more to taste if you like. Set aside.

3. Make the seasoning for the sweet potatoes and chickpeas by adding all spices to a bowl and mix until well combined. Place the sweet potato cubes on a baking sheet. Sprinkle with half the seasoning. Add 1 tablespoon water to glaze the potatoes and place in the oven. Bake for 10 minutes.

4. Toss the chickpeas to the other half of the seasoning, and then add the chickpeas to the potatoes on the baking sheet. Bake an additional 15 to 20 minutes until the sweet potatoes are soft and the chickpeas crunchy.

5. Serve over quinoa, Cauliflower Rice (page 224) or as nachos and eat with plantain or tortilla chips. Top with your favorite chipotle sauce, Taco Sauce (page 312) or Fresh Fermented Salsa (page 306), fresh cilantro, sliced avocado, broccoli sprouts, and a squeeze of lime. Enjoy!

Tip:

You can soak and cook your own black beans and chickpeas if you prefer that to using canned. Always go for food in a BPA-free can.

Calories: 442.1 | Protein: 20.9g | Carbs: 71g | Dietary Fiber: 25.3g | Fat: 9.1g | Vitamin C: 18.3mg | Vitamin D: 0 IU | Vitamin E: 1.54mg | Calcium: 144.3mg | Iron: 4.9mg | Magnesium: 49.7mg | Potassium: 1,488mg

---

DR. OZ'S SAUTÉED PORTOBELLO MUSHROOMS

Mushrooms are one of the top 20 anticancer foods! They are full of good stuff. They have proven to slow down the progression of carcinogenesis (formation of cancer cells) and are said to be useful both to prevent cancer and during conventional cancer treatments.[1] This recipe is from the ever-so-helpful DoctorOz .com website, which is full of cancer-fighting recipes.

Total time: 15 minutes

Makes 2 servings

Ingredients:

½ cup vegetable broth

½ small onion, diced

2 garlic cloves, minced

3 tablespoons balsamic vinegar

1 tablespoon organic red wine or grape juice

1 teaspoon dried thyme

½ teaspoon dried basil

2 portobello mushrooms, stems removed

Actions:

1. Line a large frying pan with a thin layer of broth, making sure it covers the entire pan surface. Add the onion and garlic and sauté over high heat for 2 minutes.

2. Add 1 cup filtered water or broth, vinegar, wine, and herbs and reduce the heat to medium. Add the mushrooms, cover, and cook for 5 minutes.

3. Gently flip the mushrooms over and cook for 5 minutes more, adding additional water or broth as necessary to prevent sticking or burning.

4. Flip the mushrooms a third time, if desired (cook until mushrooms are fork tender and juicy).

5. Plate the mushrooms, spooning the pan juices over the top.

Calories: 64.5 | Protein: 2.6g | Carbs: 11.6g | Dietary Fiber: 1.7g | Fat: 0.3g | Vitamin C: 2.4mg | Vitamin D: 953.4 IU | Vitamin E: 0.1mg | Calcium: 36.3mg | Iron: 1.4mg | Magnesium: 18.2mg | Potassium: 392.8mg

BEAN BURGERS

Beans are way underrated and we need to hype them up! They are so incredibly good for us and something everyone could incorporate more into their diet. In fact, beans have been proven to reduce the risk of breast cancer.[2]

Total time: 20 minutes

Makes 4 servings

Ingredients:

One 15-ounce can organic beans (butter beans or black beans work best; or you can soak dry beans overnight, then boil them for an hour or until soft instead of using canned)

½ cup almond meal (blended almond)

1 small yellow onion, chopped

1 tablespoon nutritional yeast

2 tablespoons broccoli sprouts, diced

1 teaspoon black seeds

½ teaspoon cumin

¼ teaspoon garlic powder

¼ teaspoon fennel

¼ teaspoon thyme

¼ teaspoon sage

¼ teaspoon sea salt

¼ teaspoon black pepper

⅛ teaspoon turmeric

Pinch of cayenne pepper

1 Flax Egg Alternative (page 315)

2 tablespoons extra-virgin coconut oil

Actions:

1. Drain the beans. Mash the beans in a bowl and mix in the remaining ingredients, except for the oil. Taste the mixture and add more spices or sea salt to your liking. Divide the mixture into 4 equal parts and shape into 4 patties.

2. Heat the oil in a large pan over medium heat. Fry the patties until golden, about 4 to 5 minutes on each side.

3. Serve on Gluten Free Tortillas (page 294), or Teff Crepes (page 295) kale, collard greens, or lettuce. The burgers taste great with herbs like fresh parsley, cilantro, and basil.

Tips:

- Nonvegans can use 1 egg in this recipe instead of the Flax Egg Alternative.

- This meal goes great with Ketchup (page 318).

Variations:

- Add extra cayenne pepper for Spicy Bean Burgers.

- Roll the mixture into 10 balls for Bean Balls. Serve on brown rice pasta, Pasta Primavera (page 230), or Zucchini Pasta (page 213).

- You can make this recipe without nutritional yeast for a less cheesy flavor. Just replace the nutritional yeast with more almond meal.

- For a nut-free version of this recipe, replace the almond meal with pumpkin seed meal.

Calories: 278.4 | Protein: 11.7g | Carbs: 25.9g | Dietary Fiber: 10.8g | Fat: 15.2g | Vitamin C: 9.1mg | Vitamin D: 0 IU | Vitamin E: 4.4mg | Calcium: 94.9mg | Iron: 2.9mg | Magnesium: 45.7mg | Potassium: 529.1mg

CHICKPEA BURGERS

Chickpea is a protein-rich, edible legume with several bioactive compounds. It includes lectin as well. Studies of the effect of lectin in fighting cancer cells suggest that it expresses anti-tumor activity and could be exploited as a treatment for breast cancer.[3]

Total time: 15 minutes

Makes 4 servings

Ingredients:

One 14-ounce can chickpeas, drained

2 teaspoons crushed garlic

1 teaspoon sea salt

1 teaspoon onion powder

¼ teaspoon cumin seeds

½ teaspoon cumin powder

¼ teaspoon turmeric

¼ teaspoon fennel

¼ teaspoon sage

¼ teaspoon rosemary

⅛ teaspoon oregano

¼ cup brown rice flour

1 tablespoon flax meal

For cooking:

2 tablespoons extra-virgin olive oil, for cooking

¼ teaspoon turmeric

¼ teaspoon black pepper

Actions:

1. Place the chickpeas in a bowl and mash them so there are no chunks.

2. Add the rest of the ingredients to the chickpeas and mix well. You can use your hands for this. Make sure the mixture is well combined.

3. Form 4 patties.

4. Heat the pan to medium with olive oil and sauté the remaining ¼ teaspoon turmeric and black pepper for 1 minute or until sizzling until it becomes a thicker paste. Spread the paste out over the pan and then add the patties. Cook for 4 minutes on each side or until golden brown.

Calories: 210.6 | Protein: 6.1g | Carbs: 23.6g | Dietary Fiber: 5.6 | Fat: 10.2g | Vitamin C: 1.1mg | Vitamin D: 0 IU | Vitamin E: 0.9mg | Calcium: 49mg | Iron: 2mg | Magnesium: 2.3mg | Potassium: 24.5mg

ANITA MOORJANI'S COCONUT CURRY!

The story of Anita Moorjani is known worldwide. Anita is the epitome of what is possible, that it truly is never too late to be healed from cancer. I had the opportunity to talk to Anita about her rock-bottom experience, which turned into a transformation. After four years of battling cancer, and with a body riddled with tumors, some the size of lemons, Anita lay dying in the intensive care unit in the hospital, where she dropped into a coma. The doctors told her husband it was too late, there was nothing more they could do for her.

During the coma, Anita had a near-death experience. She recalls, "I experienced the state of love and realized we are truly love." This led her to reenter her body and initiate the healing of her cancer. As her tumors rapidly shrank, the doctors could barely believe it. A mere four days later, Anita left the hospital. She has been cancer-free and living ever so happily since then. Her explanation for what occurred? *Love heals cancer.*

This curry is delicious for both vegetarians or fish and meat eaters. What's her secret ingredient? Love.

Ingredients:

½ red onion, coarsely chopped

4 garlic cloves, minced

1 tablespoon coconut oil or ghee

6 whole cloves

1 pound meat protein (chicken, beef, lamb), fish, or shrimp (optional)

4 cups vegetables of your choice, diced (squash, eggplant, zucchini, carrots, broccoli, string beans, baby corn, cauliflower, peas, or whatever else your favorites are!)

1 teaspoon turmeric powder

1 heaping teaspoon curry powder

1 cup coconut cream

1 stock cube dissolved in ¼ cup of warm filtered water (your choice of either chicken or vegetable stock, or freshly made stock)

1 ton love

Actions:

1. Stir-fry the onions and garlic in the coconut oil or ghee until tender.

2. Add the cloves (and if you are adding meat, this is the point to do so).

3. Add the vegetables and stir-fry everything for another 2 to 3 minutes.

4. Add the turmeric powder and curry powder. Continue to stir-fry for another 2 to 3 minutes to allow the flavors to absorb. If you have added meat, continue to stir-fry until the meat is fully cooked.

5. Add the coconut cream, bring to boil, and allow to simmer for about 5 minutes.

6. Add ¼ cup stock and allow to simmer for another 15 minutes or longer. Anita says the longer you leave the curry to simmer, the better it tastes.

7. Serve on a bed of white or brown rice or quinoa, and add sea salt to taste.

Tips:

• If you like your curry hot and spicy, add 1 coarsely chopped serrano pepper.

• One more thing: Don't eat the cloves. They enhance the flavor of the curry but are not great when chewed. Take them out before serving or just avoid them when eating the curry.

• This curry tastes even better the next day, so the leftovers are fabulous!

Calories: 345.1 | Protein: 2.7g | Carbs: 49.8g | Dietary Fiber: 3.1g | Fat: 16.1g | Vitamin C: 26.3mg | Vitamin D: 0 IU | Vitamin E: 0.6mg | Calcium: 42.8mg | Iron: 1mg | Magnesium: 34.9mg | Potassium: 459.6mg

CAULIFLOWER POPCORN

Cauliflower is a cruciferous vegetable and one of the top anticancer foods on the planet! Studies suggest that a diet that includes cruciferous vegetables like cauliflower could be an important modifiable risk factor for ovarian cancer.[4]

Total time: 25 minutes

Makes 4 servings

Ingredients:

2 ½ tablespoons extra-virgin olive oil

½ cup nutritional yeast

¾ teaspoon sea salt

1 head of cauliflower, chopped into bite-size pieces

Actions:

1. Preheat the oven to 325°F.
2. Mix the olive oil, nutritional yeast, and sea salt thoroughly in a large bowl.
3. Add the cauliflower pieces to the bowl and toss until well coated.
4. Place the cauliflower on a baking sheet and bake for 20 minutes until golden brown and crispy.

Tip:

Add 1 tablespoon sesame seeds for extra flavor.

Variations:

- If you want a cleaner dish, roast the cauliflower without any other ingredients for Plain Roasted Cauliflower—deliciously simple!
- Use broccoli for Broccoli Popcorn.

Calories: 144.4 | Protein: 6.6g | Carbs: 10g | Dietary Fiber: 4.4g | Fat: 9.4g | Vitamin C: 70.8mg | Vitamin D: 0 IU | Vitamin E: 1.2mg | Calcium: 35.3mg | Iron: 1mg | Magnesium: 33.1mg | Potassium: 571.5mg

CAULIFLOWER RICE

Use a vegetable dicer or food processor for this to make it quicker. You may also dice the cauliflower by hand, but it will take longer. This recipe goes great with spicy food, curries, soups, and salads.

Total time: 10 minutes

Makes 4 servings

Ingredients:

1 head of cauliflower

1 tablespoon coconut oil

Sea salt and pepper, to taste

Actions:

1. Use a food processor to dice the cauliflower into tiny rice-size pieces.

2. Heat the oil in a pan, add the cauliflower, and sauté for 9 minutes. Season with sea salt and pepper.

Tip:

Add 1 small diced yellow onion for extra flavor.

Calories: 66.7 | Protein: 2.8g | Carbs: 7.3g | Dietary Fiber: 2.9g | Fat: 3.6g | Vitamin C: 70.8mg | Vitamin D: 0 IU | Vitamin E: 0.1mg | Calcium: 32.3mg | Iron: 0.6mg | Magnesium: 22.5mg | Potassium: 439.5mg

---

CAJUN SPICE PASTA WITH OAT CREAM

This recipe was created by Diane Gray, breast cancer survivor, certified health coach, and proud mom of Kyle.

Total time: 45 minutes

Makes 4 servings

Ingredients:

4 small chicken breasts

2 tablespoons extra-virgin olive oil plus more for the chicken breasts

5 teaspoons Cajun spice (a mix of garlic, paprika, sea salt, black pepper, cayenne pepper, onion, thyme, and Italian seasoning [parsley, oregano, rosemary, thyme]), divided

2 cups gluten-free pasta (brown rice, lentil, chickpea, or bean)

1 red pepper, sliced

1 brown onion, sliced

2 garlic cloves, sliced

2 cups vegetable stock

1 cup oat cream or milk (can also use coconut cream)

¼ teaspoon chili pepper

Salad:

2 cups mixed greens

2 cups fresh spinach

Actions:

1. Preheat the oven to 350°F. Place the chicken breasts on a baking sheet. Drizzle each with oil and then sprinkle a teaspoon of Cajun spice on each along with a dash of sea salt and pepper. Bake for 25 to 30 minutes or until chicken is cooked through.

2. Meanwhile, make the brown rice pasta according to package instructions.

3. Sauté the pepper, onion, and garlic in olive oil. Once cooked, stir in the vegetable stock and oat milk. Add the chili and the remaining 1 teaspoon Cajun spice. Add the pasta and stir to combine well for a couple of minutes. Divide the mixture among 4 plates and place 1 chicken breast atop each.

4. Serve with a crisp salad drizzled with olive oil, sea salt, and pepper.

Tip:

If you want to make this a vegan dish, use zucchinis and broccoli instead of the chicken! Bake in the oven with Cajun spice.

Calories: 565.6 | Protein: 51.9g | Carbs: 48.4g | Dietary Fiber: 1.8g | Fat: 18.3g | Vitamin C: 51.4mg | Vitamin D: 26.7 IU | Vitamin E: . 3.1mg | Calcium: 175.7mg | Iron: 5mg | Magnesium: 65.4mg | Potassium: 749.4mg

---

BROCCOLI IN CREAMY PEA PESTO

This recipe was created by Maria Marlowe author of *The Real Food Grocery Guide.*

Ingredients:

Pea Pesto:

1 ½ cups frozen peas

1 ½ cups basil leaves

2 small garlic cloves (or 1 large)

2 tablespoons almond flour

3 tablespoons olive oil

½ teaspoon sea salt

¼ teaspoon cayenne powder (optional)

Broccoli:

4 cups broccoli florets (just the top ¾ inch)

Pinch of sea salt

Garnish:

Broccoli sprouts

Basil leaves

Red pepper flakes

Actions:

1. Combine all the pesto ingredients in a blender, and blend on high speed until the mixture is smooth. Set aside.

2. Bring a large pot of water with a pinch of sea salt to a boil. Fill a large bowl with water and 2 cups of ice and place on the side.

3. Add the broccoli florets to the pot of boiling water, cook for 90 seconds to 2 minutes, until bright green. Use a slotted spoon to transfer the broccoli to the ice bath to cool down and stop cooking.

4. After 2 minutes, drain the broccoli, then add to a dry bowl along with the pesto and mix well.

5. You can enjoy this dish at room temperature or gently warm the pesto broccoli in a dry pan over low heat, if desired.

6. Top with or stir in broccoli sprouts, basil leaves, and red pepper flakes, if desired, before serving.

Calories: 183.4 | Protein: 6.5g | Carbs: 12.4g | Dietary Fiber: 4.7g | Fat: 12.9g | Vitamin C: 87.1mg | Vitamin D: 0 IU | Vitamin E: 2.4mg | Calcium: 103mg | Iron: 2.3mg | Magnesium: 55.4mg | Potassium: 404.3mg

MAC 'N' CHEESE

This is a healthy spin on the traditional Mac 'n' Cheese, but without the dairy or gluten. So, you can feel much lighter after enjoying this dish! It's the method of cooking with the exact amount of 3 ¼ cups of water and then not draining it out afterward, along with the nutritional yeast, that gives it a creamy, cheesy flavor and texture. Nutritional yeast is a popular replacement for cheese for vegans and vegetarians. In Australia, the same ingredient might be known as savory yeast flakes. You can also use nutritional yeast in mashed potatoes, hash browns, on eggs, in soups, and on roasted cauliflower (see the Cauliflower Popcorn recipe, page 223).

Nutritional yeast is a byproduct of the production of sugar cane or beet molasses. It has 16 amino acids and a full spectrum of B vitamins.

Total time: 20 minutes

Makes 3 servings

Ingredients:

2 cups uncooked gluten-free pasta (chickpea, lentil, or brown rice)

3 ¼ cups water

3 tablespoons nutritional yeast

1 teaspoon sea salt

Actions:

1. Place the pasta and water in a pot and bring to a boil over high heat. Stir the pasta and reduce the heat to medium-low. Keep stirring until the pasta is soft, 10 to 20 minutes. As it cooks, the pasta will soak up the water and begin to take on a creamy appearance. Note: Usually when we cook pasta, there is much more water in the pot and then the pasta is drained. But for this dish to succeed and achieve a natural creaminess, we need the pasta to soak up the water. The residual liquid in the pot will become the base for the creamy sauce, so do not drain it.

2. Add the nutritional yeast and the sea salt to the pot of pasta and stir until well combined with the water to form the sauce.

Tips:

- Add 1 to 2 teaspoons thyme for flavor.
- Add 1 tablespoon coconut oil for extra smoothness and additional health benefits.
- Use extra nutritional yeast if you like a cheesier taste, or if needed to soak up some liquid.

Variation:

Stir in 1 tablespoon pepper at the end for Peppery Mac 'n' Cheese.

Calories: 284.4 | Protein: 16.7g | Carbs: 48.6g | Dietary Fiber: 0.7g | Fat: 3.5g | Vitamin C: 0mg | Vitamin D: 0 IU | Vitamin E: 0mg | Calcium: 63.2mg | Iron: 3.8mg | Magnesium: 8.1mg | Potassium: 66mg

---

MEATBALL CURRY

You can make this with ground beef, lamb, chicken, or turkey. If you are up for it, this is a fun, soothing, and healing dish to make at your own leisure. It can be done in one hour, but if you want to put on some music and sip on some wine, you can stretch it out to two hours—and it will be well worth the wait and the work! It's loaded with all the anticancer superspices, including turmeric, ginger, garlic, and black pepper.

Serve over Cauliflower Rice (see page 224), quinoa, or a bed of salad with broccoli.

Total time: 60 minutes

Makes 4 servings

Ingredients:

Curry sauce:

¼ cup olive oil

1 large yellow or brown onion, diced

2 garlic cloves, crushed

1 tablespoon curry powder

¾ teaspoon sea salt

¼ teaspoon black pepper

1 teaspoon turmeric

1 teaspoon cumin

1 teaspoon coriander

1 tablespoon fresh ginger, diced

2 carrots, sliced into circles

One 13.5 ounce can coconut milk

¾ cup tomato sauce (1 ¼ cup cherry tomatoes if you want to blend your own)

½ tablespoon coconut sugar

Meatballs:

1 pound ground organic grass-fed beef (or lamb, chicken, or turkey)

1 teaspoon curry powder

Dash of chili powder (more if you like it hot)

1 garlic clove, crushed

2 teaspoons ginger, diced fresh (or 1 teaspoon ginger powder)

1 teaspoon coriander

½ teaspoon turmeric

1 teaspoon fresh or dried fennel

1 teaspoon black pepper

½ teaspoon sea salt

2 tablespoons tomato paste

1 egg

½ teaspoon flax meal

2 tablespoons olive oil for cooking

Actions:

1. Start by making the curry sauce. Heat the oil in a fry pan over medium-high heat. Add the onions, garlic, and dry spices. Cook for 3 minutes, then add the ginger. Let all the flavors combine for a few more minutes, then add the carrots. Lower the heat and sauté for 10 minutes so the flavors can merge.

2. Add the coconut milk, tomato sauce, and coconut sugar. Stir well. Sauté for another 10 minutes.

3. While the curry sauce is simmering, make the meatballs. Add all the ingredients to a bowl and use your hands to ensure the mixture is well combined. Form the mixture into approximately 16 1-inch meatballs. Heat the oil in a fry pan over medium heat. When the oil is hot, add the meatballs. Turn using tongs when one side goes golden brown. Once the meatballs are almost cooked through, add them to the curry sauce and cook together for 10 minutes.

Calories: 680.4 | Protein: 27.9g | Carbs: 18.4g | Dietary Fiber: 4g | Fat: 57g | Vitamin C: 13.5mg | Vitamin D: 10.2 IU | Vitamin E: 5.2mg | Calcium: 93.6mg | Iron: 7.8mg | Magnesium: 96.5mg | Potassium: 1,019mg

PASTA PRIMAVERA

This colorful dish literally bounces in your mouth! It's a great combo of a nutrient-dense pasta—choose from brown rice, lentil, or chickpea pasta—and a vibrant array of vegetables. Packed with protein and nutrient-richness, it's bound to leave you feeling satisfied.

Total time: 30 minutes

Makes 4 servings

Ingredients:

2 cups uncooked gluten-free pasta (brown rice, lentil, or chickpea)

½ cup extra-virgin coconut oil

1 yellow onion, chopped

2 garlic cloves, diced

½ head of broccoli, including stems, chopped into bite-size pieces (2 to 3 cups)

1 cup fresh or frozen peas

2 carrots, chopped in thick slices

½ cup broccoli sprouts

Cracked black pepper and sea salt, to taste

Actions:

1. Place the pasta in a large pot and cover with 5 cups of filtered water. Bring to a boil over high heat. Stir the pasta, then reduce the heat to medium-low. Cook until the pasta is tender, but not mushy. This will take 10 to 15 minutes.

2. While the pasta is cooking, heat the coconut oil in a frying pan over medium heat. Add the onion and garlic and fry, stirring frequently, until these turn golden brown.

3. Add the broccoli to the frying pan. Continue frying, stirring frequently, until the broccoli is just tender.

4. Add the cooked pasta to the pan with the vegetables and toss to combine. Immediately after, add the peas, carrots, and broccoli sprouts and toss again for a few minutes until the flavors and oils are combined.

5. Season with sea salt and pepper to taste.

Variation:

Add 1 teaspoon cayenne pepper for Spicy Pasta Primavera.

Calories: 521.9 | Protein: 15.9g | Carbs: 50.4g | Dietary Fiber: 4.9g | Fat: 29.1g | Vitamin C: 85.1mg | Vitamin D: 0 IU | Vitamin E: 0.7mg | Calcium: 123.7mg | Iron: 4.1mg | Magnesium: 34mg | Potassium: 465.8mg

TURMERIC CUMIN QUINOA BOWL

All the anticancer superpower spices are in this recipe: turmeric, pepper, sea salt, cayenne pepper, and cumin, combined with a whole grain: quinoa. Quinoa is packed with the goodness of protein and bioactive peptides—17 types! One study concluded that the protein in quinoa could be utilized to reduce oxidative stress-associated diseases, including cancer.[5]

Total time: 25 minutes

Makes 3 servings

Ingredients:

1 cup uncooked quinoa

1 tablespoon cumin

½ teaspoon turmeric powder

1 teaspoon sea salt

1 teaspoon extra-virgin coconut oil (or extra-virgin olive oil)

1 teaspoon black pepper

Dash cayenne pepper, if you like a little kick

One avocado, chopped into cubes

One large cucumber, chopped into cubes

½ cup cilantro

¼ cup broccoli sprouts

½ lemon

Actions:

1. Add the quinoa and 2 ½ cups of filtered water to a pot. Bring to a boil over high heat.

2. Reduce the heat to low, cover, and simmer for 15 minutes. The quinoa will absorb the water during the process.

3. Add the remaining ingredients and continue to cook, stirring occasionally, for another 3 minutes, or until the quinoa is soft and all the flavors are well combined. Add the quinoa to bowls.

4. Place the avocado and cucumber alongside the quinoa in a bowl. Sprinkle with cilantro and broccoli sprouts. Squeeze lemon over each bowl and it's ready to enjoy!

Tip:

Serve with strawberries.

Variation:

Try using sesame seed oil instead of coconut oil for a different flavor.

Calories: 236.1 | Protein: 8.6g | Carbs: 38.4g | Dietary Fiber: 4.5g | Fat: 5.5g | Vitamin C: 0mg | Vitamin D: 0 IU | Vitamin E: 1.4mg | Calcium: 64.5mg | Iron: 4.8mg | Magnesium: 115.6mg | Potassium: 390.4mg

COCONUT BASIL SWEET POTATO FRIES

A healthy and delicious way to satisfy those fries cravings!

Total time: 20 minutes

Makes 3 servings

Ingredients:

½ cup extra-virgin coconut oil

2 large sweet potatoes, cut into the shape of French fries

1 cup fresh basil, chopped (or ¼ cup dried basil)

1 cup dried shredded coconut

Actions:

1. When the oil is sizzling, add the sweet potato fries, stirring until each is coated with oil.

2. Let the fries cook, flipping periodically, until they are golden brown (3 to 5 minutes).

3. After the fries have browned, gradually add the basil and coconut. Continue cooking until desired crunchiness (or softness) is achieved.

Tips:

• To get closer to nature, shred your own coconut from the meat of a fresh coconut.

• Sprinkle 1 tablespoon sea salt over the cooked fries.

• Sprinkle 2 tablespoons curry powder over the cooked fries.

Calories: 553 | Protein: 2.7g | Carbs: 32.5g | Dietary Fiber: 4.2g | Fat: 45.8g | Vitamin C: 4.8mg | Vitamin D: 0 IU | Vitamin E: 0.4mg | Calcium: 55.6mg | Iron: 1.5mg | Magnesium: 46.2mg | Potassium: 438.2mg

SATTVIC (PURE) KITCHARI

This recipe comes from Sahara Rose Ketabi's book on ayurvedic foods, *Eat Feel Fresh*. Ayurveda is the world's oldest medicine and closely associated with yoga. A holistic system that originated in India more than 5,000 years ago, it is based on a desire to bring the body into balance. The ayurvedic treatment for cancer might include abstinence from dietary and lifestyle elements that would cause a *tridosha* (vata, pitta, kapha) imbalance, herbal supplementation, and elimination of toxins through therapeutic practices known collectively as *panchakarma*. Ayurvedic preparations can be used as adjuncts to chemotherapy or radiation therapy.

In *The Idiot's Guide to Ayurveda*, Sahara explains the ayurvedic view that the emergence of cancer is just the body's way of letting you know that you are imbalanced. The goal then is to restore balance.

There are only three bodily constitutions, or *doshas*, and every person on earth fits in to one of these types, which are associated with elements from nature. Everybody possesses some of every dosha, but with one or two being predominant. The three doshas are:

- Vata = air + space
- Pitta = fire + water
- Kapha = earth + water

Nutritionally speaking, each dosha has somewhat different requirements to remain in balance. Those are foods that make people with a specific dosha feel their best. In a nutshell:

- Vata should emphasize grounding root vegetables and cooked foods.
- Pitta should emphasize a combination of raw and cooked foods.
- Kapha should emphasize steamed foods, sprouts, raw foods, and bitter foods.

Sahara says that if you eat the wrong foods for your body type it can cause many health issues. I am pitta-vata and therefore need a combination of raw, living foods and warming foods. If I eat too many raw foods, I become too airy and feel cold. Fortunately, Sahara has included modifications in her Kitchari recipe for each of the doshas. Kitchari literally means grabbing items from the kitchen and throwing it all in to make a tasty, nourishing meal.

Total time: 40 minutes

Serves 4

Ingredients:

2 tablespoons sesame oil (vata/ kapha) or coconut oil (pitta)

1 to 2 teaspoons cumin seeds (less for pitta, more for vata/ kapha)

2 teaspoons fennel seeds

1 teaspoon mustard seeds

2 teaspoons ground coriander

½ to 1-inch piece of fresh ginger, grated (less for pitta, more for vata/kapha)

1 teaspoon turmeric powder

¼ teaspoon asafetida (optional)

4 cups filtered water

1 cup basmati rice, soaked overnight, rinsed, and drained

1 cup split yellow mung beans (dhal), soaked overnight, rinsed, and drained

1 teaspoon chopped fresh cilantro

Juice of 1 lime

For Vata:

½ cup diced sweet potato

1 cup chopped mustard greens

For Pitta:

½ cup chopped kale

½ cup diced butternut squash

For Kapha:

½ cup cauliflower florets

1 cup chopped dandelion greens

Actions:

1. Heat the oil over medium heat in a Dutch oven. Add the cumin, fennel, and mustard seeds and cook for 3 minutes or until the mustard seeds begin to pop. Add the coriander, ginger, turmeric, and asafetida, if using. Stir to combine.

2. Stir in the water, rice, mung beans, and vegetables for your dosha. Bring the mixture to a boil, then reduce the heat and simmer, stirring occasionally, until the rice and mung beans are cooked and the vegetables are soft, about 40 minutes.

3. Serve warm, topped with fresh cilantro and lime juice. Kitchari can be refrigerated in an airtight container for up to 4 days.

Calories: 427.9 | Protein: 18.6g | Carbs: 71g | Dietary Fiber: 13.7g | Fat: 10.2g | Vitamin C: 14mg | Vitamin D: 0 IU | Vitamin E: 0.5mg | Calcium: 132.6mg | Iron: 6.3mg | Magnesium: 162.8mg | Potassium: 693.1mg

---

MUNG BEAN SWEET POTATO SPICED RICE

Beans are a staple comfort food of India and used in ayurveda. This is a favorite of cancer survivor Pasha Hogan, author of *Third Time Lucky: A Creative Recovery*. It's her go-to dish for protein. She says, "As a vegetarian, mung beans are great! I also like to make a big pot of this dish and have it in the fridge for a few days or freeze a few portions for later. It is lovely with a light salad or a piece of brown bread toasted and smeared with tahini and avocado. It's very nourishing." The Indian spices give it a savory, delicious taste.

Total time: 3 hours

Makes 6 servings

Ingredients:

¾ cup split yellow mung beans

1 ½ cups basmati rice

2 ½ tablespoons freshly grated ginger root

2 ½ tablespoons ghee or coconut oil

½ teaspoon black mustard seeds

1 teaspoon fennel seeds

1 ½ teaspoons cumin seeds

1 teaspoon turmeric powder

2 teaspoons coriander powder

1 teaspoon black pepper

1 cup chopped beets

1 cup chopped carrots

1 cup chopped sweet potatoes

1 cup green peas

2 ½ teaspoons sea salt

Actions:

1. Soak the beans and rice together in plenty of water so they are well covered for 4 hours, then rinse.

2. Boil 8 cups of filtered water in a large pot, then add the beans, rice, and ginger. Cover, reduce the heat to low, and cook for about 20 minutes.

3. Meanwhile, set a frying pan over low heat and add the ghee, mustard, fennel, and cumin seeds. Sauté until the mustard seeds pop and the other seeds brown slightly. Then add the turmeric, coriander, and pepper, and fry for 1 minute.

4. Transfer the contents of the frying pan to the pot with the beans, rice, and ginger (after they have cooked for 20 minutes). Then add all the vegetables and the sea salt. Cover and cook on low heat for another 20 to 25 minutes, stirring often.

5. Turn off the heat and let the mixture sit for at least 10 minutes before serving.

Calories: 360.9 | Protein: 13.1g | Carbs: 62.1g | Dietary Fiber: 10.7g | Fat: 8.6g | Vitamin C: 12.8mg | Vitamin D: 0 IU | Vitamin E: 0.6mg | Calcium: 74.8mg | Iron: 4.1mg | Magnesium: 97.1mg | Potassium: 570.1mg

---

TURMERIC RICE

One way to spice up rice is by adding some turmeric along with the ginger, garlic, and black pepper. This makes for a delicious and comforting meal or side dish.

Total time: 20 minutes

Makes 4 servings

Ingredients:

2 cups dry brown rice

2 tablespoons extra-virgin coconut oil

1 brown onion, chopped

2 tablespoons chopped garlic

1 tablespoon chopped ginger

2 tablespoons turmeric powder

⅛ teaspoon black pepper

1 carrot, cut in finely sliced rounds

Actions:

1. Boil the rice in 4 cups of filtered water until it is slightly tender but not entirely cooked.

2. Heat the coconut oil in a frying pan over medium heat. Add the onion, garlic, ginger, turmeric, black pepper, and carrots, and fry until they are golden brown and well combined.

3. Add the semicooked rice to the frying pan and stir-fry it with the carrot mixture for a couple of minutes until the rice is done and has turned yellow from the turmeric.

Tips:

- Wrap a scoop of turmeric rice in a piece of lettuce or bok choy for a rice taco!

- Always drain your rice a few times until the water becomes clear to remove arsenic.

Calories: 438.9 | Protein: 8.1g | Carbs: 80.2g | Dietary Fiber: 4.9g | Fat: 9.2g | Vitamin C: 4.3mg | Vitamin D: 0 IU | Vitamin E: 0.2mg | Calcium: 63.2mg | Iron: 3.7mg | Magnesium: 151.3mg | Potassium: 435.2mg

ANTICANCER VEGGIE STIR-FRY

Who said veggie stir-fries are boring? Not with this rainbow assortment of vegetables and freshly squeezed orange juice.

Total time: 35 minutes

Makes 4 servings

Ingredients:

¼ cup extra-virgin coconut oil

1 small yellow onion, chopped

4 large garlic cloves, chopped

1-inch piece of ginger, chopped

1 teaspoon turmeric powder

½ teaspoon cumin

½ teaspoon thyme

¼ teaspoon sea salt

3 leeks, chopped

4 brussels sprouts, chopped

1 large carrot, chopped

½ head of broccoli, chopped

½ cup bok choy, chopped

½ head of cauliflower, chopped

1 cup spinach

1 cup green beans

2 oranges

1 teaspoon sesame seeds

2 teaspoons black seeds

½ cup broccoli sprouts

Actions:

1. Heat the oil in a wok or frying pan, then add the onion and garlic. Sauté for 2 minutes, then add the ginger. Sauté for another minute, then add the turmeric, cumin, thyme, and sea salt.

2. Add the vegetables to the wok or pan and stir-fry until they become tender, about 10 to 15 minutes. Add the juice of the 2 oranges (hand squeezed is okay).

3. Sprinkle the sesame seeds, black seeds, and broccoli sprouts over each serving, along with salt and pepper to taste.

Tips:

- Serve with rice or quinoa.

- Add other vegetables, like peppers, snow peas, zucchini, beets, or peas.

- Add your favorite spices for different flavors and added health benefits.

- Add a squeeze of lemon right before serving for added health benefits.

Variations:

- Add 1 ½ cups cooked brown rice pasta for Vegetable Pasta Stir-Fry.

- Add 1 cup cooked rice for Vegetable Rice Stir-Fry.

- Use sesame seed oil instead of coconut oil for Sesame Vegetable Stir-Fry.

- Add ½ teaspoon cayenne pepper for Spicy Vegetable Stir-Fry.

- Add 1 tablespoon or more honey or maple syrup when adding the vegetables for Sweet Vegetable Stir-Fry.

- If you are a meat eater, you could add chicken, beef, or scrambled eggs to this dish.

Calories: 269.2 | Protein: 7.9g | Carbs: 28.5g | Dietary Fiber: 8g | Fat: 15.5g | Vitamin C: 155.5mg | Vitamin D: 0 IU | Vitamin E: 1.8mg | Calcium: 183.2mg | Iron: 4.4mg | Magnesium: 76.7mg | Potassium: 950mg

---

DAIRY-FREE MASHED POTATOES

Total time: 20 minutes

Makes 2 servings

Ingredients:

2 large potatoes

3 tablespoons extra-virgin coconut oil (or extra-virgin olive oil)

Sea salt and ground black pepper, to taste

Actions:

1. Boil the potatoes (skins on or off, your choice) until they are completely soft.

2. Drain the water, add the oil to the pot, and mash the potatoes.

3. Season to taste with salt and pepper.

Tips:

- For even creamier mashed potatoes, replace the oil with Almond Milk (page 159) or Seed Milk (page 158).
- If you want the mash to be smoother, add more oil or milk.

Variations:

- Replace the white potatoes with sweet potatoes for Mashed Sweet Potatoes.
- Add ⅛ teaspoon or more cayenne pepper for Spicy Mashed Potatoes.

Calories: 464.1 | Protein: 7.5g | Carbs: 64.5g | Dietary Fiber: 7.7g | Fat: 19.8g | Vitamin C: 72.6mg | Vitamin D: 0 IU | Vitamin E: 0.04mg | Calcium: 44.2mg | Iron: 2.9mg | Magnesium: 84.8mg | Potassium: 1,568mg

---

MASHED CAULIFLOWER

Mashed cauliflower is delicious and creamy just like potato mash, but a bit lighter, and it will give you a nice energy increase. You could also do half and half—half potatoes and half cauliflower—as a cheeky way to still get some potatoes but compromise with some cauliflower too.

Total time: 15 minutes

Makes 4 servings

Ingredients:

1 head of cauliflower, cut into bite-size pieces

1 tablespoon olive oil or coconut oil

Sea salt and pepper, to taste

Actions:

1. Bring a large pot of water to boil. Add the cauliflower and cook until very tender, about 10 minutes.

2. Drain the water, then transfer the cauliflower to a food processor. Add the oil, sea salt, and pepper and process until a smooth consistency is reached. (You could also mash the cauliflower by hand the traditional way, but a food processor will make sure the mash is extremely creamy.)

Tip:

Add filtered water, more oil, or almond milk if you want an even creamier mash.

Variation:

Replace half the cauliflower with 1 to 2 white potatoes for Potato-Cauliflower Mash.

Calories: 68.2 | Protein: 2.8g | Carbs: 7g | Dietary Fiber: 2.9g | Fat: 3.9g | Vitamin C: 70.8mg | Vitamin D: 0 IU | Vitamin E: 0.5mg | Calcium: 32.3mg | Iron: 0.6mg | Magnesium: 22mg | Potassium: 439.5mg

CHAPTER 14

SUPER SALADS AND DELICIOUS DRESSINGS

We should all have a goal to eat at least one raw, living food each day, like a salad made with fresh lettuce. Granted, a juice is raw and so is a smoothie, but eating a salad every single day will provide you with many vital nutrients and enzymes you need to boost your immune system and kill cancer cells. Making a salad can be as simple as going out to your backyard and picking some lettuce, kale, cilantro, and parsley and mixing it in a bowl with a simple dressing like olive oil and lemon. Add some avocado, chickpeas, black beans—or Almond Turmeric Crusted Chicken Tenders (page 287)—for some more substance. Alternatively, you can buy a premade organic salad mix from the supermarket and pour some of it into a bowl. Please make sure this is part of your shopping list each week: Always have fresh salad ingredients in your home and aim to have one salad a day if you want to change your health and life.

I hope you will learn to love salads if you don't love them yet. You just need to discover your soul salad—heehee! I am certain you can find it here. I refused to eat salads for years because I thought they were boring, then the Superfood Kale Salad (page 245) converted me. Another benefit is that it takes time to eat a salad; all that chewing is helpful for your digestion and metabolism.

Eating a salad can be like eating straight from God's garden!

FIVE-INGREDIENT GREEN SALAD

Total time: 10 minutes

Makes 1 serving

Ingredients:

1 avocado

1 cup fresh parsley leaves

1 cup broccoli sprouts

1 cup fresh cilantro leaves

1 lemon

Actions:

1. Chop the avocado into cubes.

2. Place the avocado, parsley, sprouts, and cilantro in a bowl. Squeeze the lemon over the salad.

Tips:

• Add sea salt and pepper to taste.

• Include the stems from the parsley and cilantro for added nutrients.

Variation:

Add 1 chopped cucumber for Six-Ingredient Green Salad.

Calories: 396.9 | Protein: 10.7g | Carbs: 24.7g | Dietary Fiber: 16g | Fat: 31.9g | Vitamin C: 247.7mg | Vitamin D: 0 IU | Vitamin E: 5mg | Calcium: 348.2mg | Iron: 7.3mg | Magnesium: 122.8mg | Potassium: 1,873mg

SUPERFOOD KALE SALAD

Total time: 10 minutes

Makes 3 servings

Ingredients:

1 bunch of kale, center ribs and stems removed (save the stems and ribs for juicing or eating later)

1 avocado

1 tablespoon apple cider vinegar

1 ½ tablespoons flaxseed oil

¾ teaspoon sea salt

4 tablespoons nutritional yeast

4 tablespoons sunflower seeds

3 tablespoons black seeds

Actions:

1. Tear the kale leaves into small pieces and place in a large bowl.
2. Massage the avocado into the pieces of kale with your fingers, covering the kale with avocado.
3. Add the remaining ingredients to the bowl and stir, or continue to massage the mixture with your fingers, until everything is well combined.

Tips:

- Add more of any of the ingredients to taste.
- Increase the amount of nutritional yeast if you would like the salad to have a cheesy flavor.

Variations:

- Wrap the salad in a brown rice tortilla for a portable Kale Wrap.
- Add 2 teaspoons garlic powder for Garlic Kale Salad.

Calories: 340.2 | Protein: 10.2g | Carbs: 17.7g | Dietary Fiber: 10.2g | Fat: 29g | Vitamin C: 32.4mg | Vitamin D: 0 IU | Vitamin E: 5.8mg | Calcium: 51.2mg | Iron: 2.6mg | Magnesium: 74.7mg | Potassium: 596.6mg

TACO SALAD

This is a great hybrid dish, good for when you are craving something light and healthy, but also meaty and fulfilling as a delicious combo of salad and taco mix. This creates a vegan taco mix using walnuts, sundried tomatoes, herbs, and spices. You can also use the Grass-Fed Beef Burrito meat recipe to add to the salad.

Total time: 10 minutes

Makes 4 servings

Ingredients:

Taco mix:

1 ½ cups walnuts

1 cup sundried tomatoes

2 tablespoons extra-virgin olive oil

1 teaspoon sage

1 teaspoon cumin

1 teaspoon fennel seeds

1 teaspoon thyme

1 teaspoon rosemary

1 teaspoon oregano

Pinch of black pepper

Pinch of cayenne pepper

Pinch of sea salt

Salad:

8 cups mixed greens including kale, spinach, and lettuce

1 cup broccoli sprouts

1 avocado, sliced

1 tablespoon nutritional yeast

Actions:

1. Place all the ingredients for the taco mix in a blender and blend until well combined.

2. Divide the salad greens and broccoli sprouts among 4 bowls.

3. Sprinkle the taco mix over each salad.

4. Top each salad with avocado slices.

5. Finish by sprinkling nutritional yeast on top of each salad.

Tips:

- Serve with Vegan Sour Cream (page 318).

- Drizzle olive oil and lemon over each salad.

- Substitute the Grass-Fed Beef Burritos filling for a meat-eater's Taco Salad (page 246).

Calories: 536.5 | Protein: 13g | Carbs: 28.5g | Dietary Fiber: 10.6g | Fat: 43.9g | Vitamin C: 65.9mg | Vitamin D: 0 IU | Vitamin E: 2.9mg | Calcium: 182.7mg | Iron: 5mg | Magnesium: 122.7mg | Potassium: 836.7mg

---

MANGO AVOCADO SALAD

A delicious combination of sweet, savory, creamy, and crunchy, this salad is a tropical dream as well as being anticancer, especially with the black seeds.

Total time: 10 minutes

Makes 2 servings

Ingredients:

Salad:

4 cups mixed greens (best for this salad is a combination of arugula, spinach, and kale)

Dressing:

3 tablespoons olive oil

½ small purple onion, chopped

Juice of 1 lime

¼ teaspoon sea salt

1 ripe mango, peeled, pitted, then sliced into cubes

1 avocado, peeled, pitted, then sliced into cubes

Cracked white pepper or black pepper, to taste

½ tablespoon sesame seeds

½ tablespoon black seeds

Actions:

1. Divide the greens into 2 bowls.

2. Mix together the olive oil, onion, lime, and sea salt for the dressing. Pour ¾ of the dressing over the greens.

3. Arrange the mango and avocado on top of each salad, then drizzle with the remaining dressing.

4. Top with the pepper and seeds.

Tip:

Serve the salad with a sprinkle of broccoli sprouts on top. This salad also goes well with Vegan Yogurt (page 203).

Calories: 494.9 | Protein: 4.8g | Carbs: 39g | Dietary Fiber: 10.7g | Fat: 39g | Vitamin C: 79.3mg | Vitamin D: 0 IU | Vitamin E: 6.2mg | Calcium: 59.6mg | Iron: 1.4mg | Magnesium: 57.4mg | Potassium: 832.2mg

CROWD-PLEASING ASIAN SALAD

This recipe is by Charlene Bollinger, co-founder of TheTruth AboutCancer.com. It is one of their family favorites, it's enjoyed by all and it is so healthy! It's packed with antioxidants and leaves you feeling refreshed but also extremely satisfied from all the protein from the nuts and sensational dressing.

Total time: 10 minutes

Serves 4

Ingredients:

Salad:

1 head romaine lettuce, cleaned and chopped

1 package organic broccoli coleslaw (or slice your own, 1 cup of cabbage, 1 cup broccoli stalks, and 1 cup carrots)

1 red pepper, sliced and diced
4 green onions, chopped
1 cup raw cashews
¾ organic sliced almonds

Dressing:

¾ cup extra-virgin olive oil

⅓ cup raw apple cider vinegar

½ cup raw honey (you may also use grade B maple syrup)

1 teaspoon sea salt

Pinch of fresh ground black pepper to taste

Actions:

1. In small bowl, mix dressing ingredients. Whisk it to make it super smooth.

2. In large bowl, place salad ingredients. Toss salad dressing ingredients over salad and mix well.

Calories: 840 | Protein: 14g | Carbs: 63g | Dietary Fiber: 10g | Fat: 64g | Vitamin C: 91.47mg | Vitamin D: 0 IU | Vitamin E: 11.88mg | Calcium: 156.64mg | Iron: 5.5mg | Magnesium: 183.43mg | Potassium: 1102.75mg

ORANGE ARUGULA AVOCADO SESAME SEED SALAD

Sesame seeds are high in iron, so if your iron levels are low, sprinkle them on your salads, soups, and eggs.

Total time: 10 minutes

Makes 2 servings

Ingredients:

Salad:

1 orange, peeled and sliced

2 cups arugula, torn into pieces

1 slice of purple onion, in wafts

1 avocado, peeled and sliced

¾ cup snap peas

1 tablespoon roasted sesame seeds

½ teaspoon black seeds

Garnish with fresh parsley, cilantro, and ½ cup broccoli sprouts

Dressing:

1 teaspoon sesame seed oil

2 teaspoons olive oil

Dash of sea salt and pepper

Juice of ½ lemon

1 tablespoon orange juice

Actions:

1. Layer the salads on 2 plates, starting with the orange slices. Then add the arugula, followed by the onion, the avocado, and the snap peas.

2. Make the dressing by whisking the ingredients together in a bowl and pour over each salad.

3. Finish by sprinkling the salads with the seeds, fresh herbs, and broccoli sprouts.

Calories: 331.6 | Protein: 6.8g | Carbs: 24.6g | Dietary Fiber: 11g | Fat: 25.1g | Vitamin C: 108.4mg | Vitamin D: 0 IU | Vitamin E: 3mg | Calcium: 208.3mg | Iron: 3.7mg | Magnesium: 74.3mg | Potassium: 897.5mg

SUPER DETOX BROCCOLI SPROUT GREEN SALAD

If you are missing a couple of ingredients for this recipe, don't worry; you can still make a salad that will be full of greens.

Total time: 25 minutes

Makes 4 servings

Ingredients:

1 head of any kind of lettuce, torn into small pieces

1 bunch of kale, including the stems and ribs, torn into small pieces

½ cup watercress, torn into pieces

½ bok choy, torn into pieces

1 cup broccoli sprouts

½ cup finally chopped broccoli

8 asparagus stalks, halved (don't include the bottom inch or so, which can be tough)

1 avocado, cut into cubes or slices

1 cucumber, chopped into cubes

1 garlic clove, diced

1-inch piece of ginger, diced

1 purple onion, chopped into thin slices

1 cup sunflower sprouts or alfalfa sprouts

1 radish, sliced

1 green apple, thinly sliced

1 celery stalk, chopped into cubes

¼ cup extra-virgin olive oil

Juice of 1 lemon

Actions:

1. Combine all the ingredients, except the oil and lemon juice, in a bowl and toss.

2. Drizzle with olive oil and lemon juice.

Variations:

- Add 1 green chili, chopped into small pieces, for a Spicy Green Salad.

- Add ½ cup walnuts to make a crunchy Nutty Green Salad.

- Add 3 tablespoons raw honey or maple syrup for a Sweet Green Salad.

- Add 2 bell peppers (any color), chopped in small pieces, for a Crunchy Green Salad.

- Add ¾ cup any type of beans for a Bean Green Salad.

Calories: 329.6 | Protein: 8.6g | Carbs: 28g | Dietary Fiber: 10.7g | Fat: 22.6g | Vitamin C: 152.1mg | Vitamin D: 0 IU | Vitamin E: 3.96mg | Calcium: 297.9mg | Iron: 4.2mg | Magnesium: 98.4g | Potassium: 1,409mg

GRATED BEET AND CARROT SALAD WITH SUNBUTTER DRESSING

This is an extremely powerful recipe to reduce your risk of getting cancer. This was the very first recipe to be featured on the news when word about this book spread! It was filmed on News 12 as host Mary Mucci wanted to feature it for cancer awareness month. If you eat this salad a few times a week you can be assured you are consuming a concoction of ingredients that have many anticancer effects. A study done provided evidence for a reduced postmenopausal breast cancer risk associated with increased consumption of sunflower seeds.[6]

Total time: 10 minutes

Makes 2 servings

Ingredients:

Salad:

4 carrots, peeled and grated

1 small beet, peeled and grated

1 tablespoon fresh basil, diced

Dressing:

3 tablespoon apple cider vinegar

1 tablespoon Sunbutter (sunflower seed butter)

Actions:

1. Grate the carrots and beet. Add to a bowl along with the basil.

2. Mix the apple cider vinegar and Sunbutter in a separate bowl, and mix until thick and creamy. Pour over the salad and toss until well coated.

Tip:

Use a food processor to save time.

Calories: 85.6 | Protein: 1.8g | Carbs: 19.8g | Dietary Fiber: 4.5g | Fat: 0.3g | Vitamin C: 9.4mg | Vitamin D: 0 IU | Vitamin E: 0.8mg | Calcium: 51.4mg | Iron: 0.8mg | Magnesium: 25.9mg | Potassium: 543.8mg

ASIAN BOK CHOY CABBAGE SALAD

Total time: 10 minutes

Makes 4 servings

Ingredients:

Salad:

2 cups shredded raw cabbage

2 carrots, grated or shredded

1 cup bok choy, diced

Dressing:

1 tablespoon rice vinegar

½ teaspoon sesame oil

2 tablespoons coconut sugar or maple syrup

½ teaspoon sea salt

¼ teaspoon black pepper

¼ cup olive oil

1 teaspoon amino acids, optional

Toppings:

1 tablespoon roasted sesame seeds

1 tablespoon black seeds

Handful of broccoli sprouts

Actions:

1. Place the cabbage, carrots, and bok choy in a large bowl and toss.

2. Combine all the ingredients together for the dressing and pour over the salad. Toss until thoroughly coated. Top with some sesame seeds, black seeds, and broccoli sprouts.

Calories: 206 | Protein: 2.4g | Carbs: 11.6g | Dietary Fiber: 2.8g | Fat: 17.4g | Vitamin C: 32.1mg | Vitamin D: 0 IU | Vitamin E: 1.9mg | Calcium: 81.9mg | Iron: 1.2mg | Magnesium: 23.5mg | Potassium: 314.8mg

CHICKPEA CUCUMBER CUMIN SALAD

You can use chickpeas from a can or Chickpea Fries (page 302).

Total time: 5 minutes

Makes 4 servings

Ingredients:

Salad:

1 cup chopped kale

¼ cup chopped spinach

¼ cup chopped broccoli sprouts

1 large cucumber, cubed

One 14-ounce can organic BPA-free chickpeas

Seasoning:

1 teaspoon cumin

¼ teaspoon sea salt

Cracked black pepper, to taste

Smidgen of turmeric powder

1 tablespoon black seeds

Dressing:

Juice of 1 lemon   2 tablespoons olive oil

Actions:

1. Divide the kale, spinach, broccoli sprouts, and cucumber among 4 salad bowls. Drain the chickpeas and add those on top of the greens.

2. Mix the seasonings in a bowl and sprinkle evenly over each salad.

3. Mix the lemon juice and olive oil for the dressing. Pour over the salads and serve.

Calories: 254.5 | Protein: 8.5g | Carbs: 27g | Dietary Fiber: 7.2g | Fat: 13.9g | Vitamin C: 26.2mg | Vitamin D: 0 IU | Vitamin E: 1.5mg | Calcium: 92.1mg | Iron: 2.4mg | Magnesium: 41mg | Potassium: 349.8mg

---

STRENGTH-BUILDING PROTEIN SALAD

You can make this salad without the chicken and it will still be high in protein! Buying chicken precut into tenders will save you time in the kitchen.

Total time: 10 minutes

Makes 4 servings

Ingredients:

Salad:

7 cups mixed greens including kale, lettuce, and spinach

Batch of Almond Turmeric Crusted Chicken Tenders (page 287)

½ cup chickpeas

1 cup broccoli sprouts

2 tablespoons hemp seeds

2 tablespoons sunflower seeds

2 tablespoons pumpkin seeds

Dressing:

1 lemon

2 tablespoons extra-virgin olive oil

Garnish:

Fresh parsley   Fresh dill

Fresh thyme

Actions:

1. Divide the mixed greens among 4 salad bowls. Add the Almond Turmeric Crusted Chicken Tenders and chickpeas. Sprinkle the sprouts and seeds over each salad.

2. Mix the lemon juice and olive oil for the dressing. Pour over each salad.

3. Garnish with fresh parsley, thyme, and/or dill.

Calories: 940 | Protein: 43.9g | Carbs: 19.4g | Dietary Fiber: 8.5g | Fat: 77g | Vitamin C: 54mg | Vitamin D: 21.6 IU | Vitamin E: 13.3mg | Calcium: 237.6mg | Iron: 6.6mg | Magnesium: 246.3mg | Potassium: 1,218mg

---

TABBOULEH

This is a very simple salad with finely chopped vegetables. It is so light and literally can bounce around in your mouth with the zing of fresh lemon.

Total time: 20 minutes

Makes 6 servings

Ingredients:

4 tomatoes, finely chopped

1 cucumber, finely chopped

2 bunches of parsley, finely chopped

12 fresh mint leaves, finely chopped

4 green onions, finely chopped

4 tablespoons lime or lemon juice

3 tablespoons extra-virgin olive oil

Actions:

1. Drain the excess liquid from the tomatoes.

2. Combine all the ingredients in a bowl and mix until well combined. Season with sea salt and pepper.

3. The tabbouleh is now ready to serve, although if you set it aside in the fridge for 30 minutes, the flavors will have a chance to absorb together.

Tips:

- This goes great with Hummus (page 298) and Guacamole (page 297).
- Use lettuce leaves and place a spoonful of the mixture inside to make a lettuce wrap.
- Add cooked quinoa to make this a hybrid dish.
- Add hemp seeds for some more nutty flavor.

Calories: 102.1 | Protein: 2.1g | Carbs: 8.5g | Dietary Fiber: 2.5g | Fat: 7.4g | Vitamin C: 58mg | Vitamin D: 0 IU | Vitamin E: 1.6mg | Calcium: 67.4mg | Iron: 2.4mg | Magnesium: 33.7mg | Potassium: 477.4mg

---

MASON JAR SALADS

When talking about salads, Christiane Northrup, M.D., advises: "Think color and you'll be on the right path, because the deep pigments in these foods contain powerful antioxidants. Go for broccoli; green leafy vegetables; berries; red, yellow, and green peppers; and tomatoes, and vary your choices through the seasons."

Salad in a jar 101: Grab your mason jar and fill it up with your salad of choice. You can make up seven of these once a week and then grab one from the fridge each day as you go off to work. Salad keeps fresh in a mason jar! See the story about James Lechmanski (page 126), who ate salads for breakfast.

Have fun with these and create vibrant layers. Inspire others with your art. Post a picture on Instagram or Pinterest and tag it #saladinajar #masonjarsalad #saladselfie #theearthdiet.

How to Build a Mason Jar Salad

1. Start with the "wet ingredients" on the bottom. First choose your salad dressing. Then add things like cucumbers, red peppers, and tomatoes. You can also incorporate fruits like strawberries and blackberries.

2. Then add your solid vegetables: carrots, broccoli, snap peas, beans, or cauliflower.

3. Add your dry ingredients, including any nuts and seeds.

4. Lastly, add your protein: pasta, meat, chicken, or egg.

5. When you are ready to eat, shake it up and you'll have a salad in a jar! You can either dump it into a bowl or eat it straight from the jar.

Fruit Jar Salad

Layer 1: Lemon juice (for dressing) and watermelon

Layer 2: Strawberries, blueberries, and grapes

Layer 3: Cantaloupe

Layer 4: Sunflower seeds, pumpkin seeds, hemp seeds, chia seeds, and flaxseeds

Fruit and Vegetable Jar Salad

Layer 1: Dressing of olive oil, flax oil, and lemon juice mixed with strawberries and cantaloupe

Layer 2: Carrots

Layer 3: Walnuts and almonds

Layer 4: Spinach and lettuce

Mediterranean Jar Salad

Layer 1: Balsamic vinegar

Layer 2: Artichokes, black olives, tomatoes, cucumber, and white cannellini beans

Layer 3: Nutritional yeast, organic feta (or the cheese of your choice), and pine nuts

Layer 4: Mixed greens and a sprinkle of oregano and thyme

High-Protein Jar Salad

Layer 1: Lemon-olive oil dressing

Layer 2: Chickpeas

Layer 3: Broccoli

Layer 4: Cooked quinoa, cooked chicken, hemp seeds, pumpkin seeds, and spinach

Detox Jar Salad

Layer 1: Lemon, garlic, ginger, and olive oil dressing

Layer 2: Pineapple, blueberries, and strawberries

Layer 3: Cooked quinoa

Layer 4: Sprouts, kale, and dandelion greens

MAKE YOUR OWN HOMEMADE SALAD DRESSING . . . FOREVER!

The basic premise of a salad dressing is combining oil and vinegar. If you have those two ingredients, you can always make your own homemade dressing. I love adding lemon to make a three-ingredient salad dressing. Make up a large batch and keep it in your fridge so you always have some on hand.

Refrigerated in an airtight container or jar, this base salad dressing lasts for up to two months.

Total time: 5 minutes

Makes ¼ cup dressing (for 1 large salad serving approximately 4 people)

Ingredients:

¼ cup extra-virgin olive oil (you can also use MCT oil, tigernut oil, or avocado oil)

3 tablespoons apple cider vinegar (you can also use balsamic vinegar; just make sure it doesn't contain white sugar or sulfites)

Action:

Add all the ingredients to a bowl and mix until well combined. Pour on salad.

Variations:

Add any of the following ingredients to your base salad dressing for extra flavors:

Garlic Salad Dressing: 2 cloves garlic, minced

Ginger Salad Dressing: 1-inch piece of ginger, minced

Lemon Salad Dressing: juice of 1 lemon

Turmeric Salad Dressing:1 teaspoon turmeric powder for extra health benefits

Sweet Salad Dressing: 1 tablespoon honey or maple syrup

Spicy Salad Dressing: ⅛ teaspoon cayenne pepper

Cheesy Dressing: 1 tablespoon nutritional yeast

Hummus Salad Dressing: 2 tablespoons Hummus (page 298)

Calories: 126 | Protein: 0g | Carbs: 0g | Dietary Fiber: 0g | Fat: 14g | Vitamin C: 0mg | Vitamin D: 0 IU | Vitamin E: 1.7mg | Calcium: 0mg | Iron: 0mg | Magnesium: 0mg | Potassium: 8.2mg

TANGY GINGER-GARLIC DRESSING

Refrigerated in an airtight container or jar, this salad dressing lasts for up to two months.

Total time: 5 minutes

Makes 4 servings

Ingredients:

2 teaspoons minced garlic

1-inch piece of ginger, minced

Juice of 1 lemon

⅓ cup extra-virgin olive oil

2 tablespoons apple cider vinegar

Actions:

Add all the ingredients to a bowl and mix until well combined. Pour on salad.

Calories: 258 | Protein: 0.1g | Carbs: 1.5g | Dietary Fiber: 0.1g | Fat: 28g | Vitamin C: 4.9mg | Vitamin D: 0 IU | Vitamin E: 3.5mg | Calcium: 3.5mg | Iron: 0.04mg | Magnesium: 1.8mg | Potassium: 30.5mg

CREAMY TAHINI SALAD DRESSING

A high protein creamy dressing that goes so well on kale!

Total time: 5 minutes

Makes 2 servings

Ingredients:

3 tablespoons tahini

1 teaspoon lemon juice

¼ cup extra-virgin olive oil

2 tablespoons apple cider vinegar

Actions:

Add all the ingredients to a bowl and mix until well combined. Pour on salad.

Calories: 385.7 | Protein: 3.9g | Carbs: 5g | Dietary Fiber: 1g | Fat: 39.9g | Vitamin C: 1.9mg | Vitamin D: 0 IU | Vitamin E: 3.4mg | Calcium: 31.8mg | Iron: 1mg | Magnesium: 21.5mg | Potassium: 116.8mg

---

CREAMY AVOCADO SALAD DRESSING

Total time: 4 minutes

Makes 4 servings

Ingredients:

Juice of 1 lemon

⅓ cup avocado oil

3 tablespoons apple cider vinegar

1 avocado, seeded and peeled

Actions:

Place all the ingredients in a bowl and mash until the avocado is smooth and everything is well combined. Pour on, or massage into, salad.

Calories: 247.9 | Protein: 1g | Carbs: 5g | Dietary Fiber: 3.4g | Fat: 26g | Vitamin C: 9.4mg | Vitamin D: 0 IU | Vitamin E: 1mg | Calcium: 6.7mg | Iron: 0.29mg | Magnesium: 15.2mg | Potassium: 263.7mg

---

CAESAR SALAD DRESSING

This dressing captures the Caesar flavor without the raw egg.

Total time: 3 minutes

Makes 4 servings

Ingredients:

Juice of 1 lemon

⅓ cup extra-virgin olive oil

¼ teaspoon mustard powder

2 tablespoons nutritional yeast

½ teaspoon honey

1 teaspoon minced garlic

¼ teaspoon sea salt

⅛ teaspoon pepper

Actions:

Add all the ingredients to a bowl and mix until well combined. Pour on salad.

Calories: 182.2 | Protein: 1g | Carbs: 2.5g | Dietary Fiber: 0.4g | Fat: 18.8g | Vitamin C: 4.6mg | Vitamin D: 0 IU | Vitamin E: 2.3mg | Calcium: 3.4mg | Iron: 0.1mg | Magnesium: 4.2mg | Potassium: 49.9mg

SWEET PURPLE GRAPE DRESSING

Total time: 2 minutes

Makes 4 servings

Ingredients:

2 tablespoons purple grape juice

1 tablespoon apple cider vinegar

1 tablespoon organic balsamic vinegar

1 teaspoon manuka or local honey

Actions:

Add all the ingredients to a bowl and mix until well combined. Pour on salad.

Calories: 11.5 | Protein: 0.03g | Carbs: 3.1g | Dietary Fiber: 0.02g | Fat: 0.01g | Vitamin C: 0.02mg | Vitamin D: 0 IU | Vitamin E: 0mg | Calcium: 0.9mg | Iron: 0.03mg | Magnesium: 0.8mg | Potassium: 11.8mg

CITRUS SALAD DRESSING

Total time: 3 minutes

Makes 4 servings

Ingredients:

Juice of 1 lemon

Juice of 1 orange

Juice of 1 grapefruit

2 tablespoons olive oil

Smidgen of turmeric powder

Actions:

Add all the ingredients to a bowl and mix until well combined. Pour on salad.

Calories: 96.6 | Protein: 0.4g | Carbs: 8g | Dietary Fiber: 0.07g | Fat: 7.1g | Vitamin C: 35.6mg | Vitamin D: 0 IU | Vitamin E: 0.8mg | Calcium: 7.9mg | Iron: 0.1mg | Magnesium: 9.8g | Potassium: 143.1mg

SESAME-GINGER DRESSING

Total time: 3 minutes

Makes 4 servings

Ingredients:

Juice of 1 lemon

¼ cup extra-virgin olive oil

3 tablespoons sesame seed oil

1 tablespoon apple cider vinegar

1 tablespoon toasted sesame seeds

1 teaspoon black seeds

1 tablespoon grated ginger

Actions:

Add all the ingredients to a bowl and mix until well combined. Pour on salad.

Calories: 237.4 | Protein: 0.6g | Carbs: 2g | Dietary Fiber: 0.6g | Fat: 25.7g | Vitamin C: 4.5mg | Vitamin D: 0 IU | Vitamin E: 1.9mg | Calcium: 3.5mg | Iron: 0.2mg | Magnesium: 8.2mg | Potassium: 28.8mg

HONEY MUSTARD VINAIGRETTE

Total time: 3 minutes

Makes 4 servings

Ingredients:

1 teaspoon minced garlic

1 tablespoon mustard

1 tablespoon manuka honey

1 ½ teaspoons apple cider vinegar

⅓ cup extra-virgin olive oil

Dash black pepper

Dash sea salt

Actions:

Add all the ingredients to a bowl and mix until well combined. Pour on salad.

Calories: 187.4 | Protein: 0.2g | Carbs: 4.8g | Dietary Fiber: 0.1g | Fat: 18.8g | Vitamin C: 0.2mg | Vitamin D: 0 IU | Vitamin E: 2.3mg | Calcium: 4.2mg | Iron: 0.1mg | Magnesium: 2.2mg | Potassium: 13.6mg

CHAPTER 15

COMFORTING SOUPS AND BROTHS

Soup can be incredibly calming, warming, and nourishing at the same time. By definition, a soup is a water-based dish for which a number of ingredients are stirred into a pot, seasoned with herbs and spices, and heated over a flame. And you can also add meats. If you are pressed for time or not feeling energetic enough to make a broth from scratch, you can buy a premade broth and use that as a base for your soup.

Soup is an opportunity to stock your fridge for a week or longer with convenience foods. Make a big batch and freeze some in individual portions. Add fresh ingredients as you reheat it. Fresh parsley, cilantro, cucumbers, and avocados are excellent additions to make a frozen soup come alive again.

Regarding the cooked soups: I prefer to cook and reheat my soups on the stovetop, as this preserves more of their nutritional value. Don't use a microwave for reheating your soups, as it changes the nutritional structure.

Some of the recipes that follow are raw soups and some are cooked. The raw soups are vegan. Some of the cooked soups call for meat. For extra protein, you can always add a boiled egg, beans, quinoa, or chickpeas to your soup.

Any of these soups can be pureed after cooking to make them smoother and easier to swallow and digest.

A broth and a stock are generally the same thing: a liquid created from either animal bones or vegetables. Stock is often called for in recipes that have a base, like a soup, but you can also use a broth as a base for soup.

VEGETABLE SOUP

Total time: 10 minutes

Makes 4 servings

INGREDIENTS:

5 cups filtered water

½ teaspoon dried thyme or 1 tablespoon fresh thyme

½ teaspoon dried parsley or 1 tablespoon fresh parsley

½ teaspoon dried oregano

½ teaspoon cumin powder

1 teaspoon sea salt

¼ teaspoon black pepper

½ head of cauliflower

½ head of broccoli

1 carrot

2 celery stalks

Dash of cayenne pepper, optional

Actions:

1. Place the water, herbs, and spices in a large pot over high heat and bring to a boil. Meanwhile, chop the vegetables into small pieces.

2. Add the vegetables to the pot and allow the mixture to boil for 7 minutes more. Transfer the soup to bowls and add a dash of cayenne pepper, if desired, for some kick.

Calories: 56.2 | Protein: 3.9g | Carbs: 11.2g | Dietary Fiber: 4.3g | Fat: 0.6g | Vitamin C: 104.8mg | Vitamin D: 0 IU | Vitamin E: 0.8mg | Calcium: 83mg | Iron: 1.4mg | Magnesium: 35mg | Potassium: 573.6mg

IMMUNE-BOOSTING SOUP

Did you know onions are high in vitamin C? This might be why you crave them when you're feeling run-down. This soup is incredibly immune boosting because it combines onion and tomato with garlic and spices. This recipe uses a combination of fresh herbs and dried spices. If you can go into the garden and pick them fresh, that is the ultimate for immune-boosting properties. If you do not have access to fresh herbs, you can just as easily make this recipe with dried herbs only.

Make a large batch and keep it in your freezer, then just defrost in a pot and add some fresh herbs to freshen it up!

Total time: 10 minutes

Makes 2 servings

INGREDIENTS:

1 tablespoon extra-virgin olive oil

1 small yellow onion

8 fresh basil leaves or 1 teaspoon dried basil

1 tablespoon fresh thyme or 1 teaspoon dried thyme

1 tablespoon fresh parsley or 1 teaspoon dried parsley

1 tablespoon fresh cilantro or 1 teaspoon dried coriander

3 fresh sage leaves or 1 teaspoon dried sage

1 teaspoon cumin powder

1 teaspoon turmeric powder

1 teaspoon sea salt

½ teaspoon cracked black pepper

Pinch or 2 of cayenne pepper

1 tablespoon minced garlic

3 medium juice tomatoes

2 cups filtered water

Actions:

1. Heat the oil in a medium pot over medium heat. Chop the onion and add it to the pot. Cook for 2 minutes until the onion begins to soften. Gather up all your herbs and spices.

2. When the onion is soft, add the herbs, spices, and garlic and mix well.

3. Squeeze the tomatoes into the pot. Chop up the tomato skins and add them to the pot as well.

4. Add the water and let the soup cook for 7 minutes.

5. Season with more sea salt and pepper, if desired. Top with broccoli sprouts and additional fresh herbs like basil, parsley, and cilantro, if desired.

Calories: 130.6 | Protein: 2.9g | Carbs: 14.2g | Dietary Fiber: 3.7g | Fat: 7.9g | Vitamin C: 34mg | Vitamin D: 0 IU | Vitamin E: 1.9mg | Calcium: 75.8mg | Iron: 2.6mg | Magnesium: 36mg | Potassium: 591.9mg

ENERGY SOUP

Ann Wigmore, an early proponent of raw food and blended soups taught a lot of her students to create an energy soup by blending vegetables and sprouts. She looked at soups as a complete meal. My variation of her soup follows her tradition. Ann said, "Let me share my vision with you: I see a world without sickness, sorrow or mental disturbance in which we are living in perfect balance with abundant health and harmony. Reconnect with nature and your body will take care of the rest. This is the beauty of self-healing."[1]

Ingredients:

1 ½ cups coconut water or fermented probiotic beverage (kombucha or green tea kombucha)

1 teaspoon dulse flakes

1 to 2 apples, coarsely chopped

1 cup baby spinach leaves

1 green onion

¼ to ½ cup broccoli sprouts (or sunflower sprouts or alfalfa sprouts)

1 avocado

Actions:

1. Blend all the ingredients in a high-powered blender until the mixture is smooth.

2. Serve the soup with fresh herbs like cilantro.

Tips:

- Use a high-powered blender, such as a Vitamix, with a variable-speed dial, to prepare this recipe.

- The soup can be an acquired taste. Tweak the ingredients and amounts to your liking. If you like savory seasonings, add cayenne, garlic, and sea salt to taste.

- The soup will keep for 7 to 10 days. Store in a glass, not plastic, container.

Calories: 525.8 | Protein: 8.9g | Carbs: 62.9g | Dietary Fiber: 23.4g | Fat: 30.8g | Vitamin C: 78.1mg | Vitamin D: 0 IU | Vitamin E: 4.5mg | Calcium: 207.2mg | Iron: 4.2mg | Magnesium: 166.2mg | Potassium: 2,301mg

REFRESHING CUCUMBER SOUP

This soup is so hydrating. It is keto, and there is no cooking involved—just blend all the ingredients together for a surprisingly delicious and fulfilling soup. This recipe comes from my good friend Dr. David Jockers.

Total time: 40 minutes

Makes 2 servings

Ingredients:

1 large cucumber, peeled and seeded

2 avocados, pitted

6 to 7 green onions

2 large garlic cloves

¼ cup lemon juice

¾ cup filtered water

½ teaspoon sea salt

½ teaspoon black pepper

1 tablespoon minced chives

Actions:

1. Place all the ingredients in a blender or powerful food processor for 1 to 2 minutes or until creamy.

2. Put the soup into a container and chill in the refrigerator for 20 to 30 minutes. Serve with sea salt, black pepper, and minced chives sprinkled on top.

Tip:

Serve with Dehydrated Crackers (page 293).

Calories: 365.8 | Protein: 6g | Carbs: 27g | Dietary Fiber: 15.9g | Fat: 29.8g | Vitamin C: 46.6mg | Vitamin D: 0 IU | Vitamin E: 4.5mg | Calcium: 89.9mg | Iron: 2.2mg | Magnesium: 89.1mg | Potassium: 1,344mg

CREAMY CARROT TURMERIC SOUP

This recipe comes from Vani Hari, author of *The Food Babe Way: Break Free from the Hidden Toxins in Your Food and Lose Weight, Look Years Younger, and Get Healthy in Just 21 Days!*

Total time: 30 minutes

Makes 2 servings

Ingredients:

1 teaspoon coconut oil

½ yellow onion, diced

1 garlic clove, minced

5 large carrots, chopped

1 cup vegetable or chicken stock

½ cup filtered water

3 Truvani turmeric tablets (or 1 teaspoon ground turmeric)

1 bay leaf

¼ cup coconut milk

Sea salt and black pepper, to taste

Actions:

1. Heat the oil in a soup pot over medium heat.

2. Add the onion, garlic, and carrots and cook for 2 to 3 minutes.

3. Add the stock, water, turmeric, and bay leaf. Cover and simmer on low for 20 to 25 minutes or until the carrots are tender.

4. Remove the pot from the heat and blend the soup using an immersion or counter blender. Place the pot back over the heat and stir in the coconut milk. Season with sea salt and pepper.

5. Serve with desired toppings. Enjoy!

Calories: 122.2 | Protein: 2.1g | Carbs: 22.8 | Dietary Fiber: 5.9g | Fat: 3.2g | Vitamin C: 13.1mg | Vitamin D: 15 IU | Vitamin E: 1.2mg | Calcium: 85.4mg | Iron: 1.3mg | Magnesium: 31.7mg | Potassium: 650.6mg

THAI SOUP

Total time: 20 minutes

Makes 4 servings

Ingredients:

1 tablespoon coconut oil

2 tablespoons grated fresh ginger

1 tablespoon red or green curry paste

4 cups chicken broth

1 cup vegetable broth

3 tablespoons coconut sugar or maple syrup

½ teaspoon sea salt

1 teaspoon amino acids

One 14-ounce can coconut milk

2 tablespoons fresh lime juice

1 teaspoon minced lemongrass

¼ cup fresh cilantro, chopped

4 tablespoons broccoli sprouts, chopped

1 cup bean sprouts

Actions:

1. Heat the oil in a large pot over medium-high heat. Add the ginger and curry paste and cook for 1 minute. Pour in the rest of the ingredients, except for the cilantro and bean sprouts. Bring to a boil and continue boiling for 8 minutes.

2. Serve with fresh cilantro, broccoli, and bean sprouts.

Tip:

Add organic chicken, beef, fish, or shrimp if you want to add protein.

Calories: 281.4 | Protein: 4.3g | Carbs: 14.6g | Dietary Fiber: 0.5g | Fat: 24.5g | Vitamin C: 7.4mg | Vitamin D: 0 IU | Vitamin E: 0.08mg | Calcium: 24mg | Iron: 3.6mg | Magnesium: 55.4mg | Potassium: 357.2mg

CHICKEN NOODLE SOUP

Total time: 10 minutes

Makes 4 servings

Ingredients:

1 tablespoon coconut oil

2 celery stalks, chopped

1 tablespoon onion powder

1 teaspoon garlic powder

½ teaspoon dried basil

½ teaspoon dried oregano

½ teaspoon dried thyme

¼ teaspoon sea salt

¼ teaspoon pepper

56 ounces Chicken Broth (page 280) or four packets of Ancient Nutrition Bone Broth Pure

14 ounces Vegetable Broth (page 279) or carton of vegetable broth

½ pound chicken strips

2 packets organic ramen noodles

Broccoli sprouts

Actions:

1. Place the oil, celery, onion powder, and garlic powder in a large pot and cook for 1 minute over medium-high heat. Pour in the rest of the ingredients, except for the ramen noodles.

2. Bring to a boil and allow to cook for 7 minutes.

3. Add the ramen noodles and cook for another minute until the ramen noodles and chicken are cooked through.

4. Serve and top with broccoli sprouts.

Calories: 199 | Protein: 17g | Carbs: 17.9g | Dietary Fiber: 1.8g | Fat: 5.5g | Vitamin C: 1.1mg | Vitamin D: 0.5 IU | Vitamin E: 0.4mg | Calcium: 37.2mg | Iron: 1.2mg | Magnesium: 23.8mg | Potassium: 362.4mg

RAW TOMATO SOUP

Total time: 7 minutes

Serves 3

Ingredients:

One 28-ounce can whole tomatoes in juice

1 rib of celery, roughly chopped

1 cup filtered water

¼ small onion

1 garlic clove

1 teaspoon dried parsley

1 teaspoon dried thyme

1 bay leaf

1 tablespoon pure maple syrup

Juice from 1 lemon

¼ teaspoon sea salt

¼ teaspoon black pepper

Actions:

1. Puree all the ingredients in a blender until smooth.

2. Taste. Season with more sea salt and pepper, if desired, and serve.

Tips:

• Add ¼ cup Vegan Sour Cream (page 318) for a creamy tomato soup!

• For a hot soup, transfer the mixture to a pot. Bring to a boil, then simmer for 7 minutes.

• Serve and top with broccoli sprouts.

Calories: 67.1 | Protein: 2.2g | Carbs: 15.5g | Dietary Fiber: 4g | Fat: 0.7g | Vitamin C: 37.7mg | Vitamin D: 0 IU | Vitamin E: 1.5mg | Calcium: 107.4mg | Iron: 1.9mg | Magnesium: 31.2mg | Potassium: 545.5mg

KIDNEY BEAN SOUP WITH WATERCRESS AND KALE

Total time: 15 minutes

Makes 4 servings

Ingredients:

1 ½ tablespoons coconut oil

1 brown onion, chopped

1 teaspoon garlic powder

3 cups filtered water

1 cup vegetable broth

Two 15-ounce cans organic kidney beans, rinsed and drained

2 cups kale, diced

2 cups watercress, diced

¼ teaspoon cumin

Black pepper to taste

Broccoli sprouts

Actions:

1. Heat the oil in a large saucepan over medium-high heat. Add the onion and garlic powder and cook for 1 ½ minutes.

2. Add the remaining ingredients and cook for another 12 minutes. Season to taste with cracked black pepper.

3. Serve and top with broccoli sprouts.

Calories: 233.4 | Protein: 11.8g | Carbs: 33.6g | Dietary Fiber: 8.3g | Fat: 6.4g | Vitamin C: 19.2mg | Vitamin D: 0 IU | Vitamin E: 0.3mg | Calcium: 122.9mg | Iron: 2.3mg | Magnesium: 53.3mg | Potassium: 519.3mg

TOMATO, BASIL, AND WHITE BEAN SOUP

Total time: 10 minutes

Makes 4 servings

Ingredients:

One 14-ounce container broth

2 teaspoons chili powder

1 teaspoon ground cumin

One 16-ounce can navy beans, drained and rinsed

1 medium chili (your choice of heat), halved and seeded

1 small yellow onion

1 pint grape tomatoes

½ cup fresh basil, plus additional for garnish

¼ cup fresh cilantro

2 tablespoons fresh lime juice

1 tablespoon extra-virgin olive oil

½ teaspoon sea salt

Broccoli sprouts

Actions:

1. Combine the broth, chili powder, cumin, and beans in a medium pot over medium-high heat.

2. Meanwhile, place the chili, onion, tomatoes, basil, and cilantro in a food processor and process until smooth. Transfer the mixture to the pot and boil for 8 minutes.

3. Remove the pot from over the heat and stir in the lime juice, olive oil, and sea salt. Garnish the soup with fresh basil and broccoli sprouts.

Calories: 202.4 | Protein: 10.3g | Carbs: 36.2g | Dietary Fiber: 7.8g | Fat: 4.4g | Vitamin C: 14.9mg | Vitamin D: 0 IU | Vitamin E: 1.9mg | Calcium: 80.5mg | Iron: 3mg | Magnesium: 62mg | Potassium: 427.4mg

LENTIL SOUP

Total time: 45 minutes

Makes 4 servings

Ingredients:

5 tablespoons extra-virgin coconut oil

1 yellow onion, chopped

3 garlic cloves, chopped

½-inch piece of ginger, chopped

2 teaspoons cumin

1 teaspoon dried thyme

1 teaspoon sage

1 teaspoon oregano

1 teaspoon turmeric powder

1/8 teaspoon cayenne pepper or more to taste

1 teaspoon sea salt

¼ teaspoon black pepper

6 cups filtered water

1 ½ cups lentils

3 celery stalks, cut into ¼-inch slices

1 cup broccoli sprouts, plus additional for garnish

1 carrot, cut into ¼-inch slices

Juice of 1 lemon

4 tablespoons chopped fresh cilantro

Actions:

1. Heat the coconut oil in a large pot and add the onion and garlic. Sauté until golden brown (about 4 minutes). Add the ginger and stir-fry for 1 minute. Add the cumin, thyme, sage, oregano, and turmeric powder and stir-fry for 1 minute more. Add the cayenne pepper, sea salt, and black pepper. Stir-fry for another minute until the spices are fragrant.

2. Stir in the water, lentils, celery, broccoli sprouts, and carrot. Bring to a boil over high heat, then reduce to medium-low, cover, and simmer for 30 minutes or until the lentils are soft.

3. Stir in the lemon and cilantro. Drizzle with olive oil and sprinkle with more sea salt or cayenne pepper to taste. Top with broccoli sprouts and serve.

Tips:

- Serve with Teff Crepes (page 295).

- Serve with rice or quinoa.

- If you want a smoother, less chunky soup, puree the soup in a blender once it's cooked.

- Some lentils are smaller than others and will require less cooking time.

- For a busy lifestyle, this is a good recipe to freeze and take out the day you need it.

Variations:

- Add 2 chopped tomatoes and 1 tablespoon tomato paste when adding the water for Tomato Lentil Soup.

- Add 1 ½ tablespoons curry powder for Curry Lentil Soup.

Calories: 456.3 | Protein: 19.6g | Carbs: 53.6g | Dietary Fiber: 9.8g | Fat: 18.7g | Vitamin C: 41.9mg | Vitamin D: 0 IU | Vitamin E: 0.3mg | Calcium: 155.1mg | Iron: 7.8mg | Magnesium: 65.3mg | Potassium: 831.9mg

---

MUSHROOM SOUP

Total time: 35 minutes

Makes 4 servings

Ingredients:

4 tablespoons Vegan Butter (page 313) or coconut oil

2 yellow onions, chopped

1 pound any kind of fresh mushrooms, sliced

4 cups filtered water

2 teaspoons dill

1 tablespoon paprika

1 teaspoon sea salt

1 teaspoon thyme

1 cup almond milk

1 tablespoon diatomaceous earth

¼ teaspoon black pepper

2 teaspoons lemon juice (from ½ lemon)

¼ cup fresh parsley, chopped

Vegan Sour Cream (page 318)

Fresh squeeze of lemon

Broccoli sprouts

Actions:

1. Melt the butter in a large pot. Add the onions and sauté for 3 minutes. Add the mushrooms and sauté for another 5 minutes.

2. Stir in the water, dill, paprika, sea salt, and thyme and continue cooking.

3. Whisk the almond milk and diatomaceous earth together in a separate bowl. Pour into the soup, stirring well to blend ingredients. Cover and simmer for 15 minutes, stirring occasionally.

4. Reduce the heat to low and stir in the black pepper, lemon juice, parsley, and sour cream. Mix together and allow to cook for another 5 minutes. Serve with broccoli sprouts.

Tips:

*   If you want a smoother, less chunky soup, puree the soup in a blender once it's cooked.

*   Serve over quinoa.

Calories: 249.9 | Protein: 6g | Carbs: 13.8g | Dietary Fiber: 3.7g | Fat: 20.3g | Vitamin C: 5.4mg | Vitamin D: 3.4 IU | Vitamin E: 0.7mg | Calcium: 88.1mg | Iron: 1.8mg | Magnesium: 52.6mg | Potassium: 726.3mg

---

GROUNDING VEGETABLE POTATO SOUP

Total time: 2 hours

Makes 4 servings

Ingredients:

1 yellow onion

2 large potatoes

2 large carrots

2 celery stalks

1 pound pumpkin or sweet potato

½ head of broccoli

2 zucchinis

1 tablespoon extra-virgin olive oil

6 garlic cloves, crushed

5 cups filtered water

½ tablespoon sea salt

1 tablespoon fresh sage or 1 teaspoon dried sage

Broccoli sprouts

Actions:

1. Dice the onion, potatoes, carrots, celery, pumpkin, broccoli, and zucchini into ½-inch cubes and set aside.

2. Heat the olive oil in a large saucepan over medium heat. Add the onions, celery, and garlic, and sauté until the onions become translucent.

3. Add the remainder of the diced vegetables to the saucepan, along with the water, sea salt, and sage, and bring to a boil. Simmer over medium heat for 90 minutes until the vegetables are broken down.

4. Season with additional sea salt and pepper to taste, and top with broccoli sprouts.

Tip:

For more protein, add 2 cups dried beans of any kind (soaked for at least 12 hours).

Calories: 281.8 | Protein: 9.3g | Carbs: 55.9g | Dietary Fiber: 9.1g | Fat: 4.5g | Vitamin C: 138mg | Vitamin D: 0 IU | Vitamin E: 2.6mg | Calcium: 143.5mg | Iron: 3.6mg | Magnesium: 103.8mg | Potassium: 1,892mg

---

BASIC BONE BROTH

Making bone broth is as simple as placing the bones from a grass-fed animal in a pot or slow cooker, and adding water and apple cider vinegar. The vinegar leaches the minerals out of the bones, which takes at least an hour. It is recommended to cook the bones longer, more like eight hours, to get the most minerals out of the bones.

If you are pressed for time, you can add some bone broth powder (like Ancient Nutrition Bone Broth Protein Pure) to water and boil that for a superquick recipe.

If bone broth doesn't sound appealing to you, don't force yourself to like it. Some people resonate with it and others don't. Trust your body, and if you are curious or excited to try it, that is a strong indicator that it would be right for your body. The process for creating a bone broth is:

1. Add bones to a crock pot or pot. Add filtered water to fully cover the bones.

2. Add apple cider vinegar.

3. Add vegetables and bring to a boil, then reduce the heat to low. The skin from the bones will float to the top. Once the broth is cooked, discard.

VEGETABLE BROTH

You can make your vegetable broth in double and triple batches and keep it in the fridge or in the freezer, so you always have it on hand for recipes.

Total time: 10 minutes

Makes 4 servings

Ingredients:

4 cups filtered water

1 tablespoon onion powder

1 tablespoon garlic powder

1 tablespoon celery powder

1 tablespoon coriander powder

1 tablespoon fresh parsley

1 tablespoon fresh thyme

2 bay leaves

1 teaspoon sea salt

¼ teaspoon black pepper

Actions:

1. Place all the ingredients in a large pot over high heat and bring to a boil. Allow to boil for 8 minutes.

2. When cooled, transfer the broth to an airtight jar or container and store in the fridge or freezer. Unlike a bone broth, vegetable broth will store in the fridge for up to 14 days.

Calories: 27.9 | Protein: 1.1g | Carbs: 4.7g | Dietary Fiber: 1.8g | Fat: 0.6g | Vitamin C: 2.7mg | Vitamin D: 0 IU | Vitamin E: 0.03mg | Calcium: 54.5mg | Iron: 1.1mg | Magnesium: 8mg | Potassium: 56.8mg

CHICKEN BONE BROTH

When making bone broth, you're allowing the collagen to leak out of the bones and form an incredibly nutrient-rich broth that is an anti-inflammatory, helps heal leaky gut, and helps to clear chemo brain.

Total time: 30 minutes prep, 24 hours cooking

Makes 9 cups

Ingredients:

Bones from 2 chickens (approx. 2 ½ pounds of chicken bones)

2 tablespoons apple cider vinegar

1 teaspoon sea salt

1 teaspoon turmeric

½ teaspoon black pepper

½-inch piece of ginger root, peeled and chopped

1 medium onion, peeled and quartered

½ head of broccoli, chopped into chunks

2 celery stalks, cut into thirds

2 carrots, peeled and halved

2 garlic cloves, smashed

1 bay leaf

2 rosemary sprigs

1 tablespoon dried oregano or oregano essential oil

20 cups filtered water

Actions:

1. Add all ingredients to a large pot and bring to a boil. Once the liquid is boiling vigorously, lower the heat, cover, and simmer for 24 hours.

2. Check the broth every few hours and stir.

3. You will know it's cooked when you poke the bones with a fork and they fall apart and break. When cooked, strain the broth through mesh so you are left with just the liquid. Discard the solids.

Tips:

- You can also put the ingredients into a slow cooker and let the broth cook for 8 to 12 hours.

- Some people like to roast their chicken bones before boiling them for a smoky flavor. You can also buy two organic rotisserie chickens instead of roasting your own.

- If you store chicken broth in the fridge, it will set hard, which is a good sign that the marrow nutrients came out of the bones. It will go to liquid again once heated.

- Store in the fridge for up to 6 days or in the freezer for up to 4 months. If freezing, just allow extra room in the container or jar as it will expand when frozen.

Variation:

Use beef bones for Beef Bone Broth.

Calories: 26.8 | Protein: 1.4g | Carbs: 5.7g | Dietary Fiber: 1.8g | Fat: 0.2g | Vitamin C: 32.3mg | Vitamin D: 0 IU | Vitamin E: 0.4mg | Calcium: 50.5mg | Iron: 0.6mg | Magnesium: 18.2mg | Potassium: 209.5mg

CHAPTER 16

STRENGTH-BUILDING MEALS FOR FISH AND MEAT EATERS

Whether or not you choose to have fish and meat in your healing protocol is entirely up to you. Go deep within and ask yourself if it feels right to have animal protein in your diet, or not. And if so, how much? For me, it felt right to include fish or meat around every third day or a few times a week. For others, especially those with blood type O, they tend to feel better if they eat meat once a day. Others thrive on being vegetarian and vegan. It really is a personal choice, and no one should pressure you into eating meat or giving up meat if it doesn't feel right for you.

This chapter features recipes for people who want to include fish and meat in their diet, or who have been advised they need it in their healing regimen. Just make sure your meat always comes from a good source, a farm you trust or that is grass-fed and organic. I interviewed patients who did only vegan and then some who incorporated some meat during their healing period and that worked for them.

The indigenous people also want us to know that when they killed an animal, they did it with intention—an intention to nourish and strengthen their bodies. They thanked the animal for its sacrifice. I believe they hunted in an incredibly admirable and sustainable way that worked well to support their health and the environment. Then grateful, they would enjoy the meat and let its nutrients seep into their muscles over the next few days, really allowing that protein to work in their body. Once they felt like they had used it all up, they would prepare to go and hunt again.

If we could adapt a similar philosophy in our modern society today, we would all eat meat only when we really need to, as well as get the most out of the spirit of the animal and the protein it provided.

If you are healing cancer, this is the best type of meat that can go through your body:

- Organic
- Grass-fed
- Non-GMO
- Local from a farm you trust
- Wild-caught

GRASS-FED BEEF BURRITOS

Total time: 25 minutes

Makes 6 servings (1 burrito each)

Ingredients:

2 tablespoons extra-virgin olive oil

½ teaspoon turmeric powder

¼ teaspoon black pepper

1 pound ground grass-fed beef

1 small yellow onion, chopped

2 large garlic cloves, diced

1 ½ teaspoons ground cumin

½ teaspoon turmeric powder

¼ teaspoon sea salt

¼ teaspoon pepper

1 teaspoon chili powder or ¼ teaspoon cayenne pepper, optional (if you want it a little spicy)

6 brown rice tortillas/wraps or Quick Bread (page 294)

Fillings of your choice:

¾ cup Vegan Sour Cream
(page 318)

1 cup nutritional yeast

½ cup grated carrot

Diced lettuce

1 avocado, cubed

1 pepper, diced

Fresh cilantro, chopped

Broccoli sprouts

16 ounces black beans (soaked, cooked, soft)

Actions:

1. Heat a large frying pan with oil over medium heat. Add the turmeric and black pepper. Sauté for 1 minute or until sizzling. Add the beef and cook for 3 to 4 minutes or until it turns brown, stirring frequently.

2. Add the onion, garlic, cumin, turmeric powder, sea salt, pepper, and chili powder, if using, to the meat and stir. Cook for 7 minutes or until the vegetables are tender and the flavors are well combined.

3. Place ¼ cup of meat into each tortilla and then add your fillings of choice.

Tips:

- If you want to take it a step further, heat the oven to 375°F, fully assemble your burrito and then place on parchment paper and bake for 12 minutes, until the burritos have turned golden brown.

- Add ¼ cup Raw Tomato Sauce (page 311) to the beef.

Variations:

- Use chicken for Chicken Burritos.

- Use fish for Fish Burritos.

- Use beans and Vegetable Stir-Fry for Veggie Burritos.

Calories: 353.5 | Protein: 17.1g | Carbs: 26.3g | Dietary Fiber: 0.5g | Fat: 19.2g | Vitamin C: 1.1mg | Vitamin D: 0 IU | Vitamin E: 1mg | Calcium: 23.5mg | Iron: 3mg | Magnesium: 17.5mg | Potassium: 366.8mg

GRASS-FED BEEF BURGERS

Total time: 20 minutes

Makes 4 servings

Ingredients:

1 pound ground grass-fed beef

2 eggs, beaten

1 cup almond meal

1 tablespoon fresh sage or 1 teaspoon dried sage

1 teaspoon sea salt

1 teaspoon turmeric powder

½ teaspoon black pepper

¼ cup extra-virgin coconut oil

Actions:

1. Place all the ingredients, except the coconut oil, in a bowl. Mix until thoroughly combined.

2. Form 4 patties by hand.

3. Heat a large frying pan with the coconut oil over medium heat. When the pan is hot, place the patties in it.

4. Allow the patties to cook until the undersides have browned, then flip over. Cook until desired doneness is achieved.

Tips:

- Serve with lettuce as the wrap, or on Gluten-Free Rolls (page 294).

- Top with Ketchup (page 318).

Calories: 543.3 | Protein: 31.2g | Carbs: 6.8g | Dietary Fiber: 3.2g | Fat: 43.8g | Vitamin C: 0mg | Vitamin D: 20.5 IU | Vitamin E: 7.7mg | Calcium: 92.8mg | Iron: 4.1mg | Magnesium: 106.9mg | Potassium: 379.4 mg

---

MEATBALLS

These make a great quick protein snack on their own, or you can add them to pasta, pizza, salad, or soup.

Total time: 10 minutes

Makes 4 servings

Ingredients:

2 tablespoons extra-virgin coconut oil

2 eggs

1 pound ground grass-fed beef

1 teaspoon sea salt

½ teaspoon pepper

1 teaspoon cumin

½ teaspoon dried sage

½ teaspoon dried oregano

½ teaspoon dried parsley

¼ teaspoon turmeric

Actions:

1. Heat the oil in a fry pan over medium heat. Meanwhile, beat the eggs in a bowl and add the ground beef. Use your hands to combine the ingredients.

2. Add the spices and mix until well combined. Roll the meat mixture into balls.

3. Add the meatballs to the fry pan and cook for 8 minutes or until done.

Tip:

Serve with Raw Tomato Sauce (page 311).

Calories: 324 | Protein: 25.3g | Carbs: 0.7g | Dietary Fiber: 0.3g | Fat: 23.4g | Vitamin C: 0.09mg | Vitamin D: 20.5 IU | Vitamin E: 0.7mg | Calcium: 35.1mg | Iron: 2.9mg | Magnesium: 25.9mg | Potassium: 372.1mg

ALMOND TURMERIC CRUSTED CHICKEN TENDERS

This recipe is absolutely divine, the crunch and crispiness with the soft succulent meat can win anyone over to the "healthier" side. Unlike the toxic conventional version, a crust of turmeric and black pepper make it anti-inflammatory and anticancer—a major upgrade for when you want to enjoy chicken tenders!

Total time: 30 minutes

Makes 4 servings

Ingredients:

1 cup whole almonds

2 tablespoons turmeric powder

1 teaspoon sea salt

¼ teaspoon black pepper

1 pound boneless, skinless chicken breasts

2 eggs

¾ cup extra-virgin coconut oil

Broccoli sprouts

Actions:

1. Place the almonds, turmeric powder, salt, and pepper in a blender and blend until the mixture has the consistency of a fine flour meal. Some chunks are okay. Transfer the mixture to a plate.

2. Cut the chicken breast into tender slices or nugget-size pieces.

3. Crack the eggs into a bowl and whisk with a fork.

4. Dip the chicken in the egg, coating well.

5. Dredge the chicken in the flour meal, coating well on all sides.

6. Heat the coconut oil in a frying pan over medium heat. When the oil is hot, carefully place the chicken pieces in the pan 1 by 1. Let 1 side of the chicken cook until golden brown and crispy. Flip the chicken and cook the other side.

7. Carefully remove the chicken from the pan. Place on a paper towel to absorb the excess oil if you like, then serve with a sprinkle of broccoli sprouts.

Tip:

Serve with Coconut Basil Sweet Potato Fries (page 233) and Five-Ingredient Green Salad (page 244).

Variation:

For extra heat, add 1 tablespoon cayenne pepper to the flour meal mixture for Spicy Chicken Tenders.

Calories: 749.4 | Protein: 36.5g | Carbs: 10g | Dietary Fiber: 5.2g | Fat: 62.3g | Vitamin C: 0.02mg | Vitamin D: 21.6 IU | Vitamin E: 10.2mg | Calcium: 122mg | Iron: 4mg | Magnesium: 138.3mg | Potassium: 745.8mg

WHOLESOME SAGE FISH

Total time: 15 minutes

Makes 1 serving

Ingredients:

1 tablespoon extra-virgin coconut oil

1 piece of fish, such as tuna steak, swordfish steak, salmon steak, or fillet just less than ½-inch thick

1 ½ teaspoons dried sage, divided

Juice from 1 lemon, divided

Sea salt and ground black pepper, to taste

Broccoli sprouts

Actions:

1. Heat the coconut oil in a frying pan over medium heat. Add the fish.

2. While the fish is cooking, sprinkle ½ of the sage and ½ of the lemon juice over the fish.

3. Once you see that ½ of the fish is turning from raw to white from the bottom up, turn the fish over. Sprinkle the remainder of the sage over the fish and cook through.

4. Transfer the fish to a plate. Squeeze the remaining lemon juice onto the fish. Season with sea salt and pepper to taste, and garnish with broccoli sprouts.

Tip:

Serve with Five-Ingredient Green Salad (page 244), or Mashed Potatoes (page 240).

Variations:

- Add 2 teaspoons garlic powder instead of sage for Simple Garlic Fish.

- Add ½ teaspoon thyme and oregano for Simple Herb Fish.

- Add a dash of cayenne pepper on each side for Simple Spicy Fish.

Calories: 336.3 | Protein: 22.8g | Carbs: 3.7g | Dietary Fiber: 05g | Fat: 25g | Vitamin C: 22.2mg | Vitamin D: 0 IU | Vitamin E: 1.4mg | Calcium: 32.2mg | Iron: 0.3mg | Magnesium: 110.4mg | Potassium: 493.9mg

SAUTÉED SCALLOPS

Scallops are great for blood cancers because they are high in B12, magnesium, and potassium, which relaxes blood vessels, lowers blood pressure, improves circulation, improves your mood, and provides a very lean source of protein with more than 80 nutrients.

Total time: 10 minutes

Makes 2 servings

Ingredients:

1 tablespoon chicken broth or vegetable broth

½ pound scallops

1 ½ teaspoons minced garlic

2 tablespoons olive oil

1 tablespoon lemon juice

Sea salt and pepper, to taste

Fresh or dried dill

Broccoli sprouts

Actions:

1. Heat the broth in a pan over medium heat. When it is steaming, add the scallops and garlic and sauté for 1 ½ minutes. Turn the scallops over and cook on the other side for 1 ½ minutes.

2. Remove from the heat. Serve the scallops dressed with olive oil, lemon, sea salt, pepper, and dill, and a sprinkle of broccoli sprouts.

Tip:

For larger scallops, you may have to cook for an additional minute. Don't cook them for too long, however, as they can get tough.

Calories: 209.4 | Protein: 13.8g | Carbs: 4.8g | Dietary Fiber: 0.07g | Fat: 14.5g | Vitamin C: 3.6mg | Vitamin D: 1.1 IU | Vitamin E: 1.7mg | Calcium: 11.1mg | Iron: 0.4mg | Magnesium: 25.9mg | Potassium: 248.8mg

BAKED WALNUT-CRUSTED SALMON

Total time: 35 minutes

Makes 4 servings

Ingredients:

1 cup walnuts, blended to a meal

1 teaspoon sage

½ teaspoon sea salt

1 teaspoon thyme

1 egg

1 ½ pounds of skinless salmon, cut into 4 pieces

Broccoli sprouts

Actions:

1. Preheat the oven to 380°F.

2. Prepare a baking sheet with parchment paper or thin coating of coconut oil.

3. Mix the walnut meal, sage, sea salt, and thyme in a bowl. Beat the egg in a separate bowl and dip each salmon fillet into the egg. Press each fillet into the walnut mixture to coat on both sides. Place the salmon on the baking sheet.

4. Bake for 7 minutes. Turn the salmon over and bake for another 7 minutes, or to your desired doneness.

5. Serve with a sprinkle of broccoli sprouts.

Tips:

- Serve the salmon with roasted potatoes, Five-Ingredient Green Salad (page 244), and/or Mashed Potatoes (page 240).

- To make this recipe without the egg, brush the salmon with oil instead and then dip it into the walnut mixture.

- For fewer calories, place the salmon on the baking sheet, sprinkle your desired amount of walnut mixture on top, and bake.

Variations:

- Sprinkle with mustard seeds before serving for Honey Mustard Baked Walnut-Crusted Salmon.

- Drizzle with honey once cooked for Sweet Baked Walnut-Crusted Salmon.

- For a fried version, heat a frying pan with extra-virgin coconut oil and cook for Fried Walnut-Crusted Salmon.

- Use almonds, pecans, Brazil nuts, or macadamia nuts instead of the walnuts.

- For a nut-free version, use ground hemp seeds, sunflower seeds, or pumpkin seeds instead of the walnuts.

Calories: 514.8 | Protein: 39.9g | Carbs: 4.3g | Dietary Fiber: 2.1g | Fat: 38g | Vitamin C: 7.3mg | Vitamin D: 10.2 IU | Vitamin E: 2.4mg | Calcium: 84.6mg | Iron: 1.8mg | Magnesium: 209.8mg | Potassium: 818.4mg

CHAPTER 17

FUN SIDES AND SAVORY SNACKS

Quick and easy sides and snacks can be incredibly useful, especially if you have cancer that is making you lack energy or motivation. If you always have some healthy, nourishing, delicious snacks on standby it may just uplift your mood right away knowing they are there.

A snack or a side dish can also become a meal! Enjoy the following recipes.

CANCER'S GONE CRACKERS

Total time: 20 minutes to assemble, 12 hours to set in refrigerator, and 15 to 20 hours to dehydrate

Makes 20 servings (4 crackers each)

Ingredients:

3 cups ground flaxseeds

1 cup sunflower seeds

2 tablespoons minced onion or 3 tablespoons onion powder

2 tablespoons sesame seeds

1 tablespoon minced garlic or 2 tablespoons garlic powder

2 teaspoons cumin powder

1 teaspoon chili powder

1 teaspoon sea salt

1 teaspoon cayenne pepper

½ teaspoon turmeric

½ cup filtered water

Actions:

1. Put all the dry ingredients in the bowl of a food processor and blend until a fine, flourlike consistency is achieved.

2. Add the water and mix until a batter forms. Cover and allow the batter to set in the fridge for 12 hours.

3. Spread a 1/8-inch layer of batter on nonstick dehydrator sheets and dehydrate at 100°F for 15 to 20 hours. (Use a dehydrator kitchen appliance, or for an oven alternative see Tips below.)

4. Cut or break the cracker sheet into pieces the size of your choice and store in an airtight container at room temperature or in the fridge for up to 8 weeks.

Tips:

- For an oven alternative to using a dehydrator, spread a layer of batter on nonstick baking paper or a baking sheet lightly greased with coconut oil and place in the oven at 180°F for 2 to 4 hours. The batter becomes a base when it is crisp and dry; check frequently. Cut into cracker squares.

- Serve these crackers with Hummus (page 298), Tahini (page 317), Pesto Sauce (page 212), and/or Cashew Cheese (page 303).

- This can be the base of the Raw Pizza (page 214) as well as Raw Tacos (page 246).

Calories: 138.7 | Protein: 4.8g | Carbs: 6.9g | Dietary Fiber: 5.4g | Fat: 11.2g | Vitamin C: 0.4mg | Vitamin D: 0 IU | Vitamin E: 2.6mg | Calcium: 61.7mg | Iron: 1.7mg | Magnesium: 92.4mg | Potassium: 200mg

GLUTEN-FREE TORTILLAS

Total time: 15 minutes

Makes 6 servings

Ingredients:

1 ½ cups rice flour

½ cup tigernut flour

1 cups buckwheat flour

1 cup warm filtered water

2 teaspoons apple cider vinegar

1 tablespoon Flax Egg Alternative (page 315)

Actions:

1. Combine the rice, tigernut, and buckwheat flours in a large bowl. Slowly add the water and vinegar, stirring constantly to combine. Add the Flax Egg Alternative, mixing well to form the dough.

2. Knead the dough for 2 minutes until it feels tougher and form into a ball.

3. Roll out the ball of dough with a rolling pin to make six 6-inch circles (1/3 cup of dough each).

4. Heat a cast-iron pan on the stove over medium heat. Place the dough circles in the hot pan. Cover the pan while the dough cooks. (This is important for the softness of the tortillas.) Cook for 1 to 2 minutes on each side until there is no more soft dough.

5. Once the tortillas are ready, transfer them to a plate and cover with a clean dish towel or cotton napkin to keep them soft. They are best eaten the day they're made.

Tips:

- Add 1 teaspoon sea salt for enhanced flavor.
- These can be used as wraps, sliced into pieces and dipped into hummus, or used as a pizza base.
- Add a dash of cayenne pepper to make them spicy.

Variation:

Add 1 teaspoon cayenne pepper for Spicy Quick Bread.

Calories: 248.8 | Protein: 6.8g | Carbs: 51.8g | Dietary Fiber: 5.1g | Fat: 2.3g | Vitamin C: 0mg | Vitamin D: 0 IU | Vitamin E: 0.3mg | Calcium: 20.1mg | Iron: 2mg | Magnesium: 119.9mg | Potassium: 288.4mg

---

TEFF CREPES

Made with teff, these are gluten-free. To make sweet dessert crepes, just add some maple syrup to the batter. Use as a savory side or substitute instead of bread, and fill with your favorite fillings such as beans, quinoa, Turmeric Hummus (see page 298), and/or Chickpea Fries (page 302)!

Total time: 10 minutes prep, 30 minutes to set, 16 minutes to cook

Makes 8 crepes

Ingredients:

1 cup teff flour

1 cup almond milk (Note: If the almond milk has vanilla in it, the result will taste more like a dessert crepe.)

¼ cup filtered water

3 eggs

2 tablespoons olive oil, MCT oil, or coconut oil

¼ teaspoon sea salt

Coconut oil, for frying

Actions:

1. Add all the ingredients to a blender and mix until smooth and well combined. Let the batter sit for at least 30 minutes, or set in the fridge overnight.

2. Add ½ teaspoon coconut oil to a fry pan. When the oil is hot and melted over the entire surface of the pan, pour in the batter. Cook, one crepe at a time, for 2 minutes or until the batter starts to bubble, then turn over. Cook for another 2 minutes, then serve.

Tip:

Add more water or almond milk for a thinner crepe and less for a thicker crepe.

Variations:

To make a Dessert Crepe, add 1 teaspoon vanilla extract, 1 tablespoon maple syrup, and spices like cinnamon, cardamom, and orange zest.

Calories: 167.7 | Protein: 5.8g | Carbs: 15.6g | Dietary Fiber: 3g | Fat: 9.2g | Vitamin C: 0mg | Vitamin D: 15.3 IU | Vitamin E: 0.6mg | Calcium: 53.6mg | Iron: 1.8mg | Magnesium: 14.6mg | Potassium: 58.7mg

COCONUT WRAPS

These are raw coconut tortillas. They can be used in desserts by adding a filling like Instant Ice Cream (page 330), fresh berries, or Whipped Coconut Cream (page 342), or for a savory dish like a burrito or spring roll. To make the Coconut Wraps sweet, add 2 tablespoons maple syrup to the mixture.

Total time: 15 minutes prep, 16 hours to dehydrate

Makes 2 servings (1 wrap each)

Ingredients:

2 cups raw coconut meat (from young coconuts or green coconuts), about 4 to 6 coconuts

1 tablespoon coconut water (when you open the coconut)

¼ teaspoon sea salt

Actions:

1. Add the coconut meat, coconut water, and sea salt to a food processor and process until the mixture is completely smooth. If it is too dry, add more coconut water, up to another tablespoon.
2. Spread the coconut batter to ¼-inch thickness on a dehydrator sheet (or baking paper).
3. Dehydrate the batter at 105°F for 8 to 9 hours. At the 8-hour mark the top will be dry and solid. Turn the batter over and dehydrate for another 8 to 9 hours.

VARIATIONS:

Add 1 teaspoon turmeric powder for Turmeric Coconut Wraps.

Calories: 284.6 | Protein: 2.7g | Carbs: 12.4g | Dietary Fiber: 7.2g | Fat: 26.8g | Vitamin C: 2.8mg | Vitamin D: 0 IU | Vitamin E: 0.1mg | Calcium: 13mg | Iron: 1.9mg | Magnesium: 27.4mg | Potassium: 303.5mg

---

GUACAMOLE

This recipe is a great go-to. Guacamole is so simple to make, and it can be a satisfying meal in itself. Just add some tomatoes, carrot sticks, celery, or other vegetables.

Total time: 5 minutes

Makes 1 serving

Ingredients:

1 avocado

¼ teaspoon sea salt

¼ teaspoon black pepper

Juice of ½ lemon

Actions:

1. Mash the avocado in a bowl with a fork.
2. Blend in the other ingredients.

Tips:

- Eat with carrot sticks.
- Eat with cucumber sticks.
- Add ½ small purple onion, diced.
- Add ½ small bell pepper, any color, diced.

Variation:

Add diced broccoli sprouts to the guacamole for Broccoli Sprout Guacamole.

Calories: 328 | Protein: 4.1g | Carbs: 19g | Dietary Fiber: 13.6g | Fat: 29.5g | Vitamin C: 28.9mg | Vitamin D: 0 IU | Vitamin E: 4.2mg | Calcium: 28mg | Iron: 1.1mg | Magnesium: 60.6mg | Potassium: 1,006mg

---

TURMERIC HUMMUS

Total time: 10 minutes

Makes 4 servings

Ingredients:

One 14-ounce can chickpeas

¼ cup aquafaba (water from the can of chickpeas)

2 tablespoons garlic salt

1 ½ tablespoons lemon juice

1 ½ tablespoons sesame seeds

1 ½ tablespoons turmeric powder

1 tablespoon sesame seed oil

1 tablespoon flax oil, extra-virgin olive oil, or tigernut oil

½ teaspoon sea salt

Actions:

Combine all ingredients in a food processor and process until smooth.

Tips:

- Serve with carrots, green beans, and cucumber sticks.
- Goes great with Quick Bread (page 294) and Raw Crackers (page 293).
- As an alternative to chickpeas, use almonds, sunflower seeds, or hemp seeds.

Variation:

Hummus makes a great salad dressing. It can be thinned by mixing in lemon juice and some olive oil. Or leave it as is and massage it into kale or lettuce for a thicker, creamier dressing.

Calories: 194.1 | Protein: 6.2g | Carbs: 21.9g | Dietary Fiber: 5.4g | Fat: 10.3g | Vitamin C: 2.3mg | Vitamin D: 0 IU | Vitamin E: 0.3mg | Calcium: 69.5mg | Iron: 2.8mg | Magnesium: 36.1mg | Potassium: 197.8mg

HUMMUS-STUFFED PEPPERS

Total time: 10 minutes

Makes 1 serving

Ingredients:

1 bell pepper, any color

¾ cup Turmeric Hummus (page 298)

Paprika or cayenne pepper, to taste

Actions:

1. Cut the bell pepper in half and scoop out the seeds.
2. Stuff each pepper half with hummus. Sprinkle with fresh spices like paprika and cayenne pepper.

Tip:

Use carrot or celery sticks to scoop out the dip.

Variation:

For a change of pace, stuff an avocado instead of a bell pepper. Stuff everything! Haha—just kidding.

Calories: 615 | Protein: 20g | Carbs: 71g | Dietary Fiber: 18.9g | Fat: 31.9g | Vitamin C: 138.9mg | Vitamin D: 0 IU | Vitamin E: 1.6mg | Calcium: 224.9mg | Iron: 9mg | Magnesium: 124.8mg | Potassium: 880.5mg

---

STUFFED OLIVES

This is an incredibly easy recipe, and it's delicious, packed with flavor and nutrition including iron, vitamin E, and fiber. You could also stuff each olive with half of a roasted garlic clove. Make sure to always buy organic olives, as regular olives are loaded with preservatives such as sodium benzoate and sulfites. If you buy already stuffed olives, they can contain sodium alginate, which is also a lethal preservative.

Total time: 10 minutes

Makes 4 servings

INGREDIENTS:

2 cups fresh olives, pitted

1 red pepper, diced

Actions:

Place the olives on a sheet or plate and simply insert a piece of pepper inside each olive.

Calories: 74.9 | Protein: 0.8g | Carbs: 1.7g | Dietary Fiber: 0.6g | Fat: 7.1g | Vitamin C: 37.9mg | Vitamin D: 0 IU | Vitamin E: 1.7mg | Calcium: 40.9mg | Iron: 0.7mg | Magnesium: 17.6mg | Potassium: 120.8mg

FERMENTED VEGETABLES

This food-preserving technique, which has been used for hundreds of years, has many health benefits. Fermented vegetables are a natural probiotic! They can also boost immunity. You can eat them on their own or add them to soups, salads, and main dishes. You can make all types of blends using ingredients like cabbage, beets, cauliflower, cucumbers, carrots, peppers, and onions. One of the most famous fermented dishes is sauerkraut, which is fermented cabbage.

The process of fermenting a vegetable is:

1. Chop the vegetables into tiny pieces, which allows their liquids to release faster.
2. Mix the vegetables with sea salt and herbs like thyme and oregano in a bowl.
3. Add water and then transfer the vegetables to a jar. The water should cover the vegetables by at least ½ inch.
4. Keep at room temperature for 3 to 5 days, and then in the refrigerator indefinitely. This is surprising, but fermented vegetables truly do last for years.

PROBIOTIC PICKLED CUCUMBERS

Total time: 5 minutes preparation and 3–5 days fermenting

Serves 5

Ingredients:

5 cucumbers

2 teaspoons mustard seeds

1 tablespoon dill

1 tablespoon sea salt

1 cup filtered water, room temperature

Actions:

1. Place 5 whole cucumbers in a quart-size jar. Add the remaining ingredients. The water should cover the cucumbers completely, and the top of the liquid should be at least ½ inch below the top of the jar.

2. Cover tightly and store at room temperature for 3 to 5 days before refrigerating. The pickles will keep indefinitely.

3. Serve with salads and meat meals, or mix into stir-fries!

Calories: 65 | Protein: 2.8g | Carbs: 14g | Dietary Fiber: 2g | Fat: 1g | Vitamin C: 10.7mg | Vitamin D: 0 IU | Vitamin E: 0.2mg | Calcium: 66.7mg | Iron: 1.2mg | Magnesium: 55.7mg | Potassium: 566.4mg

SIMPLE STEAMED ARTICHOKES

Total time: 40 minutes

Makes 3 servings

Ingredients:

1 lemon

2 teaspoons sea salt

3 whole artichokes

Actions:

1. Fill a large pot ¾ full of water, adding the juice of 1 lemon and 2 teaspoons salt. Bring to a boil.

2. Place the artichokes in a steamer tray inside the pot, stem side up. Cover the pot and steam the artichokes until the hearts are tender and the inner leaves pull out easily. This will take about 25 to 35 minutes.

3. Remove the artichokes from the heat and serve.

Calories: 79.5 | Protein: 5.3g | Carbs: 18g | Dietary Fiber: 8.7g | Fat: 0.2g | Vitamin C: 24.8mg | Vitamin D: 0 IU | Vitamin E: 0.3mg | Calcium: 72.1mg | Iron: 2mg | Magnesium: 98.1mg | Potassium: 615.1mg

CHICKPEA FRIES

Chickpea Fries are an excellent snack eaten hot or cold. You can take them to lunch the next day or even add them to soups and salads.

Total time: 10 minutes

Makes 1 to 2 servings

Ingredients:

1 tablespoon extra-virgin olive oil

One 14-ounce can organic chickpeas, drained of liquid

¼ teaspoon sea salt

Pepper, to taste

Actions:

1. Heat a fry pan with oil over medium heat. When hot, add the chickpeas.

2. Sprinkle with salt and pepper, then cook for 5 to 7 minutes or until the chickpeas are golden brown on the outside.

Variations:

Top your Chickpea Fries with any of the following:

- A squeeze of lemon.
- A sprinkle of dried rosemary.
- A sprinkle of dried thyme.
- A sprinkle of dried cayenne pepper or paprika.
- A sprinkle of dried cumin.
- A sprinkle of dried curry.

Calories: 238.2 | Protein: 8.9g | Carbs: 29g | Dietary Fiber: 8g | Fat: 10.1g | Vitamin C: 0.1mg | Vitamin D: 0 IU | Vitamin E: 1.2mg | Calcium: 54.6mg | Iron: 1.2mg | Magnesium: 30.4mg | Potassium: 138.4mg

CASHEW CHEESE

Serve on Raw Tacos (page 246), in Raw Lasagna (page 211), or on lettuce for Lettuce Wraps.

Total time: 10 minutes

Makes 1 serving (¼ cup each)

Ingredients:

2 cups cashews

2 tablespoons nutritional yeast

Juice of 1 small lemon (but no more than ¼ cup)

½ teaspoon sea salt

½ cup filtered water (more for a softer cheese)

Actions:

1. Put all the ingredients in a food processor.

2. Blend until the mixture is smooth, adding more water if a softer cheese is desired.

Tips:

- Soak the cashews for 4 hours for a smoother, creamier cheese.
- For a nut-free version, use hempseeds, pumpkin seeds, or sunflower seeds instead of cashews.
- This recipe also works well with almonds, macadamia nuts, walnuts, or Brazil nuts.
- For a cheesier flavor, add more nutritional yeast, to taste. You can also make this recipe without nutritional yeast.
- Add a dash of cayenne pepper or chili flakes for spice.
- Add 1 teaspoon thyme for more flavor.

Variations:

- To make Raw "Parmesan" Cheese, add additional 3 tablespoons nutritional yeast to the mixture and spread to ¼-inch thick on a dehydrator tray. Place in a food dehydrator for 12 hours. It will crumble easily when you're ready to use it.
- Add 1 garlic clove or more for Garlic Cashew Cheese.
- Add 1 cup fresh basil leaves for Pesto Cashew Cheese.

Calories: 369.5 | Protein: 12.8g | Carbs: 21g | Dietary Fiber: 2.5g | Fat: 28.6g | Vitamin C: 4.7mg | Vitamin D: 0 IU | Vitamin E: 0.6mg | Calcium: 26.4mg | Iron: 4.4mg | Magnesium: 193.7mg | Potassium: 474.1mg

HARD VEGAN CHEESE

This recipe can make eliminating dairy cheese from your diet much easier! It sets hard, like regular cheese, and comforts you during the cheese craving time. To make the cheese set hard, an ingredient called agar is used. This is a naturally gelatinous substance obtained from seaweed.

Total time: Overnight soaking, 15 minutes prep, 1 hour in fridge

Serves 4

Ingredients:

¾ cup cashews

1 ½ teaspoon agar powder

1 cup filtered water, divided

1 tablespoon nutritional yeast

1 garlic clove

1 ½ teaspoons arrowroot flour or tapioca flour

⅛ teaspoon sea salt

2 tablespoons plus 1 teaspoon lemon juice

¼ teaspoon turmeric powder

Actions:

1. Soak the cashews in filtered water overnight.

2. Mix the agar with ½ cup of filtered water in a saucepan. Do not apply heat yet; set aside.

3. Drain the cashews, then add them to a food processor with the nutritional yeast, garlic, arrowroot, sea salt, lemon juice, turmeric, and the remaining ½ cup of filtered water. Blend until the mixture is very smooth.

4. Add the cashew cheese to the agar pot and bring to a boil over low heat until it forms a thick batter consistency.

5. Transfer the mixture to a dish that you want the shape of your cheese to be in. You could divide it into cupcake holders, for example. Refrigerate the cheese for 1 hour and then enjoy.

Calories: 148.7 | Protein: 5.1g | Carbs: 10.2g | Dietary Fiber: 1.1g | Fat: 10.7g | Vitamin C: 3.8mg | Vitamin D: 0 IU | Vitamin E: 0.2mg | Calcium: 18.7mg | Iron: 2mg | Magnesium: 74.2mg | Potassium: 203.9mg

---

BAKED KALE CHIPS

Purchasing prewashed and precut kale will save you a lot of time. Simply season the kale and bake it in the oven.

Total time: 10 minutes

Makes 2 servings

Ingredients:

1 packet or bunch of prewashed, precut kale

1 tablespoon extra-virgin olive oil

1 teaspoon sea salt

Actions:

1. Preheat the oven to 400°F. Line a baking sheet with parchment paper. Lining with paper instead of oil will ensure faster bake time.

2. Add the kale to a bowl along with the oil and sea salt and massage until the leaves are well covered.

3. Bake for 9 minutes or until the edges of the kale are brown and crisp. They will dry out given time to rest after baking. Store in a dry place if you don't eat them all at once!

Tips:

*   If you begin with a bunch of whole kale, wash it and drain the water well. You don't want the kale to be wet when baking, which will result in soggy chips. Use a paper towel to take out the excess water. Tear the leaves from the stems in as big pieces as possible, keeping in mind the chips shrink as they bake. Discard the stems.

*   Add cayenne pepper if you like them spicy!

*   Add ⅓ cup nutritional yeast for a cheesy flavor.

Calories: 78.6 | Protein: 1.3g | Carbs: 2.8g | Dietary Fiber: 1.1g | Fat: 7.3g | Vitamin C: 38.4mg | Vitamin D: 0 IU | Vitamin E: 1.3mg | Calcium: 48mg | Iron: 0.4mg | Magnesium: 15mg | Potassium: 157.1mg

---

FRESH FERMENTED SALSA

This salsa by Donna Schwenk, author of *Cultured Food Life*, is loaded with health-promoting properties, not to mention lots of prebiotics (fertilizer for your good bacteria) in the onions and garlic. Tomatoes are loaded with lycopene, and garlic and onions contain organosulfur and allicin, which bring cardiovascular benefits, inflammation reduction, and cancer protection. Donna says: "The probiotics in your gut can help you greatly if you have cancer or have to undertake chemotherapy. Chemo can destroy the gut lining, but inside the human gut, a layer of epithelial cells is regenerated every four to five days, as long as you have the right gut flora. If you have healthy gut flora and include a group of healthy strains of bacteria, your body will regenerate itself. If it is not healthy, then it slows or halts the regeneration of your intestinal cells. The probiotics in your gut can help determine how well your body handles chemotherapy—making it even more crucial for those with cancer and going through chemo to add probiotics and prebiotics to their diet."[1]

Total time:

Makes 16 servings

Ingredients:

6 large ripe tomatoes

2 small onions

2 small red or green peppers

Two 4-ounce cans organic chopped green chilies with juice

2 garlic cloves

2 teaspoons paprika

2 teaspoons ground cinnamon

4 teaspoons chipotle powder

1 tablespoon coconut sugar or honey (The microbes will eat the sugar and make more probiotics.)

⅛ teaspoon Cutting Edge Starter Culture (You can find this culture on Amazon or at culturedfoodlife.com.)

Actions:

1. Place all the ingredients except the Cutting-Edge Culture in a blender or food processor and process until well combined. You can leave the mixture a little chunky if you like your salsa that way.

2. Add the Cutting-Edge Culture and stir until well combined.

3. Transfer the salsa to jars and seal with a secure lid. Let the salsa ferment at room temperature for 2 days, then store it in the refrigerator.

Storage Note: This salsa should last for at least a month in a sealed container in your refrigerator.

Calories: 25.3 | Protein: 1.3g | Carbs: 5.5g | Dietary Fiber: 1.4g | Fat: 0.2g | Vitamin C: 30.4mg | Vitamin D: 0 IU | Vitamin E: 0.6mg | Calcium: 14.1mg | Iron: 0.5mg | Magnesium: 10.4mg | Potassium: 209.4mg

PROTEIN BALLS

Total time: 10 minutes

Makes 15 servings (1 ball per serving)

Ingredients:

7 tablespoons almond butter or peanut butter

½ cup almond meal

5 tablespoons raw honey or maple syrup

6 tablespoons hemp seeds, divided

3 tablespoons pumpkin seeds

Actions:

1. Mix the ingredients together in a bowl (reserving 3 tablespoons of hemp seeds for Step 2) until well combined. If the mixture is too dry to mold, add some water.

2. Form the mixture into 15 balls, then roll the balls in the remaining hemp seeds to coat.

Calories: 119.5 | Protein: 4.1g | Carbs: 8.4g | Dietary Fiber: 1.4g | Fat: 8.7g | Vitamin C: 0.09mg | Vitamin D: 0 IU | Vitamin E: 2.81mg | Calcium: 37.8mg | Iron: 0.8mg | Magnesium: 69.1mg | Potassium: 120.5mg

HOMEMADE PROTEIN POWDER

Making your own protein powder can be fun and you save money. This batch will give you four scoops. Stored in an airtight container in the refrigerator, it will keep for up to a month.

Total time: 6 minutes

Makes 4 servings

Ingredients:

½ cup pumpkin seeds

½ cup hemp seeds

½ cup almonds

½ cup uncooked quinoa

Actions:

1. Add all the ingredients to a blender and mix until you get a fine powder.

2. Mix with ½ cup filtered water or almond milk to make a protein shake or smoothie.

Calories: 382.3 | Protein: 17.9g | Carbs: 20.9g | Dietary Fiber: 5.4g | Fat: 27.5g | Vitamin C: 0.4mg | Vitamin D: 0 IU | Vitamin E: 5.6mg | Calcium: 79.4mg | Iron: 4.6mg | Magnesium: 325.5mg | Potassium: 621.1mg

CHAPTER 18

SENSATIONAL SAUCES AND LIFE-CHANGING CONDIMENTS

We can pack a lot of extra nutrients and health benefits into the sauces, condiments, and seasonings we add to our various dishes. Made from ingredients that include fruits, vegetables, nuts, seeds, and herbs, these delectable additions to every meal are nutritious for sure, providing us with minerals such as iron, magnesium, potassium, and more! They also add an important element of pizzazz and delicious flavor to our food. This is the spice of life—the emotional and spiritual sparkle we all need when we are ready to sit down at the table and eat wholesome food. These extras enhance our quality of life.

RAW TOMATO SAUCE

Serve this sauce with the Zucchini Pasta and Walnut "Meatballs" (page 213), in the Raw Tacos (page 246), and as an extra layer on the Raw Lasagna (page 211).

Total time: 10 minutes

Makes 4 servings

Ingredients:

2 large tomatoes

1 cup sundried tomatoes

1 garlic clove

¼ red or yellow onion

1 tablespoon extra-virgin olive oil

¼ teaspoon black pepper

¼ teaspoon chili flakes or cayenne pepper

1 tablespoon fresh basil or ½ tablespoon dried basil

½ teaspoon dried thyme

½ teaspoon dried parsley

½ teaspoon dried oregano

Action:

Add all the ingredients to the blender and mix for 1 minute or until well combined.

Tip:

Soak the sundried tomatoes for 1 hour to make the blending process easier and the sauce smoother.

Calories: 123.4 | Protein: 3g | Carbs: 18.8g | Dietary Fiber: 3.4g | Fat: 3.7g | Vitamin C: 20.7mg | Vitamin D: 0 IU | Vitamin E: 1mg | Calcium: 19mg | Iron: 1.2mg | Magnesium: 12.5mg | Potassium: 239.1mg

---

TACO SAUCE

Total time: 5 minutes

Makes 9 servings

Ingredients:

1 ¼ cup ketchup

¼ cup filtered water

1 teaspoon cumin powder

1 teaspoon onion powder

1 teaspoon garlic powder

1 teaspoon chili powder

¼ teaspoon sea salt

Actions:

Mix all the ingredients in a small bowl until well combined.

Calories: 41.8 | Protein: 0.5g | Carbs: 11g | Dietary Fiber: 0.3g | Fat: 0.1g | Vitamin C: 1.6mg | Vitamin D: 0 IU | Vitamin E: 0.6mg | Calcium: 9.6mg | Iron: 0.2mg | Magnesium: 5.9mg | Potassium: 118.7mg

---

VEGAN BUTTER

This butter can be stored in an airtight container in the refrigerator for up to one month. Wrapped in plastic and stored in the freezer, this butter will last up to a year.

Total time: 25 minutes prep, plus 1 hour to set

Makes 16 servings (½ tablespoon each)

Ingredients:

¼ cup plus 2 teaspoons Almond Milk (page 159)

1 teaspoon apple cider vinegar

½ teaspoon sea salt

½ cup extra-virgin coconut oil, melted

1 tablespoon extra-virgin olive oil

Actions:

1. Place the almond milk, apple cider vinegar, and sea salt in a small cup and whisk together with a fork.
2. Let sit for 10 minutes, until the mixture curdles.
3. Place the coconut oil and olive oil in a blender and mix on high speed until well combined and smooth.
4. Add the almond milk mixture to the oil in the blender. Mix for 2 minutes until smooth and creamy.
5. Place the mixture into a mold and place in the freezer to solidify. An ice cube tray works well as a mold. It will be ready to use as butter in 1 hour.

Tips:

- To make your butter nut-free, use Seed Milk (page 158) as an alternative to almond milk.

- If you don't like the taste of dairy butter but still want to moisten toast or pancakes, use extra-virgin coconut oil, extra-virgin olive oil, or avocado oil as butter. You can also use avocado as a butter substitute.

Variations:

- Add ¼ teaspoon cinnamon and 2 teaspoons maple syrup to the oil for Cinnamon Butter.

- Make Cinnamon Toast by spreading Cinnamon Butter on Quick Bread or Gluten-Free Rolls.

Calories: 71.6 | Protein: 0.1g | Carbs: 0.1g | Dietary Fiber: 0.08g | Fat: 7.7g | Vitamin C: 0mg | Vitamin D: 0 IU | Vitamin E: 0.1mg | Calcium: 1.8mg | Iron: 0.02mg | Magnesium: 1.8mg | Potassium: 5mg

---

3-MINUTE INSTANT BUTTER

This butter is ready to use immediately. If you store it in a container in the freezer, however, it will set solid like a stick of dairy butter.

Total time: 3 minutes

Makes 1/3 cup

Ingredients:

½ cup extra-virgin olive oil

½ teaspoon sea salt

⅛ teaspoon apple cider vinegar

Actions:

Blend the ingredients until whipped.

Calories: 201.6 | Protein: 0g | Carbs: 0g | Dietary Fiber: 0g | Fat: 22.4g | Vitamin C: 0mg | Vitamin D: 0 IU | Vitamin E: 2.7mg | Calcium: 0mg | Iron: 0mg | Magnesium: 0mg | Potassium: 0.09mg

FLAX EGG ALTERNATIVE

For every egg in an original recipe, use one serving of this flax meal to keep a recipe vegan.

Total time: 10 minutes

Makes the equivalent of 1 egg

Ingredients:

3 teaspoons ground flaxseed

4 teaspoons filtered water

Actions:

1. Whisk the flaxseed and water in a bowl.
2. Let sit for 5 to 10 minutes. The mixture will become gummy, just like eggs.

Calories: 30 | Protein: 1.5g | Carbs: 2.5g | Dietary Fiber: 2g | Fat: 1.7g | Vitamin C: 0mg | Vitamin D: 0 IU | Vitamin E: 0mg | Calcium: 14mg | Iron: 0.4mg | Magnesium: 0.2mg | Potassium: 0mg

VEGAN MAYONNAISE

A blender is important in this recipe to make a thick, smooth, creamy mayonnaise.

Total time: 10 minutes

Makes 4 servings

Ingredients:

¾ cup almond milk or cashew milk

1 ½ tablespoons lemon juice

1 teaspoon mustard

¾ cup olive oil or avocado oil

⅛ teaspoon sea salt

⅛ teaspoon pepper

Actions:

1. Place the almond milk, lemon juice, mustard, sea salt, and pepper in a blender. Mix until well combined, about 1 minute.

2. Add the oil to the mixture and continue to blend until it thickens, 3 to 4 minutes. When emulsified, the mayonnaise is ready to eat and to store in a jar or airtight container in the fridge.

Calories: 419.1 | Protein: 1.4g | Carbs: 1.9g | Dietary Fiber: 0.9g | Fat: 45.4g | Vitamin C: 2.2mg | Vitamin D: 0 IU | Vitamin E: 5.2mg | Calcium: 20.8mg | Iron: 0.2mg | Magnesium: 19.6mg | Potassium: 57.9mg

---

BLUEBERRY CHIA SEED JAM

This jam will last up to two months in the refrigerator and six months in the freezer.

Total time: 20 minutes

Makes 12 servings (about 2 tablespoons per serving)

Ingredients:

2 cups blueberries (strawberries work well too)

1 cup filtered water

¼ cup chia seeds

¼ cup maple syrup or honey

Actions:

1. Place all the ingredients in a pot and bring to a boil.

2. Reduce the heat to a simmer and stir constantly so the chia seeds do not burn on the bottom of the pot.

3. When the mixture has thickened and the fruit is entirely broken down (about 10 minutes), allow to cool and then place in a glass jar and cool completely before placing in the fridge. The jam is now ready to eat, but if you refrigerate it overnight, the jam will set more. Serve on Gluten-Free Rolls (page 294) or as a garnish for any dessert.

Variations:

- Use blueberries for Blueberry Chia Seed Jam.
- Use blackberries for Blackberry Chia Seed Jam.
- Use raspberries for Raspberry Chia Seed Jam.
- Use mulberries for Mulberry Chia Seed Jam.
- Use ¼ cup each strawberries, blackberries, raspberries, and blueberries for Mixed Berry Chia Seed Jam.

Calories: 48 | Protein: 0.7g | Carbs: 9.5g | Dietary Fiber: 1g | Fat: 1.1g | Vitamin C: 2.4mg | Vitamin D: 0 IU | Vitamin E: 0.1mg | Calcium: 30.9mg | Iron: 0.3mg | Magnesium: 14.8mg | Potassium: 47.3mg

TAHINI

Total time: 10 minutes

Makes 4 to 6 servings

Ingredients:

½ cup filtered water

8 tablespoons sesame seeds

4 teaspoons sesame oil

¾ teaspoon sea salt

Action:

Place all the ingredients in the bowl of a food processor and blend until smooth.

Tips:

- Use this in the recipe for Turmeric Hummus (page 298).
- Tahini makes a great salad dressing!
- Add this to Guacamole (page 297).

Calories: 143.2 | Protein: 3.1g | Carbs: 4.2g | Dietary Fiber: 2.1g | Fat: 13.4g | Vitamin C: 0mg | Vitamin D: 0 IU | Vitamin E: 0.1mg | Calcium: 176.3mg | Iron: 2.6mg | Magnesium: 63.4mg | Potassium: 84.2mg

VEGAN SOUR CREAM

Refrigerated in an airtight container or jar, this sour cream lasts for up to two weeks.

Total time: 5 minutes

Makes 1 cup (8 2-tablespoon servings)

Ingredients:

1 cup raw cashew nuts

¼ teaspoon sea salt

1 teaspoon apple cider vinegar

Juice of 1 small lemon (no more than ¼ cup)

½ teaspoon dill

3 ½ tablespoons filtered water

Action:

Add all the ingredients to a blender and mix until the consistency is creamy. Add more water as needed if a smoother consistency is desired.

Tips:

- For a nut-free alternative, substitute sunflower seeds or hemp seeds for cashew nuts.
- For a creamier sour cream, soak the cashews for 4 hours in water. If you do soak the cashews, use half the amount of water in the recipe.
- Use this in any recipe that calls for sour cream.
- Use this sour cream on Raw Tacos and Raw Crackers.

Calories: 91.3 | Protein: 3g | Carbs: 5.3g | Dietary Fiber: 0.5g | Fat: 7.1g | Vitamin C: 2.3mg | Vitamin D: 0 IU | Vitamin E: 0.1mg | Calcium: 7.6mg | Iron: 1.1mg | Magnesium: 48.1mg | Potassium: 115.7mg

KETCHUP

This ketchup keeps well in the refrigerator for four to eight weeks, or in the freezer for three to six months.

Total time: 10 minutes

Makes 3 cups (48 1-tablespoon servings)

Ingredients:

One 14 ounce can organic tomato paste

⅓ cup filtered water

1 teaspoon apple cider vinegar

2 tablespoons maple syrup or honey

⅓ teaspoon garlic powder

⅓ tablespoon onion powder

⅓ teaspoon cayenne pepper

½ teaspoon cinnamon

Pinch of ground cloves

⅔ teaspoon sea salt

Actions:

1. Place all the ingredients in a blender and mix well.

2. Pour the ketchup into a glass container and store in the fridge. The flavors will mesh well overnight.

Tip:

Add a dash of allspice for added flavor.

Variation:

Add 1 teaspoon dried mustard powder for Mustard Ketchup.

Calories: 9.9 | Protein: 0.5g | Carbs: 2.1g | Dietary Fiber: 0.2g | Fat: 0g | Vitamin C: 1.5mg | Vitamin D: 0 IU | Vitamin E: 0mg | Calcium: 1.2mg | Iron: 0.1mg | Magnesium: 0.2mg | Potassium: 2.6mg

TACO SEASONING

A must-have staple in the kitchen for taco lovers! Keep this in the cupboard for whenever you want to have meat tacos (beef, chicken, and fish). It also makes a great seasoning for salads.

Total time: 5 minutes

Makes slightly less than ½ cup

Ingredients:

1 tablespoon sea salt

1 tablespoon cumin

1 tablespoon turmeric

1 tablespoon garlic powder

1 tablespoon onion powder

1 ½ teaspoons paprika

¾ teaspoon black pepper

3 dashes of cayenne pepper

Actions:

Mix all the spices together in a bowl. Put the seasoning in a shaker bottle.

Nutrition facts for entire recipe: Calories: 111.7 | Protein: 4.5g | Carbs: 21.8g | Dietary Fiber: 6.8g | Fat: 1.9g | Vitamin C: 2mg | Vitamin D: 0 IU | Vitamin E: 1.4mg | Calcium: 101.6mg | Iron: 6.9mg | Magnesium: 38.2mg | Potassium: 423mg

---

GARLIC SALT

Great on fries and when cooking vegetables or meat.

Total time: 1 minute

Makes 6 servings (1 tablespoon per serving)

Ingredients:

3 tablespoons sea salt

3 tablespoons garlic powder

Actions:

Add both ingredients to a spice jar and shake until well combined.

Calories: 1.2 | Protein: 0.06g | Carbs: 0.2g | Dietary Fiber: 0.03g | Fat: 0g | Vitamin C: 0mg | Vitamin D: 0 IU | Vitamin E: 0mg | Calcium: 0.3mg | Iron: 0.02mg | Magnesium: 0.3mg | Potassium: 4.6mg

---

CUMIN AND TURMERIC SEASONING

Use this as a base for soups and also as an add-on for chicken, fish, and beef.

Total time: 1 minute

Makes 5 servings (1 tablespoon per serving)

Ingredients:

2 tablespoons cumin

2 tablespoons turmeric

½ teaspoon sea salt

Actions:

Add the ingredients to a spice jar and shake until well combined.

Calories: 16.7 | Protein: 0.6g | Carbs: 2.5g | Dietary Fiber: 1.2g | Fat: 0.5g | Vitamin C: 0.06mg | Vitamin D: 0 IU | Vitamin E: 0.1mg | Calcium: 20.3mg | Iron: 2.1mg | Magnesium: 5.4mg | Potassium: 54.9mg

OREGANO SAGE SEASONING

Use this for roasted meats.

Total time: 1 minute

Makes 5 servings (1 tablespoon per serving)

Ingredients:

2 tablespoons fresh sage

2 tablespoons fresh oregano

1 teaspoon dried parsley

1 teaspoon cumin powder

½ teaspoon turmeric powder

½ teaspoon sea salt

¼ teaspoon black pepper

Dash of cayenne pepper

Actions:

Add the ingredients to a spice jar and shake until well combined.

Calories: 5.7 | Protein: 0.1g | Carbs: 0.9g | Dietary Fiber: 0.2g | Fat: 0.1g | Vitamin C: 1.1mg | Vitamin D: 0 IU | Vitamin E: 0.03mg | Calcium: 17.5mg | Iron: 0.2mg | Magnesium: 2.4mg | Potassium: 20.8mg

VEGETABLE SEASONING

Use for stir-fried vegetable dishes.

Total time: 1 minute

Makes 4 servings (1 tablespoon per serving)

Ingredients:

1 tablespoon thyme

1 teaspoon sage

1 teaspoon parsley

1 teaspoon basil

1 teaspoon coriander

½ teaspoon turmeric

½ teaspoon cumin

½ teaspoon sea salt

½ teaspoon garlic powder

¼ teaspoon ginger powder

Actions:

Add the ingredients to a spice jar and shake until well combined.

Calories: 8.7 | Protein: 0.3g | Carbs: 1.6g | Dietary Fiber: 0.8g | Fat: 0.2g | Vitamin C: 0.5mg | Vitamin D: 0 IU | Vitamin E: 0.1mg | Calcium: 28.5mg | Iron: 1.5mg | Magnesium: 5.7mg | Potassium: 30.4mg

CHAPTER 19

NUTRIENT-RICH DESSERTS AND SWEET SNACKS

You don't need to cut out desserts, sweets, and treats to be healthy. Instead, ask yourself: "How can I have my favorite dessert or treat, but in a healthier way? How can I get nutrients from chocolate? Or fulfill a craving, for example, for gummy bears, in a way that won't deteriorate my health?" The human body can actually break down natural sugars; it was designed to digest fruits (nature's candy), dates, honey, maple syrup, stevia, and so forth. It's only processed refined sugars, like white sugar, brown sugar, and corn syrup that get us into trouble.

If you've indulged a sweet tooth up to now, I promise that when you eat the Cancer-Free with Food dessert recipes you'll feel better than before. Soon the body chemistry changes, and the impulses to eat destructive, unhealthy foods disappear. It never worked when I tried to give up all sweets completely. So I gave myself permission to eat up to 20 of the Chocolate Balls (page 324) per day, and I felt no guilt about this because it was a major upgrade from processed chocolate that contains dairy, soy lecithin, and refined sugar. My immune system felt stronger and I was so excited that I could still eat chocolate that was healthy and nourishing.

Be committed to never eating refined white sugar or corn syrup ever again. With this goal set in mind you will create a new path for yourself, one where you will find you won't come across refined sugars often. Why do we need refined sugars anymore? We don't—especially when we have all these delicious alternatives that taste even better!

All the dessert recipes in this chapter are free of refined sugar, dairy, soy, gluten, and preservatives. All these dessert recipes are nutrient-rich meals in themselves, so you can enjoy getting vitamins and minerals at the same time as fulfilling your dessert desires. They are delicious, and you will experience no sense of deprivation when eating them. I recommend starting with the recipe that jumps out at you, the one that excites you the most. The recipe that gets you excited will be a winner!

One final thought: Before making a recipe and spending money and time on multiple ingredients, remind yourself that you can always simplify and focus on the "candy" that nature provides. These will always be the healthiest sugars for us. Bite into some yummy:

- Blueberries
- Blackberries
- Raspberries
- Strawberries
- Apples
- Pineapple
- Dates
- Figs
- Coconuts

CLASSIC THREE-INGREDIENT CHOCOLATE BALLS

This recipe is made with just three ingredients, so it will be easy for you to remember how to make it for the rest of your life. Making healthy chocolate is easier than you may think. This is one of the most popular recipes I offer. This chocolate can stay fresh in the fridge for 14 days and in the freezer for three months. I also love to add almond butter or peanut butter to these balls for another flavor. And you can roll them in any superfood you like—for example, coconut or goji berries. These make beautiful-looking truffles, excellent gifts to give others too! And you can shape the chocolate mixture into balls or pat them into squares to make brownies.

Total time: 10 minutes

Makes 12 balls

Ingredients:

1 cup almond flour/nut meal (finely ground almonds or other nuts)

¼ cup cacao powder

3 tablespoons maple syrup or raw honey

Actions:

1. Mix the nut meal, cacao powder, and maple syrup in a bowl.

2. Roll the mixture into 12 balls.

Tips:

- Add ¼ teaspoon sea salt and ¼ teaspoon pure vanilla extract for enhanced flavor.

- Add essential oils (therapeutic-grade only): cinnamon, orange, peppermint, tangerine—start with 1 drop and then increase to 2 to 3 drops according to your preference.

- You can use this mixture to make brownies (just form the mixture into squares) or a dessert pie (simply press into a pie plate with your fingertips).

- Roll them in superfoods including shredded coconut, goji berries, hemp seeds, or cacao nibs.

Variations:

- Add ¼ teaspoon pure vanilla extract for Chocolate-Vanilla Balls.

- Add ¼ teaspoon sea salt for Salty Chocolate Balls.

- Add 1 to 2 tablespoons almond butter or peanut butter.

- Add a dash of chlorella or spirulina powder to make Alkaline Chocolate Balls.

- Add a dash of turmeric to make Turmeric Chocolate Balls.

Calories: 73 | Protein: 2.3g | Carbs: 6.3g | Dietary Fiber: 1.3g | Fat: 4.8g | Vitamin C: 0mg | Vitamin D: 0 IU | Vitamin E: 2.3mg | Calcium: 25.1mg | Iron: 0.6mg | Magnesium: 39mg | Potassium: 36.6mg

RAW CHOCOLATE CHIP COOKIE DOUGH

This cookie dough doesn't need eggs or butter to make it delicious. It's unbelievably buttery, made with almond flour and coconut oil. You can also bake these cookies for a Melt-In-Your Mouth Chocolate Chip experience.

Total time: 10 minutes

Makes 12 balls

Ingredients:

2 cups almond meal/flour (or tigernut flour)

1 teaspoon pure vanilla extract

5 teaspoons maple syrup

¼ teaspoon sea salt

1 tablespoon coconut oil

2 tablespoons organic chocolate chips or cacao nibs

Actions:

1. Combine all the ingredients, except for the chocolate chips, in a large bowl and mix until well combined. The dough should be moist, so add a dash of water if needed.

2. Stir the chocolate chips into the dough.

3. Roll the dough into 12 balls, then press them into cookie shapes. They're ready to eat!

Tips:

- Roll the dough balls in cacao powder.
- Use tigernut flour if you have a nut allergy or want to go nut-free.
- Use medium-chain triglyceride (MCT) oil.
- Bake in the oven at 325°F for 8 minutes.

Variations:

- Use 1 cup cashew nuts blended into a flour, and 1 cup gluten-free oats for Healthy Cashew Oatmeal Cookies.

- Preheat the oven to 325°F and bake for 7 minutes for Melt-in-Your Mouth Baked Chocolate Chip Cookies.

Calories: 136 | Protein: 4.1g | Carbs: 7g | Dietary Fiber: 2g | Fat: 11g | Vitamin C: 0mg | Vitamin D: 0 IU | Vitamin E: 4.7mg | Calcium: 42.8mg | Iron: 0.8mg | Magnesium: 53.9mg | Potassium: 6.4mg

---

MINI CASHEW CHEESECAKES

You'll need 20 small paper cupcake cups for this recipe. You can also make a regular-size cheesecake (recipe to come).

Total time: 10 minutes

Makes 20 mini cheesecakes

Ingredients:

3 cups cashew nuts

½ cup lemon juice

¾ cup maple syrup

¾ cup coconut oil

1 tablespoon pure vanilla extract

⅛ teaspoon sea salt

Actions:

1. Put all the ingredients in a high-speed blender and whip until completely smooth.

2. Spoon 1 heaping tablespoon of the cheesecake mixture into each paper cupcake cup.

3. Set in the freezer for 6 minutes. Enjoy!

Tips:

- Soak the cashews for 3 hours to make them softer and easier to blend.

- You will absolutely need a high-speed blender to make these creamy and without any chunks.

- Place a pecan, walnut, or macadamia nut on the top of each cupcake for decoration and texture.

- Keep these in the freezer or fridge and they'll set harder.

- If you have a metal cupcake tray, it can help to hold the cupcakes while they are setting.

Calories: 214.2 | Protein: 3.5g | Carbs: 14.4g | Dietary Fiber: 0.6g | Fat: 16.3g | Vitamin C: 2.4mg | Vitamin D: 0 IU | Vitamin E: 0.1mg | Calcium: 19mg | Iron: 1.3mg | Magnesium: 59.9mg | Potassium: 161.4 mg

CHOCOLATE-AVOCADO MOUSSE

I recommend using a powerful blender for this recipe, to whip it up so it has the same texture as traditional mousse. When it's whipped like this, it's super smooth with no chunks, the avocado is unrecognizable, and it's unbelievably creamy and delicious.

Total time: 5 minutes

Makes 1 serving

Ingredients:

1 avocado

2 tablespoons cacao powder, or more to taste

2 tablespoons raw honey or maple syrup, or more to taste

Actions:

1. Blend all the ingredients in a food processor until smooth and creamy. Alternatively, you can mash the avocado with a fork in a bowl, and then add the cacao powder and honey.

2. Add more cacao if you want a more chocolaty mousse. Add more honey if you want a sweeter mousse.

Tips:

- Serve this mousse with fresh raspberries or strawberries.
- Add a dash of pure vanilla extract for enhanced flavor.
- Serve this mousse on top of Chocolate Brownies (page 325), ice cream, or cupcakes.
- Add a tablespoon of MCT oil for added health benefits.
- Add a drop of peppermint essential oil or extract if you like the chocolate-mint combo.

Calories: 489.2 | Protein: 6.1g | Carbs: 57.7g | Dietary Fiber: 15.5g | Fat: 30.4g | Vitamin C: 20.3mg | Vitamin D: 0 IU | Vitamin E: 4.1mg | Calcium: 26.6mg | Iron: 2.7mg | Magnesium: 127.1mg | Potassium: 1,170mg

---

CHOCOLATE SAUCE

This sauce is a true game changer! It's so creamy, smooth and thick, it's ideal as a dip for strawberries and other fruits. Chocolate Sauce also makes a great topping for Plant-Based Ice Cream (page 340), Classic Three-Ingredient Chocolate Balls (page 324), and even the Raw Cookie Dough (page 326).

Total time: 5 minutes

Makes six ¼-cup servings

Ingredients:

⅔ cup cacao powder

½ cup maple syrup

¼ cup extra-virgin coconut oil

Actions:

Combine the ingredients in a blender and blend on high speed until they become a smooth sauce.

Tips:

- For a more intense chocolate flavor, add more cacao powder.

- For a sweeter flavor, add more maple syrup.

- If you want the recipe to be raw, substitute raw honey for the maple syrup.

- You can also make this without a blender. Use a bowl and a spoon.

- Add the chocolate sauce to the inside of raspberries for Stuffed Raspberries.

Variations:

- Add ¾ cup raspberries for Chocolate Raspberry Sauce.
- Add ¾ cup cherries for Chocolate Cherry Sauce.

Calories: 184.8 | Protein: 1.7g | Carbs: 23.2g | Dietary Fiber: 1.7g | Fat: 9.5g | Vitamin C: 0mg | Vitamin D: 0 IU | Vitamin E: 0mg | Calcium: 27mg | Iron: 1.3mg | Magnesium: 66mg | Potassium: 211.2mg

---

ICE CREAM BITES WITH CHOCOLATE SAUCE

This is my favorite ice cream recipe ever! I am so excited for you to try this—particularly if you love the combo of ice cream and chocolate sauce. These bites are so nutrient-dense that they are quite satisfying.

Total time: 10 minutes

Makes 15 bites

Ingredients:

Ice cream:

1 ½ cups cashews, soaked for 4 hours

1 small lemon

½ cup maple syrup

¼ cup coconut oil

1 tablespoon vanilla extract

Dash of sea salt

2 teaspoons maca powder or lucama powder, optional

Chocolate sauce:

⅔ cup cacao powder

½ cup maple syrup

¼ cup coconut oil

Actions:

1. Combine all the ice cream ingredients in a blender and blend on high speed until they become smooth. There should be absolutely no lumps whatsoever. Scoop the ice cream mixture onto a baking tray lined with paper and place in the freezer. They will set in 1 to 2 hours. Clean the blender basin so you can use it again.

2. Once the bites are set, make the chocolate sauce by putting the ingredients in the blender and mixing them until smooth and whipped. Add a spoonful to each ice cream bite. They are ready to eat! Keep them in the freezer and they will set even harder.

Tip:

Soak the cashews for 4 hours to get a creamy, easier-to-whip ice cream.

Calories: 209.1 | Protein: 3.1g | Carbs: 20.8g | Dietary Fiber: 1.2g | Fat: 13g | Vitamin C: 2.1mg | Vitamin D: 0 IU | Vitamin E: 0.1mg | Calcium: 27.6mg | Iron: 1.4mg | Magnesium: 67mg | Potassium: 199.5mg

---

ROASTED HAZELNUT CHOCOLATE BLOCK

Total time: 1 hour

Makes 1 block, serves 8

Ingredients:

1 cup cacao butter, not melted

2 tablespoons cacao powder

3 tablespoons raw honey or maple syrup

1 cup almond meal (or hemp seeds blended into a powdered form)

½ cup roasted hazelnuts

Actions:

1. Melt the cacao butter either in the sun or over very low heat on the stove.

2. Place the melted cacao butter, cacao powder, and honey in a bowl, stirring well so the mixture is thoroughly blended.

3. Add the almond meal to the bowl and stir until the mixture is smooth.

4. Pour the mixture into chocolate molds or a baking dish, add halzenuts on top, and then let set in the freezer or fridge until hard.

Tips:

- The finer the almond meal, the smoother the chocolate will be.

- To get all the cacao butter out of the saucepan, add a tablespoon of almond meal and stir it around to soak up the cacao butter.

- Bonus to working with this ingredient: Cacao butter makes a great skin moisturizer!

Variations:

- Add raisins, blueberries, and sultanas to make a Chocolate-Fruit Block.

- Add a dash of turmeric and reishi mushroom powder to make Medicinal Healing Turmeric Chocolate.

Calories: 439.25 | Protein: 5.4g | Carbs: 12.6g | Dietary Fiber: 3.1g | Fat: 43.7g | Vitamin C: 0.94mg | Vitamin D: 0 IU | Vitamin E: 5.7mg | Calcium: 46.7mg | Iron: 0.68mg | Magnesium: 72mg | Potassium: 123.5mg

CHOCOLATE ALMOND BUTTER CUPS

This is the recipe that helped me convert my chocolate-and-peanut-butter cravings to a much healthier one. Before I created this recipe I was eating the conventional version that we all know so well, the one with sugar, non-organic dairy and preservatives . . . a dangerous combination! When I first made these I was over the moon delighted—I could enjoy my favorite chocolate-nut combination but in a much healthier way, where I was actually getting antioxidants, vitamin E, and protein. Have your chocolate cup and eat it too!

Total time: 35 minutes

Makes 13 chocolate almond butter cups

Ingredients:

¾ cup cacao butter

3 tablespoons cacao powder

½ cup almond meal

3 tablespoons maple syrup

13 teaspoons almond butter (just over ¼ cup)

13 mini (1 ⅝-inch diameter) paper baking cups

Actions:

1. Melt the cacao butter in the sun or over very low heat on the stove. Once melted, add the cacao powder, almond meal, and maple syrup, mixing well. Taste, and then add more cacao if you prefer darker chocolate, and more maple syrup if you prefer a sweeter taste.

2. Spoon 1 teaspoon of the chocolate mixture into each baking cup, filling ⅓ of the way. Reserve the other ½ of the mixture for the top of the cups.

3. Put the baking cups in the freezer for 5 minutes to set.

4. Remove the cups from the freezer and add 1 teaspoon peanut butter to each. Each cup should now be ⅔ full.

5. Add 1 ½ teaspoons of the remainder of the chocolate mixture into the baking cups.

6. Place the cups in the freezer again and allow to set for 15 minutes.

Tips:

• Use your favorite nut butter.

• Add sea salt to the nut butter, to taste.

Variations:

• Substitute peanuts for almonds for Chocolate Peanut Butter Cups.

• Substitute the peanuts and almond meal for sunflower seeds for nut-free Chocolate Sunflower Cups.

Calories: 184.7 | Protein: 2.2g | Carbs: 5.7g | Dietary Fiber: 1.2g | Fat: 18.1g | Vitamin C: 0mg | Vitamin D: 0 IU | Vitamin E: 2.3mg | Calcium: 32.4mg | Iron: 0.5mg | Magnesium: 36mg | Potassium: 69.7mg

---

FRESH FRUIT SORBET

No need for added sugar in this recipe—the fruit is sweet enough! This is great if you have a sore throat. It's very soothing when you can't eat solid food.

Total time: 5 minutes

Makes 2 servings

Ingredients:

2 cups fruit of your choice, such as strawberries, grapefruit, pitted cherries, apples, mango, pineapple, peach, blueberries, or oranges

4 cups of ice cubes

Actions:

1. Place the ingredients in a high-speed blender and blend for 1 minute or until you achieve an icy sorbet consistency.

2. Serve immediately.

Tips:

- Add 1 to 2 tablespoons honey, maple syrup, or coconut sugar if you want a sweeter sorbet.

- Add some nut milk ice for a creamier sorbet.

Calories: 46 | Protein: 0.9g | Carbs: 11g | Dietary Fiber: 2.8g | Fat: 0.4g | Vitamin C: 84.6mg | Vitamin D: 0 IU | Vitamin E: 0.4mg | Calcium: 33.2mg | Iron: 0.5mg | Magnesium: 22.1mg | Potassium: 223.7mg

BLUEBERRY CHIA SEED PUDDING

Total time: 10 minutes

Makes 2 servings

Ingredients:

1 cup fresh blueberries

2 cups almond milk

½ teaspoon vanilla extract

2 tablespoons honey or maple syrup

¼ teaspoon sea salt

½ cup chia seeds

Actions:

1. Blend all the ingredients together except the chia seeds.

2. Add the chia seeds and then set in fridge for 9 minutes so the pudding can gelatinize.

Tips:

- This also makes a great breakfast!

- If the pudding has not gelled enough for your liking after 9 minutes, let it set for an additional 20 minutes.
- Serve with fresh blueberries.

Calories: 347.2 | Protein: 10g | Carbs: 35.7g | Dietary Fiber: 13.8g | Fat: 20.6g | Vitamin C: 5.3mg | Vitamin D: 0 IU | Vitamin E: 0.4mg | Calcium: 249.4mg | Iron: 3.2mg | Magnesium: 163mg | Potassium: 335.2mg

---

VANILLA PUDDING

Total time: 10 minutes

Makes 4 servings

Ingredients:

1 cup vanilla almond milk

1 cup coconut milk

1 tablespoon maple syrup (optional)

2 seedless dates, diced

2 figs, diced

1 teaspoon vanilla extract

Dash of sea salt

½ cup chia seeds

Toppings:

¼ cup sliced almonds

Handful of walnuts

1 cup strawberries, chopped

Actions:

1. Whisk the almond milk, coconut milk, maple syrup, vanilla, and sea salt in a bowl until well combined. Stir in the chia seeds, dates, and figs. Set the pudding in the fridge for 10 minutes.

2. Transfer the pudding to individual bowls and add toppings.

Tip:

Leave in the fridge for an additional 20 minutes to set further if the chia seeds have not gelatinized to your liking.

Variations:

Use 1 tablespoon cacao powder for Chocolate Pudding.

Calories: 194.1 | Protein: 5.5g | Carbs: 18g | Dietary Fiber: 9g | Fat: 12g | Vitamin C: 0.4mg | Vitamin D: 30 IU | Vitamin E: 0.1mg | Calcium: 196mg | Iron: 2.1mg | Magnesium: 108mg | Potassium: 208mg

BLUEBERRY CRUMBLE

Total time: 30 minutes

Makes 5 servings

Ingredients:

4 ½ cups fresh blueberries

1 tablespoon extra-virgin coconut oil

1 ½ cups almond meal

⅓ cup dried, shredded coconut

2 tablespoons cinnamon powder

5 tablespoons maple syrup, divided

Actions:

Preheat the oven to 400°F.

1. Bring a pot of water to boil. Add the blueberries and cook until they are semisoft.

2. Heat the coconut oil in a small skillet over low heat. Add the almond meal, coconut, cinnamon, and 2 tablespoons maple syrup and toast the mixture. Set aside.

3. Drain the water from the blueberries and add the remaining 3 tablespoons maple syrup to the pot. Stir while continuing to cook the blueberries over medium-low heat, until the blueberries are soft. Remove from heat.

4. Combine the blueberries with the toasted nut mixture in an ovenproof dish. Bake for 10 minutes.

Tips:

• The crumble tastes delicious served with Plant-Based Ice Cream (page 340) and chunks of nuts.

• Substitute raw honey for the maple syrup if you prefer.

Variations:

- For an Apple Crumble, use 4 large apples, peeled, cored, and cut into bite-size pieces.
- Substitute pears for the blueberries for Pear Crumble.
- Substitute peaches for the blueberries for Peach Crumble.

Calories: 386.8 | Protein: 8.6g | Carbs: 43.5g | Dietary Fiber: 9.3g | Fat: 23.3g | Vitamin C: 13.1mg | Vitamin D: 0 IU | Vitamin E: 9.3mg | Calcium: 133mg | Iron: 2.1mg | Magnesium: 114.8mg | Potassium: 187.3mg

CASHEW CHEESECAKE

Total time: 3 hours to soak the cashews, 25 minutes prep, and 4 hours to freeze

Makes 16 servings

Ingredients:

For the base:

4 cups pecans (you can also use walnuts, macadamia nuts, or almond meal)

5 tablespoons maple syrup or raw honey

⅛ teaspoon vanilla extract

Smidgen of sea salt

Dash of water

For the cheesecake filling:

½ cup lemon juice (approximately 2 large lemons)

3 cups cashews, soaked in filtered water for 3 hours to soften

¾ cup maple syrup or raw honey

¾ cup coconut oil

1 tablespoon pure vanilla extract

⅛ teaspoon sea salt

Actions:

1. For the base, add the pecans in a food processor until you have a fine meal. Combine the nut meal and other ingredients in a bowl. The mixture should be dry, but moist enough to hold together.

2. Transfer the base mixture to a deep pie dish (large enough to hold 2 ½ quarts) and press it evenly to cover the bottom and sides of the dish. Set aside.

3. For the cheesecake filling, place all the ingredients in a powerful blender and blend until the mixture is very smooth and light in texture. Pour the filling into the prepared crust.

4. Freeze for 4 hours. Once the cheesecake is set, cut into slices and serve.

Variations:

Add blueberries to the whipped cashew cheesecake mixture, and then add more fresh blueberries on top for a true Blueberry Cashew Cheesecake!

Calories: 472.4 | Protein: 6.9g | Carbs: 26g | Dietary Fiber: 3.4g | Fat: 40g | Vitamin C: 3.3mg | Vitamin D: 0 IU | Vitamin E: 0.6mg | Calcium: 50.3mg | Iron: 2.3mg | Magnesium: 109.2mg | Potassium: 326.8mg

---

RAW APPLE CRUMBLE

A no-bake crumble for when you want to enjoy a traditional apple crumble in less time, and with more nutrients!

Total time: 25 minutes

Makes 4 servings

Ingredients:

For the crumble:
1 batch Almond Butter Granola (page 200)

For the filling:
4 apples, peeled and cored	1 tablespoon honey or maple syrup
½ teaspoon cinnamon powder	Dash of sea salt

For the topping:
Fresh Fruit Sorbet (page 333) or Whipped Coconut Cream (page 342). Berries for garnish, optional

Actions:

1. Create a layer of Almond Butter Granola in the bottom of each of 4 bowls.

2. Blend the filling ingredients together, leaving some chunks of apples. It should be moist and creamy. Pour into the bowls over the granola.

3. Top the bowls with Fresh Fruit Sorbet or Whipped Coconut Cream. Garnish with fresh berries.

Variations:

Use blueberries for Raw Blueberry Crumble.

Calories: 346.2 | Protein: 7.5g | Carbs: 55g | Dietary Fiber: 7.9g | Fat: 12.8g | Vitamin C: 6.5mg | Vitamin D: 0 IU | Vitamin E: 3.9mg | Calcium: 94.5mg | Iron: 1.8mg | Magnesium: 93.3mg | Potassium: 378.2mg

CHOCOLATE-COVERED STRAWBERRIES

Total time: 10 minutes

Make 4 servings

Ingredients:

1 batch Chocolate Sauce (page 329)

2 cups strawberries

Actions:

Dip the strawberries into the Chocolate Sauce and place on a tray. Let set for a few minutes in the freezer to harden the sauce or eat right away!

Variations:

Dip different kinds of nuts and fruits in the Chocolate Sauce. Try:

- Chocolate-Covered Macadamia Nuts
- Chocolate-Covered Almonds
- Chocolate-Covered Blueberries
- Chocolate-Covered Hazelnuts
- Chocolate-Covered Bananas

- Chocolate-Covered Pomegranate Clusters
- Chocolate-Filled Raspberries!

Calories: 300.3 | Protein: 3.1g | Carbs: 40.3g | Dietary Fiber: 4.1g | Fat: 14.5g | Vitamin C: 42.3mg | Vitamin D: 0 IU | Vitamin E: 0.2mg | Calcium: 52.3mg | Iron: 2.2mg | Magnesium: 108.4mg | Potassium: 426.9mg

CHOCOLATE HAZELNUTELLA

Total time: 5 minutes

Makes 1 cup (8 2-tablespoon servings)

Ingredients:

1 cup raw or roasted hazelnuts

¼ cup maple syrup

1 teaspoon vanilla extract

⅛ teaspoon sea salt (unless you're using raw nuts, then use ¼ teaspoon sea salt)

¼ cup raw cacao powder

3 tablespoons almond milk

Actions:

Blend all the ingredients in a blender until smooth.

Calories: 148.3 | Protein: 3.2g | Carbs: 11.2g | Dietary Fiber: 2.2g | Fat: 10.9g | Vitamin C: 1mg | Vitamin D: 0 IU | Vitamin E: 2.5mg | Calcium: 31.9mg | Iron: 1.2mg | Magnesium: 48.9mg | Potassium: 186.3mg

PLANT-BASED ICE CREAM

This nondairy ice cream recipe is wonderful served with fresh fruit, nuts, and/or Chocolate Sauce (page 329).

Total time: 15 minutes prep, 3 to 5 hours to freeze

Makes 2 servings

Ingredients:

1 cup cashew nuts (substitute sunflower seeds or hemp seeds if you have nut allergies)

⅔ cup Almond Milk (page 159) or filtered water

1 teaspoon vanilla extract

4 tablespoons maple syrup

¼ teaspoon sea salt

Actions:

1. Blend all the ingredients in a food processor or ice-cream maker until the mixture is as creamy and frothy as you can make it.

2. Pour the mixture into a container. Allow the ice cream to set in the freezer for 2 to 5 hours or overnight.

Tips:

- Using Almond Milk instead of water will give you a creamier ice cream. You can also use cashew milk to keep the recipe consistent with only cashews.

- If you have an ice-cream maker, make the recipe in the blender and then pour it into the ice-cream maker. Allow to churn for 30 minutes in the ice-cream maker and then it will be ready to eat.

- The more powerful your blender, the creamier your ice cream will be.

- Use 1 cup dates instead of maple syrup, if you choose.

Variations:

- Add 1 tablespoon (or more, to taste) cacao powder to make Chocolate Ice Cream.

- Add 1 tablespoon cacao powder and 3 tablespoons cacao nibs to make Chocolate Chip Ice Cream.

- Add 1 cup strawberries to make Strawberry Ice Cream.

- Add 1 tablespoon green tea to make Green Tea Ice Cream.

- Add 1 tablespoon very finely ground espresso to make Coffee Ice Cream.

- Drop raw Cookie Dough Balls (page 326) into partially frozen ice cream to make Cookie Dough Ice Cream.

- Add a handful of mint leaves and a drop of mint extract to make Mint Ice Cream.

- Add a handful of mint leaves, a drop of mint extract, or 1 to 2 drops peppermint or spearmint essential oil (therapeutic-grade only) and 1 tablespoon cacao powder to make Chocolate Mint Ice Cream.

- Add the juice of 1 to 2 lemons for Vanilla-Lemon Ice Cream.

- Add the juice of 1 to 2 limes for Vanilla-Lime Ice Cream.

Calories: 539 | Protein: 14.3g | Carbs: 49g | Dietary Fiber: 3.6g | Fat: 34.5g | Vitamin C: 0.3mg | Vitamin D: 0 IU | Vitamin E: 0.5mg | Calcium: 99.5mg | Iron: 4.8mg | Magnesium: 231.6mg | Potassium: 604.8mg

WHIPPED COCONUT CREAM

Enjoy this vegan, dairy-free alternative to whipped cream. It goes great on fruit salads, ice cream, yogurt parfaits, pies, French toast, mousse, and cake.

Total time: 10 minutes

Makes 1 cup

Ingredients:
One 14-ounce can coconut cream, chilled overnight

Actions:
1. Open the can carefully and scoop out the top layer of the hard coconut cream into a bowl with a hand mixer, or a blender. A powerful blender will work, but a hand mixer is better. Be careful not to get any liquids in the bowl at all; this will not allow the coconut cream to whip, it must be the hard part of the cream only.

2. Whip for a few minutes until the coconut cream is soft and fluffy.

Tips:
- Add a dash of vanilla extract to enhance the flavor.

- To properly chill the coconut cream, just leave it in the fridge overnight. The next day, don't shake it; just open the can and scoop out the top layer, which should be very thick. You won't need to use the runny liquid, so reserve it for another recipe, such as a curry!

- Chill your mixing bowl to help you get a nice consistency when beating.

- If you let the cream rest in the fridge, it will harden and set.

Calories: 237.4 | Protein: 0.7g | Carbs: 35.3g | Dietary Fiber: 0.1g | Fat: 10.8g | Vitamin C: 0mg | Vitamin D: 0 IU | Vitamin E: 0.09mg | Calcium: 2.6mg | Iron: 0.09mg | Magnesium: 11.3mg | Potassium: 67.1mg

GELATO

You can't get any simpler than this ice cream made with just one ingredient: frozen bananas! And then add other ingredients to make other flavors.

Total time: 5 minutes

Makes 1 to 2 servings

Ingredients:

2 frozen bananas

Actions:

Add the bananas to a blender and mix until they are smooth and fluffy, exactly like ice cream. At first your gelato will appear chunky and then it will become juicy and smooth.

Tips:

- To freeze bananas, peel them and then wrap them in plastic and put in the freezer. Grab however many you need whenever you want to make a smoothie or ice cream.

- Add other ingredients for different flavors. For example, a dash of vanilla, a vanilla bean, 2 teaspoons cacao powder, 1 tablespoon peanut butter, almond butter, or 1/3 cup strawberries, raspberries, or blueberries.

Variations:

- Add ½ cup frozen blueberries for Blueberry Gelato.
- Add 2 teaspoons cacao powder for Chocolate Gelato.
- Add 3 frozen strawberries for Strawberry Gelato.
- Add ½ a frozen mango for Mango Gelato.

Calories: 105 | Protein: 1.2g | Carbs: 26.9g | Dietary Fiber: 3g | Fat: 0.3g | Vitamin C: 10.2mg | Vitamin D: 0 IU | Vitamin E: 0.1mg | Calcium: 5.9mg | Iron: 0.3mg | Magnesium: 31.8mg | Potassium: 422.4mg

VANILLA CAKE

Use this recipe as an "upgrade" instead of baking a conventional vanilla cake. It doesn't have the gluten or unecessary white sugar!

Total time: 55 minutes

Serves 12

Ingredients:

1 cup almond milk

1 tablespoons apple cider vinegar

1 ½ cups almond flour

1 cup coconut sugar

2 teaspoons baking soda

½ teaspoon sea salt

⅓ cup coconut oil

¼ cup filtered water

1 tablespoon lemon juice

1 tablespoon vanilla extract

Actions:

1. Preheat the oven to 350°F. Grease an 8 x 8-inch baking dish.

2. Stir the almond milk and apple cider vinegar together in a large bowl. Set aside.

3. Whisk the flour, sugar, baking powder, and sea salt in a separate bowl. Set aside.

4. Whisk the coconut oil, water, lemon juice, and vanilla extract into the almond milk mixture using a fork. Add the flour mixture and whisk until it is smooth.

5. Pour the batter into the prepared baking dish.

6. Bake in the oven for 35 minutes.

Tip:

If you have a nut allergy, you could use tigernut milk and tigernut flour instead of almonds.

Variations:

For Chocolate Cake, add 2 tablespoons cacao powder to the ingredient list.

Calories: 190.2 | Protein: 3.2g | Carbs: 14.3g | Dietary Fiber: 1.8g | Fat: 13.2g | Vitamin C: 0.4mg | Vitamin D: 0 IU | Vitamin E: 0mg | Calcium: 39.6mg | Iron: 0.7mg | Magnesium: 12.3mg | Potassium: 237.8mg

CHOCOLATE HAZELNUT CAKE

Use this recipe as an "upgrade" from conventional chocolate cake. It even has flax meal, one of the top anticancer seeds we can consume!

Total time: 1 hour 10 minutes

Makes 16 servings

Ingredients:

For the cake:

1 cup almond milk or sunflower seed milk

3 teaspoons baking soda

1 teaspoon apple cider vinegar

4 tablespoons flaxseed meal

10 tablespoons filtered water

3 apples, peeled and cored

⅔ cup coconut sugar

½ cup plus 2 tablespoons maple syrup

1 teaspoon vanilla extract

½ teaspoon sea salt

½ cup coconut oil or Vegan Butter (page 313)

1 ½ cups almond meal

1 cup oat flour (or blended oats to a fine flour consistency)

½ cup tapioca flour

1 cup cacao powder

For the frosting:

½ cup almond milk

½ cup cacao powder

¼ cup maple syrup

¼ cup coconut oil or Vegan Butter (page 313)

1 ½ cups organic powdered sugar

For the topping:

1 ½ cups roasted hazelnuts

Actions:

1. Preheat the oven to 350°F.

2. Grease a 9" round cake pan.

3. Add the almond milk, baking soda, and apple cider vinegar to a large bowl. Stir, then let the mixture curdle.

4. Place the flax meal and water in a separate bowl. Whisk together well and set aside. In 5 minutes, the mixture will turn gummy like eggs.

5. Blend the apples in a food processor until you have applesauce.

6. Add the flax meal mixture, applesauce, coconut sugar, and maple syrup to the bowl with the almond milk mixture. Whisk well.

7. Add the vanilla, sea salt, and coconut oil and stir again.

8. Add the almond meal, oat flour, and tapioca flour and whisk to combine.

9. Pour the batter into the cake pan. Bake for 40 to 45 minutes. Let it cool in the tin before removing it from the pan.

10. For the frosting, combine all the ingredients in a bowl or blender and whip until the mixture is thick and smooth. When the cake is completely cooled, smooth the frosting on.

11. Top the cake with the roasted hazelnuts. Enjoy!

Calories: 449 | Protein: 7.9g | Carbs: 50.7g | Dietary Fiber: 5.7g | Fat: 25.4g | Vitamin C: 1.6mg | Vitamin D: 0 IU | Vitamin E: 4.3mg | Calcium: 69.3mg | Iron: 2.3mg | Magnesium: 116.3mg | Potassium: 367.5mg

RAW HIGH-PROTEIN GRANOLA BARS WITH CHOCOLATE CHIP ALMOND BUTTER

Total time: 8 minutes

Makes 21 bars

Ingredients:

1 ½ cups almond butter

1 cup oats

1 cup organic chocolate chips or cacao nibs

¼ cup maple syrup

¼ cup chia seeds

¼ cup hemp seeds

Actions:

1. Mix all the ingredients until they are moist enough to stick together.

2. Pat the mixture into a 9 x 13-inch glass baking dish.

3. Cut into squares.

Calories: 213.5 | Protein: 6.1g | Carbs: 15.5g | Dietary Fiber: 3g | Fat: 16.5g | Vitamin C: 0.04mg | Vitamin D: 0 IU | Vitamin E: 4.4mg | Calcium: 82.9mg | Iron: 1.6mg | Magnesium: 78.6mg | Potassium: 192.7mg

FRUIT LEATHERS

Satisfy your candy cravings and feel fulfilled as a cook in the process by making homemade Fruit Leathers. Basically, to make one you simply puree your favorite fruits and flavors and then dehydrate them in flat sheets until they are sticky and sweet like candy. *Note*: Although these take less than 10 minutes to prepare, they need to be dehydrated overnight. It is also possible to use your oven if it's set on very low (150°F) heat.

I put this recipe in the book for candy lovers! If you squish the leather together or make a roll-up with it, this can fulfill gummy bear cravings. The Cherry Leather is my favorite fruit leather!

Actions:

1. Add your fruit ingredients to a food processor and blend until smooth with no chunks.

2. Place parchment paper on the mesh screens in your dehydrator. Pour the fruit mixture on the paper to ¼-inch thick.

3. Dehydrate at 115°F for 8 to 12 hours, or until no longer wet.

Tip:

Instead of a dehydrator, bake in your oven at 150°F for 4 to 6 hours.

Calories: 201.6 | Protein: 2.7g | Carbs: 50.3g | Dietary Fiber: 5.2g | Fat: 1.2g | Vitamin C: 122.3mg | Vitamin D: 0 IU | Vitamin E: 3mg | Calcium: 36.9mg | Iron: 0.5mg | Magnesium: 33.6mg | Potassium: 564.8mg

Variations:

*   *Strawberry Banana Leather*: 3 cups strawberries and 4 peeled bananas

*   *Strawberry Banana Blueberry Leather*: 2 cups strawberries, 3 peeled bananas, and 2 cups blueberries

- *Strawberry Kiwifruit Leather*: 2 cups strawberries and 10 peeled kiwifruits
- *Strawberry Apple Leather*: 2 cups strawberries and 4 apples, cored
- *Strawberry Nectarine Leather*: 2 cups strawberries and 4 nectarines, seeded
- *Strawberry Peach Leather*: 2 cups strawberries and 4 peaches, seeded
- *Cherry Leather*: 8 cups cherries, seeded
- *Plum Leather*: 8 cups plums, seeded
- *Peach Apple Leather*: 4 apples, cored and peeled, and 4 peaches, seeded
- *Peach Goji Berry Leather*: 1 cup goji berries and 8 peaches, seeded
- *Apricot Leather*: 8 cups fresh apricots, seeded
- *Blueberry Leather*: 8 cups blueberries
- *Green Apple Leather*: 8 apples, cored
- *Apple and Pear Leather*: 4 apples, cored and peeled, and 4 pears, cored and peeled
- *Mango Leather:* 4 mangoes, peeled and seeded
- *Mango Banana Leather:* 3 mangos, peeled and seeded, and 3 peeled bananas
- *Raspberry Leather:* 6 cups raspberries
- *Sweet Potato Leather:* 3 peeled sweet potatoes, 3 apples, ½ teaspoon cinnamon powder, ¼ teaspoon nutmeg powder, 1/8 teaspoon turmeric powder, ¼ teaspoon ginger powder, pinch of ground clove

ENDNOTES

Introduction

1. Zosia Chustecka. "Cancer Strikes 1 in 2 Men and 1 in 3 Women," Medscape Medical News, February 9, 2007, https://www.medscape.com/viewarticle/551998.

Chapter 1: Seven Key Nutritional Principles for Preventing and Overcoming Cancer

1. Mark Hyman. "5 Strategies to Prevent and Heal Cancer," Dr. Hyman blog (accessed July 9, 2018), http://drhyman.com/blog/2015/08/07/5-strategies-to-prevent-and-treat-cancer.

2. Deepak Chopra. "Cancer: A Preventable Disease Is Creating a Revolution," Beliefnet (accessed June 27, 2018), http://www.beliefnet.com/columnists/intentchopra/2012/01/cancer-a-preventable-disease-is-creating-a-revolution.html.

3. Joseph Mercola. "How a High-Fat Diet Helps Starve Cancer," Mercola.com, May 30, 2016. https://articles.mercola.com/sites/articles/archive/2016/05/30/how-high-fat-diet-helps-starve-cancer.aspx.

4. Mark Hyman. "5 Strategies to Help Prevent and Treat Cancer," Huffington Post (August 17, 2015), https://www.huffingtonpost.com/dr-mark-hyman/5-strategies-to-prevent-a_b_7972340.html.

5. AICR eNews. "7 Key Nutrients: Find Them in Your Cancer-Fighting Foods," American Institute for Cancer Research (March 2, 2017), http://www.aicr.org/enews/2017/03-march/enews-7-key-nutrients-found-in-foods.html.

6. Mehmet Oz. "5 Foods That Starve Cancer," Dr. Oz Show blog (posted September 10, 2010), http://www.doctoroz.com/article/5-foods-starve-cancer.

7. Mark Hyman. "5 Strategies to Prevent and Heal Cancer."

8. Dana Cohen and Gina Bria. Quench: Beat Fatigue, Drop Weight, and Heal Your Body Through the New Science of Optimum Hydration (New York: Hachette Books, 2018), p. 4.

Chapter 2: The Top 15 Cancer-Healing Foods

1. Veronique Desaulniers. "The Landmark Johns Hopkins Sulforaphane Cancer Study Your Doctor Isn't Telling You About," Truth About Cancer blog (accessed June 30, 2018), https://thetruthaboutcancer.com/johns-hopkins-sulforaphane-cancer-study.

2. Johns Hopkins Medical Institutions. "Cancer Protection Compound Abundant in Broccoli Sprouts, Johns Hopkins Scientists Find," ScienceDaily (accessed June 26, 2018), www.sciencedaily.com/releases/1997/09/970919062654.htm. Also: Melissa Hendricks. "More Reasons to Eat Those Vegetables," Johns Hopkins Medicine, Institute for Basic Biomedical Sciences (accessed June 30, 2018), https://www.hopkinsmedicine.org/institute_basic_biomedical_sciences/news_events/articles_and_stories/cancer_disease/2010_08_eat_veggies.html.

3. "Potential for Added Medical Benefits Uncovered for Widely Used Breast Cancer Drug," Johns Hopkins Medicine News release. (November 7, 2013), https://www.hopkinsmedicine.org/news/media/releases/potential_for_added_medical_benefits_uncovered_for_widely_used_breast_cancer_drug.

4. "Broccoli Sprouts," Memorial Sloan Kettering Cancer Center (accessed June 26, 2018), https://www.mskcc.org/cancer-care/integrative-medicine/herbs/broccoli-sprouts.

5. Teresa L. Johnson. "Broccoli extract may lower blood sugar among some with diabetes, study finds," American Cancer Research Institute blog (posted June 26, 2017), http://blog.aicr.org/2017/06/26/broccoli-extract-may-lower-blood-sugar-among-some-with-diabetes-study-finds/?_ga=2.87538392.1138489825.1525817004-1726391947.1525817004.

6. "Gutsy Germs Succumb to Baby Broccoli," Johns Hopkins Medicine News release (posted April 6, 2009), https://www.hopkinsmedicine.org/news/media/releases/gutsy_germs_succumb_to_baby_broccoli.

7. Miranda Hitti. "Broccoli Sprouts vs. Bladder Cancer?" WebMD (posted February 28, 2008), https://www.webmd.com/cancer/bladder-cancer/news/20080228/broccoli-sprouts-vs-bladder-cancer.

8. Melissa Hendricks. "More Reasons to Eat Those Vegetables," Johns Hopkins Medicine, Institute for Basic Biomedical Sciences (accessed June 30, 2018), https://www.hopkinsmedicine.org/institute_basic_biomedical_sciences/news_events/articles_and_stories/cancer_disease/2010_08_eat_veggies.html

9. Mehmet Oz. "Nine Cancer-Fighting Foods," *The Doctor Oz Show* blog (posted December 16, 2016), https://www.doctoroz.com/gallery/9-cancer-fighting-foods.

10. Visit: https://www.mdanderson.org/research/departments-labs-institutes/programs-centers/center-for-cancer-prevention-by-dietary-botanicals.html.

11. Lauren Martin and Corey Schuler. "Turmeric, Curcuminoids, and Curcumin Defined," Integrative Therapeutics (September 1, 2016), https://www.integrativepro.com/Resources/Integrative-Blog/2016/Turmeric-Curcuminoids-Curcumin-Defined.

12. "Turmeric," Memorial Sloan Kettering Cancer Center (accessed June 26, 2018), https://www.mskcc.org/cancer-care/integrative-medicine/herbs/turmeric.

13. Ibid.

14. Mark Hyman. "Ingredients Archive: Turmeric," Dr. Hyman blog (accessed June 30, 2018), http://drhyman.com/blog/ingredient/turmeric.

15. Michael Greger. "Turmeric Curcumin and Colon Cancer," Care2 (posted March 6, 2015), https://www.care2.com/greenliving/turmeric-curcumin-and-colon-cancer.html.

16. M. Cruz-Correa, D.A. Shoskes, P. Sanchez, et. Al. "Combination Treatment with Curcumin and Quercetin of Adenomas in Familial Adenomatous Polyposis," *Clinical Gastroenterology and Hepatology,* vol. 4, no. 8 (August 2006), pp. 1035–8, http://www.ncbi.nlm.nih.gov/pubmed/16757216.

17. National Center for Complementary and Integrative Health. "Turmeric," U.S. Department of Health and Human Services, National Institutes of health (accessed June 30, 2018), https://nccih.nih.gov/health/turmeric/ataglance.htm.

18. Timothy J. Moynihan. "Curcumin: Can It Slow Cancer Growth?" Mayo Clinic (accessed June 30, 2018), https://www.mayoclinic.org/diseases-conditions/cancer/expert-answers/curcumin/faq-20057858.

19. M. Bayet-Robert, F. Kwiatkowski, M. Leheurteur, et al. "Phase I dose escalation trial of docetaxel plus curcumin in patients with advanced and metastatic breast cancer," *Cancer Biology & Therapy,* vol. 9, no. 1 (January 2010), pp. 8–14, https://www.ncbi.nlm.nih.gov/pubmed/19901561.

20. R. Epelbaum, M. Schaffer, B. Vizel, et al. "Curcumin and Gemcitabine in Patients with Advanced Pancreatic Cancer," *Nutrition and Cancer,* vol. 62, no. 8 (2010), pp. 1113–1141, http://www.ncbi.nlm.nih.gov/pubmed/21058202. Also: N. Dhillon, B.B. Aggarwal, R.A. Newman, et al. "Phase II Trial of Curcumin Patients with Advanced Pancreatic Cancer. *Clinical Cancer Research,* vol. 14, no. 14 (July, 15 2008), pp. 4491–9, http://www.ncbi.nlm.nih.gov/pubmed/18628464; and Kanai M, Yoshimura K, Asada M, et al. "A phase I/II study of gemcitabine-based chemotherapy plus curcumin for patients with gemcitabine-resistant pancreatic cancer." *Cancer Chemotherapy and Pharmacology,* vol. 68, no. 1 (July 2011), pp. 157–64, http://www.ncbi.nlm.nih.gov/pubmed/20859741.

21. Z.Y. He, C.B. Shi, H. Wen, et al. "Upregulation of p53 Expression in Patients with Colorectal Cancer by Administration of Curcumin," *Cancer Investigation,* vol. 29, no. 3 (March 2011), pp. 208–13, http://www.ncbi.nlm.nih.gov/pubmed/21314329. Also: A.B. Kunnumakkara, P. Diagaradjane, S. Guha, et al. "Curcumin Sensitizes Human Colorectal Cancer Xenografts in Nude Mice to Gamma-Radiation by Targeting Nuclear Factor-KappaB-Regulated Gene Products," *Clinical Cancer Research,* vol. 14, no. 7 (April 1, 2008), pp. 2128–36, http://www.ncbi.nlm.nih.gov/pubmed/18381954.

22. S.S. Lin, K.C. Lai, S.C. Hsu, et al. "Curcumin inhibits the migration and invasion of human A549 lung cancer cells through the inhibition of matrix metalloproteinase-2 and -9 and Vascular Endothelial Growth Factor (VEGF)," *Cancer Letters*, vol. 285, no. 2 (November 28, 2009), pp.127–33, http://www.ncbi.nlm.nih.gov/pubmed/19477063. Also: M.G. Alexandrow, L.J. Song, S. Altiok, et al. "Curcumin: A Novel Stat3 Pathway Inhibitor for Chemoprevention of Lung Cancer," *European Journal of Cancer Prevention*, vol. 21, no. 5 (December 7, 2011), pp. 407–12, http://www.ncbi.nlm.nih.gov/pubmed/22156994; and S.H. Wu, L.W. Hang, J.S. Yang, et al. "Curcumin Induces Apoptosis in Human Non-Small Cell Lung Cancer NCI-H460 Cells Through ER Stress and Caspase Cascade- and Mitochondria-Dependent Pathways," *Anticancer Research*, vol. 30, no. 6 (June 2010), pp. 2125–33, http://www.ncbi.nlm. nih.gov/pubmed/20651361.

23. J. Shi, Y. Wang, Z. Jia, et al. "Curcumin Inhibits Bladder Cancer Progression via Regulation of β-Catenin Expression. *Tumor Biology*, vol. 39, no. 7 (published online July 14, 2017), http://journals.sagepub.com/doi/10.1177/1010428317702548.

24. K. Selvendiran, S. Ahmed, A. Dayton, et al. "HO-3867, a Curcumin Analog, Sensitizes Cisplatin-Resistant Ovarian Carcinoma, Leading to Therapeutic Synergy Through STAT3 Inhibition," *Cancer Biology & Therapy*, vol. 12, no. 9 (November 1, 2011), pp. 837–45, http://www. ncbi.nlm.nih.gov/pubmed/21885917.

25. C.N. Sreekanth, S.V. Bava, E. Sreekumar, et al. "Molecular Evidences for the Chemosensitizing Efficacy of Liposomal Curcumin in Paclitaxel Chemotherapy in Mouse Models of Cervical Cancer," *Oncogene*, vol. 30, no. 28 (July 14, 2011), p. 3139–52, http://www.ncbi.nlm.nih.gov/pubmed/21317920.

26. Q. Qiao, Y. Jiang, G. Li. "Curcumin Improves the Antitumor Effect of X-ray Irradiation by Blocking the NF-kappaB Pathway: An In-Vitro Study of Lymphoma," *Anticancer Drugs*, vol. 23, no. 6 (January 23, 2012), pp. 597–605, http://www.ncbi.nlm.nih.gov/pubmed/22273827. Also: S. Uddin, A.R. Hussain, P.S. Manogaran, et al. "Curcumin Suppresses Growth and Induces Apoptosis in Primary Effusion Lymphoma," Oncogene, vol. 24, no. 47 (October 27, 2005), pp. 7022–30, http:// www.ncbi.nlm.nih.gov/pubmed/16044161.

27. K.W. Chang, P.S. Hung, I.Y. Lin, et al. "Curcumin Upregulates Insulin-like Growth Factor Binding Protein-5 (IGFBP-5) and C/EBPalpha During Oral Cancer Suppression," *International Journal of Cancer*, vol. 127, no. 1 (July 1, 2010), pp. 9–20, http://www.ncbi.nlm.nih.gov/pubmed/20127863.

28. "Turmeric," Memorial Sloan Kettering Cancer Center.

29. "Anticancer Properties of Blueberries," Cancer Effects (accessed June 30, 2018), http://www.cancereffects.com/Anticancer-Properties-of-Blueberries.html.

30. Delarno's blog. "Blueberries Kill Cancer Cells and Reduce Tumor Size," Cancer Survivors Network (posted October 12, 2015), https://csn. cancer.org/node/297330.

31. S.A. Johnson and B.H. Arjmandi. "Evidence for Anticancer Properties of Blueberries: A Mini-Review," *Anticancer Agents in Medicinal Chemistry,* vol. 13, no. 8 (October 2013), pp. 1142–8, https://www.ncbi.nlm.nih.gov/pubmed/23387969.

32. A. Faria, D. Pestana, D. Teixeiria, et al. "Blueberry anthocyanins and pyruvic acid adducts: anticancer properties in breast cancer cell lines," *Phytotherapy Research,* vol. 24, no. 12 (December 2010), pp. 1862-9, https://www.ncbi.nlm.nih.gov/pubmed/20564502.

33. Kristoffer T. Davidson, Ziwen Zhu, Qian Bai, et al. "Blueberry as a Potential Radiosensitizer for Treating Cervical Cancer," *Pathology & Oncology Research* (published online 2017), https://link.springer.com/article/10.1007/s12253-017-0319-y. Also: Honor Whiteman. "How Blueberries Help to Kill Cancer Cells," *Medical News Today* (January 3, 2018), https://www.medicalnewstoday.com/articles/320517.php.

34. Sylvia Booth Hubbard. "Blueberries: A Natural Weapon to Treat Alzheimer's, Heart Disease, and Cancer," Newsmax (posted Mach 29, 2016), https://www.newsmax.com/health/headline/blueberries-natural-weapon-treat/2016/03/29/id/721354.

35. "5 Foods That Help Lower Your Cancer Risk," MD Anderson Cancer Center (August 2016), https://www.mdanderson.org/publications/focused-on-health/August2016/foods-lower-cancerrisk.html.

36. AICR's Foods That Fight Cancer. "Broccoli and Cruciferous Vegetables," American Institute for Cancer Research (accessed June 30, 2018), www.aicr.org/foods-that-fight-cancer/broccoli-cruciferous.html.

37. Kellie Bramlet. "Phytochemicals and Cancer: What You Should Know," MD Anderson Cancer Center (January 2017), https://www.mdanderson.org/publications/focused-on-health/january-2017/phytochemicals-and-cancer-what-you-should-know.html.

38. Ibid.

39. A.M. Tarrazo-Antelo, A. Ruano-Ravina, J. Abal Arca, et al. "Fruit and Vegetable Consumption and Lung Cancer Risk: A Case-Control Study in Galicia, Spain," *Nutrition and Cancer,* vol. 66, no. 6 (August 2014), https://www.ncbi.nlm.nih.gov/pubmed/25085257.

40. AICR's Foods That Fight Cancer. "Broccoli and Cruciferous Vegetables."

41. "Cruciferous Vegetables and Cancer Prevention," National Cancer Institute (accessed June 23, 2018), https://www.cancer.gov/about-cancer/causes-prevention/risk/diet/cruciferous-vegetables-fact-sheet.

42. A. Tanskanen, J.R. Hibbeln, J. Tuomilehto, et al. "Fish Consumption and Depressive Symptoms in the General Population in Finland," *Psychiatric Services,* vol. 52, no. 4 (2001), pp. 529–31, https://www.ncbi.nlm.nih.gov/pubmed/11274502.

43. A. Calado, P.M. Neves, T. Santos, et al. "The Effect of Flaxseed in Breast Cancer: A Literature Review," *Frontiers in Nutrition* (February 27, 2018), https://www.frontiersin.org/articles/10.3389/fnut.2018.00004/full. Also: J. Lee, K. Cho. "Flaxseed Sprouts Induce Apoptosis and Inhibit Growth in MCF-7 and MDA-MB-231 Human Breast Cancer Cells," *In Vitro Cellular Development & Biology - Animal,* vol. 48, no. 4 (2012), pp. 244–50, https://www.ncbi.nlm.nih.gov/pubmed/22438134.

44. Ibid.

45. "Flaxseed," Memorial Sloan Kettering Cancer Center (accessed June 26, 2018), https://www.mskcc.org/cancer-care/integrative-medicine/herbs/flaxseed. Also: L.U. Thompson, J.M. Chen, T. Li, et al. "Dietary Flaxseed Alters Tumor Biological Markers in Postmenopausal Breast Cancer," *Clinical Cancer Research*, vol. 11, no. 10 (2005), pp. 3828–35, http://www.ncbi.nlm.nih.gov/pubmed/15897583. Also: S.E. McCann, L.U. Thompson, J. Nie, et al. "Dietary Lignan Intakes in Relation to Survival among Women with Breast Cancer: The Western New York Exposures and Breast Cancer (WEB) Study," *Breast Cancer Research and Treatment*, vol. 122, no. 1 (July 2010), pp. 229–35, https://www.ncbi.nlm.nih.gov/pubmed/20033482.

46. Chen, K.A. Power, J. Mann, et al. "Flaxseed alone or in combination with tamoxifen inhibits MCF-7 breast tumor growth in ovariectomized athymic mice with high circulating levels of estrogen," *Experimental Biology and Medicine*, vol. 232, no. 8 (September 2007), pp. 1071–80, https://www.ncbi.nlm.nih.gov/pubmed/17720953.

47. "Flaxseed," Memorial Sloan Kettering Cancer Center.

48. B. Liang, S. Wang, Y.J. Ye, et al. "Impact of Postoperative Omega-3 Fatty Acid-supplemented Parenteral Nutrition on Clinical Outcomes and Immunomodulations in Colorectal Cancer Patients," *World Journal of Gastroenterology*, vol. 14, no. 15 (2008), pp. 2434–9, https://www.ncbi.nlm.nih.gov/pubmed/18416476. Also: C.H. MacLean, et al. "Effects of Omega-3 Fatty Acids on Cancer Risk," JAMA, vol. 295, no. 4 (2006), pp. 403–15, http://www.ncbi.nlm.nih.gov/pubmed/16434631; and M.K. Sung, M. Lautens, L.U. Thompson. "Mammalian Lignans Inhibit the Growth of Estrogen-independent Human Colon Tumor Cells," *Anticancer Research*, vol. 18, no. 3A (May–June 1998), pp. 1405–8, https://www.ncbi.nlm.nih.gov/pubmed/9673348.

49. L.E. Rhodes, H. Shahbakhti, R.M. Azurdia, et al. "Effect of Eicosapentaenoic Acid, an Omega-3 Polyunsaturated Fatty Acid, on UVR-related Cancer Risk in Humans. An Assessment of Early Genotoxic Markers," *Carcinogenesis*, vol. 24, no. 5 (May 2003), pp. 919–25, https://www.ncbi.nlm.nih.gov/pubmed/12771037. Also: L. Yan, J.A. Yee, D. Li, et al. "Dietary flaxseed supplementation and experimental metastasis of melanoma cells in mice," *Cancer Letters*, vol. 124, no. 2 (February 1998), pp.181–6, http://www.ncbi.nlm.nih.gov/pubmed/9500208.

50. W. Demark-Wahnefried, T.J. Polascik, S.L. George, et al. "Flaxseed Supplementation (not Dietary Fat Restriction) Reduces Prostate Cancer Proliferation Rates in Men Presurgery," Cancer Epidemiology, Biomarkers & Prevention, vol. 17, no. 12 (December 2008), pp. 3577–87, http://www.ncbi.nlm.nih.gov/pubmed/19064574.

51. "Flaxseed," Memorial Sloan Kettering Cancer Center.

52. O. Azarenko, M.A. Jordan, and L. Wilson. "Erucin, the Major Isothiocyanate in Arugula (*Eruca Sativa*), Inhibits Proliferation of MCF7 Tumor Cells by Suppressing Microtubule Dynamics," *PLoS One*, vol. 9, no. 6 (June 2014), p. e100599, https://www.ncbi.nlm.nih.gov/pubmed/24950293.

53. H. Akasaka, R. Sasaki, K. Yoshida. "Monogalactosyl diacylglycerol, a replicative DNA polymerase inhibitor, from spinach enhances the anti-cell proliferation effect of gemcitabine in human pancreatic cancer cells," *Biochimica et Biophisica Acta*, vol. 1830, no. 3 (March 2013), pp. 2517–25, https://www.ncbi.nlm.nih.gov/pubmed/23174220.

54. D.M. Jiménez-Aguilar and M.A. Grusak. "Evaluation of Minerals, Phytochemical Compounds and Antioxidant Activity of Mexican, Central American, and African Green Leafy Vegetables," *Plant Foods for Human Nutrition*, vol. 70, no. 4 (December 2015), pp. 357–64, https://www.ncbi.nlm.nih.gov/pubmed/26490448.

55. N.I. Park, J.K. Kim, W.T. Park. "An Efficient Protocol for Genetic Transformation of Watercress (*Nasturtium officinale*) Using Agrobacterium Rhizogenes," *Molecular Biology Reports*, vol. 38, no. 8 (November 2011), pp. 4947–53, https://www.ncbi.nlm.nih.gov/pubmed/21161399.

56. G. Schäfer and C.H. Kaschula. "The immunomodulation and anti-inflammatory effects of garlic organosulfur compounds in cancer chemoprevention," *Anticancer Agents in Medicinal Chemistry*, vol. 14, no. 2 (February 2014), pp. 233–40, https://www.ncbi.nlm.nih.gov/pubmed/24237225.

57. H.L. Nicastro, S.A. Ross, J.A. Milner, et al. "Garlic and Onions: Their Cancer Prevention Properties," *Cancer Prevention Research*, vol. 8, no. 3 (March 2015), pp. 181–9, https://www.ncbi.nlm.nih.gov/pubmed/25586902.

58. W.H. Talib. "Consumption of Garlic and Lemon Aqueous Extracts Combination Reduces Tumor Burden by Angiogenesis Inhibition, Apoptosis Induction, and Immune System Modulation," *Nutrition*, vol. 43–44 (November–December 2017), pp. 89–97, https://www.ncbi.nlm.nih.gov/pubmed/28935151.

59. A. Muhammad, M.A. Ibrahim, O.L. Erukainure, et al. "Spices with Breast Cancer Chemopreventive and Therapeutic Potentials: A Functional Foods Based-Review," *Anticancer Agents in Medicinal Chemistry*, vol. 18, no. 2 (2018), pp. 182–94, https://www.ncbi.nlm.nih.gov/pubmed/28901261.

60. W.T. Kim, S.P. Seo, Y.J. Byun, et al. "The Anticancer Effects of Garlic Extracts on Bladder Cancer Compared to Cisplatin: A Common Mechanism of Action via Centromere Protein M," *American Journal of Chinese Medicine*, vol. 46, no. 3 (March 2018), pp. 689–705, https://www.ncbi.nlm.nih.gov/pubmed/29595070.

61. S. Patel and A. Goyal. "Recent Developments in Mushrooms as Anticancer Therapeutics: A Review," *3 Biotech*, vol. 2, no. 1 (March 2012), pp. 1–15, http://www.ncbi.nlm.nih.gov/pmc/articles/pmc3339609.

62. D. Akramiene, A. Kondrotas, J. Didziapetriene, et al. "Effects of Beta-Glucans on the Immune System," *Medicina (Kaunas)*, vol. 43, no. 8 (2007), pp. 597–606, https://www.ncbi.nlm.nih.gov/pubmed/17895634.

63. J. Li, L. Zou, W. Chen, et al. "Dietary mushroom intake may reduce the risk of breast cancer: evidence from a meta-analysis of observational studies," *PloS One*, vol. 9, no. 4 (April 2-014), pp. e93437, https://www.ncbi.nlm.nih.gov/pubmed/24691133.

64. J.H. Kang, J.E. Jang, S.K. Mishra, et al. "Ergosterol Peroxide from Chaga Mushroom (Inonotus Obliquus) Exhibits Anticancer Activity by Down-regulation of the β-catenin Pathway in Colorectal Cancer," *Journal of Ethnopharmacology*, vol. 173 (September 2015), pp. 303–12, https://www.ncbi.nlm.nih.gov/pubmed/26210065.

65. "Eating Mushrooms Daily 'May Cut Breast Cancer Risk by Two Thirds,'" *Telegraph* (March 16, 2009), as cited in Ocean Robbins. *31-Day Food Revolution: Heal Your Body, Feel Great, and Transform Your World* (New York: Grand Central Life & Style, 2019), advance copy provided by the author prior to publication.

66. M. Zhang, et al., "Dietary Intake of Mushrooms and Green Tea Combine to Reduce the Risk of Breast Cancer in Chinese Women," *International Journal of Cancer*, vol. 124, no. 6 (March 15, 2009), pp. 1404–8, as cited by Ocean Robbins.

67. Joel Fuhrman. "Mighty Mushrooms: Boost Immune Function and Guard Against Cancer," Dr. Fuhrman blog (May 31, 2017), as cited by Ocean Robbins.

68. S.A. Oyeleke, A.M. Ajayi, S. Umukoro. "Anti-inflammatory Activity of Theobroma Cacao L. Stem Bark Ethanol Extract and Its Fractions in Experimental Models," *Journal of Ethnopharmacology*, vol. 222 (August 2018), pp. 239–48, https://www.ncbi.nlm.nih.gov/pubmed/29733944.

69. Z. Baharum, A.M. Akim, T.Y. Hin, et al. "Theobroma Cacao: Review of the Extraction, Isolation, and Bioassay of Its Potential Anticancer Compounds," *Tropical Life Sciences Research*, vol. 27, no. 1 (February 2016), pp. 21–42, https://www.ncbi.nlm.nih.gov/pubmed/27019680.

70. N. Sugimoto, S. Miwa, Y. Hitomi, et al. "Theobromine, the Primary Methylxanthine Found in Theobroma cacao, Prevents Malignant Glioblastoma proliferation by Negatively Regulating Phosphodiesterase-4, Extracellular signal-regulated Kinase, Akt/mammalian Target of Rapamycin Kinase, and Nuclear factor-kappa B," *Nutrition and Cancer*, vol. 66, no. 3 (February 2014), https://www.ncbi.nlm.nih.gov/pubmed/24547961.

71. "Caffeine Has Positive Effect on Memory," Johns Hopkins Medicine (accessed July 3, 2018), https://www.hopkinsmedicine.org/news/stories/caffeine_memory.html.

72. M. Hashibe, C. Galeone, S.S. Buys, et al. "Coffee, Tea, Caffeine Intake, and the Risk of Cancer in the PLCO Cohort," *British Journal of Cancer*, vol. 113, no. 5 (September 2015), pp. 809–16, https://www.ncbi.nlm.nih.gov/pubmed/26291054.

73. R. Franco, A. Oñatibia-Astibia, E. Martínez-Pinilla. "Health Benefits of Methylxanthines in Cacao and Chocolate," *Nutrients*, vol. 5, no. 10 (October 2013), pp. 4159–73, https://www.ncbi.nlm.nih.gov/pubmed/24145871.

74. R. Latif. "Chocolate/Cocoa and Human Health: A Review," *Netherlands Journal of Medicine*, vol. 71, no. 2 (March 2013), pp. 63–8, https://www.ncbi.nlm.nih.gov/pubmed/23462053.

75. S.J. Kim, S.H. Park, H.W. Lee, et al. "Cacao Polyphenols Potentiate Anti-Platelet Effect of Endothelial Cells and Ameliorate Hypercoagulatory States Associated with Hypercholesterolemia," *Journal of Nanoscience and Nanotechnology*, vol. 17, no. 4 (April 2017), pp. 2817–823, https://www.ncbi.nlm.nih.gov/pubmed/29668171.

76. H. Kord-Varkaneh, E. Ghaedi, A. Nazary-Vanani. "Does cocoa/dark chocolate supplementation have favorable effect on body weight, body mass index and waist circumference? A systematic review, meta-analysis and dose-response of randomized clinical trials," *Critical Reviews in Food Science and Nutrition* (March 19, 2018), pp. 1–14, https://www.ncbi.nlm.nih.gov/pubmed/29553824.

77. A.K. Pandurangan, Z. Saadatdoust, N.M. Esa. "Dietary cocoa protects against colitis-associated cancer by activating the Nrf2/Keap1 pathway," *Biofactors*, vol. 41, no. 1 (January 2015), pp. 1–14, https://www.ncbi.nlm.nih.gov/pubmed/25545372.

78. Z. Saadatdoust, A.K. Pandurangan, S.K. Ananda Sadagopan, et al. "Dietary cocoa inhibits colitis associated cancer: a crucial involvement of the IL-6/STAT3 pathway," *Journal of Nutritional Biochemistry*, vol. 26, no. 12 (December 2015), pp. 1547–58, https://www.ncbi.nlm.nih.gov/pubmed/26355019.

79. X. Li, J. Fu, Y. Wang. "Preparation of Low Digestible and Viscoelastic Tigernut (Cyperus Esculentus) Starch by Bacillus Acidopullulyticus Pullulanase," *International Journal of Biological Macromolecules*, vol. 102 (September 2017), pp. 651–7, https://www.ncbi.nlm.nih.gov/pubmed/28433770.

80. N.O. Onuoha, N.O. Ogbusua, A.N. Okorie, et al. "Tigernut (*Cyperus esculentus* L.) 'Milk' as a Potent 'Nutri-drink' for the Prevention of Acetaminophen-induced Hepatotoxicity in a Murine Model," *Journal of Intercultural Ethnopharmacology*, vol. 6, no. 3 (June 2017), pp. 290–5, https://www.ncbi.nlm.nih.gov/pubmed/28894628.

81. A.A. Tahir, N.F. Sani, N.A. Murad, et al. "Combined Ginger Extract and Gelam Honey Modulate Ras/ERK and PI3K/AKT Pathway Genes in Colon Cancer HT29 Cells," *Nutrition Journal*, vol. 14 (April 1, 2015), p. 31, https://www.ncbi.nlm.nih.gov/pubmed/25889965.

82. S. Prasad and A.K. Tyagi. "Ginger and Its Constituents: Role in Prevention and Treatment of Gastrointestinal Cancer," *Gastroenterology Research and Practice*, epub March 2015, https://www.ncbi.nlm.nih.gov/pubmed/25838819.

83. S. Paramee, S. Sookkhee, C. Sakonwasun, et al. "Anticancer Effects of Kaempferia parviflora on Ovarian Cancer SKOV3 Cells," *BMC Complementary and Alternative Medicine*, vol. 18, no. 1 (June 2018), p. 178, https://www.ncbi.nlm.nih.gov/pubmed/29891015.

84. A. Saha, J. Blando, E. Silver, et al. "6-Shogaol from dried ginger inhibits growth of prostate cancer cells both in vitro and in vivo through inhibition of STAT3 and NF-κB signaling," *Cancer Prevention Research*, vol. 7, no. 6 (June 2014), p. 627-38, https://www.ncbi.nlm.nih.gov/pubmed/24691500.

85. Andrew Weil. "Ginger," Dr. Weil blog (accessed July 4, 2018), https://www.drweil.com/vitamins-supplements-herbs/herbs/ginger.

86. "Ginger," Memorial Sloan Kettering Cancer Center blog (accessed July 4, 2018), https://www.mskcc.org/cancer-care/integrative-medicine/herbs/ginger.

87. M. Kaur, C. Agarwal, and R. Agarwal. "Anticancer and Cancer Chemopreventive Potential of Grape Seed Extract and Other Grape-based Products," *Journal of Nutrition*, vol. 139, no. 9 (September 2009, pp. 1806S–12S, https://www.ncbi.nlm.nih.gov/pmc/articles/PMC2728696.

88. MD Anderson Cancer Center, "5 Foods That May Help Lower Your Cancer Risk," (August 2016), https://www.mdanderson.org/publications/focused-on-health/August2016/foods-lower-cancerrisk.html.

89. A.J. Braakhuis, P. Campion, and K.S. Bishop. "Reducing Breast Cancer Recurrence: The Role of Dietary Polyphenolics," *Nutrients*, vol. 8, no. 9 (September 2016), p. ii: E547, https://www.ncbi.nlm.nih.gov/pubmed/27608040.

90. S.R. Lee, H. Jin, W.T. Kim, et al. "Tristetraprolin Activation by Resveratrol Inhibits the Proliferation and Metastasis of Colorectal Cancer Cells," *International Journal of Oncology*, epub ahead of print (June 25, 2018), pp. 1269–1278, https://www.ncbi.nlm.nih.gov/pubmed/29956753.

91. J.R. Heo, S.M. Kim, K.A Hwang, et al. "Resveratrol Induced Reactive Oxygen Species and Endoplasmic Reticulum Stressmediated Apoptosis, and Cell Cycle Arrest in the A375SM Malignant Melanoma Cell Line," *International Journal of Molecular Medicine*, epub ahead of print (June 25, 2018), https://www.ncbi.nlm.nih.gov/pubmed/29916532.

92. "Prostate Cancer, Nutrition, and Dietary Supplements (PDQ®)–Health Professional Version," National Cancer Institute (accessed July 1, 2018), http://www.cancer.gov/about-cancer/treatment/cam/hp/prostate-supplements-pdq.

93. V. Er, J.A. Lane, R.M. Martin, et al. "Adherence to Dietary and Lifestyle Recommendations and Prostate Cancer Risk in the Prostate Testing for Cancer and Treatment (ProtecT) Trial," *Cancer Epidemiology, Biomarkers & Prevention*, vol. 23, no. 10 (October 2014), pp. 2066–77, https://www.ncbi.nlm.nih.gov/pubmed/25017249.

94. M. Friedman, C.E. Levin, H.J. Kim, et al. "Tomatine-containing Green Tomato Extracts Inhibit Growth of Human Breast, Colon, Liver, and Stomach Cancer Cells," *Journal of Agricultural and Food Chemistry*, vol. 57, no. 13 (July 2009), pp. 5727–33, https://www.ncbi.nlm.nih.gov/pubmed/19514731.

95. V. Er, J.A. Lane, R.M. Martin, et al.

96. MD Anderson Cancer Center, "5 Foods That May Help Lower Your Cancer Risk," (August 2016), https://www.mdanderson.org/publications/focused-on-health/August2016/foods-lower-cancerrisk.html.

97. T. Fang, D.D. Liu, H.M. Ning, et al. "Modified citrus pectin inhibited bladder tumor growth through downregulation of galectin-3," *Acta Pharmacologia Sinica*, epub ahead of print May 16, 2018, https://www.ncbi.nlm.nih.gov/pubmed/29769742.

98. S. Cirmi, M. Navarra, J.V. Woodside, et al. "Citrus Fruits Intake and Oral Cancer Risk: A Systematic Review and Meta-analysis," *Pharmacological Research*, vol. 133 (May 2018), pp. 187–94, https://www.ncbi.nlm.nih.gov/pubmed/29753688.

99. S.K. Jaganathan, M.V. Vellayappan, G. Narasimhan, et al. "Role of Pomegranate and Citrus Fruit Juices in Colon Cancer Prevention," *World Journal of Gastroenterology*, vol. 20, no. 16 (April 2014), pp. 4618–25, https://www.ncbi.nlm.nih.gov/pubmed/24782614.

100. A. Wang, C. Zhu, L. Fu, et al. "Citrus Fruit Intake Substantially Reduces the Risk of Esophageal Cancer: A Meta-Analysis of Epidemiologic Studies," *Medicine*, vol. 94, no. 39 (September 2015), p. e1390, https://www.ncbi.nlm.nih.gov/pubmed/26426606.

101. MD Anderson Cancer Center, "5 Foods That May Help Lower Your Cancer Risk," (August 2016), https://www.mdanderson.org/publications/focused-on-health/August2016/foods-lower-cancerrisk.html.

102. R. Vilcacundo, B. Miralles, W. Carrillo, et al. "In Vitro Chemopreventive Properties of Peptides Released from Quinoa (*Chenopodium Quinoa Willd.*) Protein under Simulated Gastrointestinal Digestion," *Food Research International*, vol. 105 (March 2018), pp. 403–11, https://www.ncbi.nlm.nih.gov/pubmed/29433229.

103. Ibid.

104. Food Tank staff. "25 Indigenous Fruits and Vegetables Promoting Health All Over the World," Food Tank blog (accessed July 1, 2018), https://foodtank.com/news/2015/01/twenty-five-indigenous-fruits-and-vegetables-promoting-health-all-over-the.

105. Kathryn Gorman-Lovelady. "An Aboriginal Approach to Fighting Cancer," Alive (posted April 24, 2015), https://www.alive.com/health/an-aboriginal-approach-to-fighting-cancer.

Chapter 3: Top Anticancer Supplements

1. M.M. Dias, H.S. Martino, G. Noratto, et al. "Anti-inflammatory Activity of Polyphenolics from Açai (Euterpe oleracea Martius) in Intestinal Myofibroblasts CCD-18Co Cells," Food & Function, vol. 6, no. 10 (October 2015), pp. 3249–56, https://www.ncbi.nlm.nih.gov/pubmed/26243669.

2. Fact sheet: "Laetrile/Amygdalin (PDQ®)–Patient Version," National Cancer Institute (accessed July 3, 2018), https://www.cancer.gov/about-cancer/treatment/cam/patient/laetrile-pdq#link/_23.

3. L. Qian, B. Xie, Y. Wang, et al. "Amygdalin-mediated Inhibition of Non-small Cell Lung Cancer Cell Invasion in Vitro," International Journal of Clinical and Experimental Pathology, vol. (May 2015), pp. 5363–70, https://www.ncbi.nlm.nih.gov/pubmed/26191238.

4. Z. Song and X. Xu. "Advanced Research on Anti-tumor Effects of Amygdalin," Journal of Cancer Research and Therapeutics, vol. 10, supplement 1 (August 2014), pp. 3–7, https://www.ncbi.nlm.nih.gov/pubmed/25207888.

5. J. Hantash. "The Use of Polysulfated Polysaccharides Heparin-like Compounds, Glycosaminoglycans, and Vitamin B17 as a Possible Treatment for Prostate Cancer," Medical Hypotheses, vol. 112 (March 2018), pp. 1–3, https://www.ncbi.nlm.nih.gov/pubmed/29447928.

6. B.M. Biswal, S.A. Sulaiman, H.C. Ismail, et al. "Effect of Withania Somnifera (Ashwagandha) on the Development of Chemotherapy-induced Fatigue and Quality of Life in Breast Cancer Patients," Integrative Cancer Therapies, vol. 12, no. 4 (July 2013), pp. 312–22, https://www.ncbi.nlm.nih.gov/pubmed/23142798.

7. R. Wadhwa, R. Singh, R. Gao, et al. "Water Extract of Ashwagandha Leaves Has Anticancer Activity: Identification of an Active Component and Its Mechanism of Action," PloS One, vol. 8, no. 10 (October 10, 2013), p. e77189, https://www.ncbi.nlm.nih.gov/pubmed/24130852.

8. S.R. Fauce, B.D. Jamieson, A.C. Chin, et al. "Telomerase-Based Pharmacologic Enhancement of Antiviral Function of Human CD8+ T Lymphocytes," Journal of Immunology, vol. 181, no. 10 (November 15, 2008), pp. 7400–6, http://www.jimmunol.org/content/181/10/7400.

9. Andrew Weil. "Astragalus," Dr. Weil blog (accessed July 9, 2018), https://www.drweil.com/vitamins-supplements-herbs/herbs/astragalus.

10. Webster Kehr. "Jim Kelmun Protocol Supplemental," Cancer Tutor (accessed July 7, 2018), https://www.cancertutor.com/kelmun.

11. "Nigella sativa," Memorial Sloan Kettering Cancer Center blog (accessed July 3, 2018), https://www.mskcc.org/cancer-care/integrative-medicine/herbs/nigella-sativa. Also: R. Agbaria, A. Gabarin, A. Dahan, et al. "Anticancer activity of Nigella sativa (black seed) and its relationship with the thermal processing and quinone composition of the seed," Drug Design, Development, and Therapy, vol. 9 (June 2015), pp. 3119-24, https://www.ncbi.nlm.nih.gov/pubmed/26124636.

12. Samantha Davis. "Black Cumin Oil Is the Most Important Oil You Can Put in Your System," Natural News, January 11, 2013, https://www.naturalnews.com/038644_black_cumin_oil_immune_system_NK_cells.html.

13. E.S. Al-Sheddi, N.N. Farshori, M.M. Al-Oqail, et al. "Cytotoxicity of Nigella Sativa Seed Oil and Extract Against Human Lung Cancer Cell Line," Asian Pacific Journal of Cancer Prevention, vol. 15, no. 2 (2014), pp. 983–7, https://www.ncbi.nlm.nih.gov/pubmed/24568529.

14. S.J. Ichwan, I.M. Al-Ani, H.G. Bilal, et al. "Apoptotic Activities of Thymoquinone, an Active Ingredient of Black Seed (Nigella sativa), in Cervical Cancer Cell Lines," Chinese Journal of Physiology, vol.57, no. 5 (October 2014), pp. 249–55, https://www.ncbi.nlm.nih.gov/pubmed/25241984.

15. C.C. Woo, A.P. Kumar, G. Sethi, et al. "Thymoquinone: Potential Cure for Inflammatory Disorders and Cancer," Biochemical Pharmacology, vol. 83, no. 4 (February 2012), pp. 443–51, https://www.ncbi.nlm.nih.gov/pubmed/22005518.

16. "Black Cumin Seed Oil Targets Cancer," Gene Changer blog (accessed July 4, 2018), https://genechanger.com/black-cumin-seed-oil-targets-cancer/. Also: M.L. Salem. "Immunomodulatory and Therapeutic Properties of the Nigella sativa L. Seed," International Immunopharmacology, vol. 5, no 13–14 (December 2005), pp. 1749–70, https://www.ncbi.nlm.nih.gov/pubmed/16275613.

17. "Nigella sativa," Memorial Sloan Kettering Cancer Center blog.

18. "Blue-Green Algae," WebMD (accessed July 9, 2018), https://www.webmd.com/vitamins/ai/ingredientmono-923/blue-green-algae.

19. A. Felczykowska, A. Pawlik, H. Mazur-Marzec, et al. "Selective Inhibition of Cancer Cells' Proliferation by Compounds Included in Extracts from Baltic Sea Cyanobacteria," Toxicon, vol. 108 (December 2015), pp. 1–10, https://www.ncbi.nlm.nih.gov/pubmed/26410109.

20. R. Koníčková, K. Vaňková, J. Vaníková, et al. "Anticancer Effects of Blue-green Alga Spirulina platensis, a Natural Source of Bilirubin-like Tetrapyrrolic Compounds," Annals of Hepatology, vol. 13, no. 2 (March–April 2014), pp. 273–83, https://www.ncbi.nlm.nih.gov/pubmed/24552870.

21. Y.S. Chan, L.N. Cheng, J.H. Wu, et al. "A Review of the Pharmacological Effects of Arctium lappa (Burdock)," Inflammopharmacology, vol. 19, no. 5 (October 2011), pp. 245–54, https://www.ncbi.nlm.nih.gov/pubmed/20981575.

22. L.N. Urazova, T. Kuznetsova, R.S. Boev, et al. "Efficacy of Natural L-asparagine in the Complex Therapy for Malignant Tumors in Experimental Studies," Experimental Oncology, vol. 33, no. 2 (June 2011), pp. 90–3, https://www.ncbi.nlm.nih.gov/pubmed/21716205.

23. M. Chu, H. Li, Q. Wu, et al. "Pluronic-encapsulated Natural Chlorophyll Nanocomposites for in Vivo Cancer Imaging and Photothermal/photodynamic Therapies," Biomaterials, vol. 35, no. 29 (September 2014), pp. 8357–73, https://www.ncbi.nlm.nih.gov/pubmed/25002262.

24. Edward Group. "5 Things You Must Know about Colloidal Silver," Global Healing Center (posted October 5, 2015), https://www.globalhealingcenter.com/natural-health/5-things-must-know-colloidal-silver.

25. Robert Scott Bell and Ty Bollinger. Unlock the Power to Heal (updated edition). Infinity 510 Squared Partners, 2014.

26. K. Morrill, K. May, D. Leek, et al. "Spectrum of Antimicrobial Activity Associated with Ionic Colloidal Silver," Journal of Alternative and Complementary Medicine, vol. 19, no. 3 (March 2013), https://www.ncbi.nlm.nih.gov/pubmed/23017226.

27. M.A. Franco-Molina, E. Mendoza-Gamboa, R.A. Gómez-Flores, et al. "Antitumor Activity of Colloidal Silver on MCF-7 Human Breast Cancer Cells," Journal of Experimental & Clinical Cancer Research, vol. 29 (November 2010), p.148, https://www.ncbi.nlm.nih.gov/pubmed/21080962.

28. D. Guo, J. Zhang, Z. Huang, et al. "Colloidal Silver Nanoparticles Improve Anti-Leukemic Drug Efficacy via Amplification of Oxidative Stress," Colloids and Surfaces B: Biointerfaces, vol. 126 (February 2015), pp. 198–203, https://www.ncbi.nlm.nih.gov/pubmed/25576804.

29. S. Kirste, M. Treier, S.J. Wehrle, et al. "Boswellia serrata acts on cerebral edema in patients irradiated for brain tumors: a prospective, randomized, placebo-controlled, double-blind pilot trial," Cancer, vol. 117, no. 16 (August 2011), pp. 3788–95, https://www.ncbi.nlm.nih.gov/pubmed/21287538.

30. M. Takahashi, B. Sung, Y. Shen,et al. "Boswellic acid exerts antitumor effects in colorectal cancer cells by modulating expression of the let-7 and miR-200 microRNA family," Carcinogenesis, vol. 33, no. 12 (December 2012), pp. 2441–9, https://www.ncbi.nlm.nih.gov/pubmed/22983985.

31. From a private meeting with Dr. David Steuer in New York City on April 21, 2018.

32. D. Dibaba, P. Xun, K. Yokota, et al. "Magnesium intake and incidence of pancreatic cancer: the VITamins and Lifestyle study," British Journal of Cancer, vol. 113, no. 11 (December 2015), pp. 1615–21, https://www.ncbi.nlm.nih.gov/pubmed/26554653.

33. H.J. Ko, C.H. Youn, H.M. Kim, "Dietary Magnesium Intake and Risk of Cancer: A Meta-analysis of Epidemiologic Studies," Nutrition and Cancer, vol. 66, no. 6 (2014), pp. 915–23, https://www.ncbi.nlm.nih.gov/pubmed/24910891.

34. L. Yang, X. Song, T. Gong, et al. "Enhanced Anti-tumor and Anti-metastasis Efficacy Against Breast Cancer with an Intratumoral Injectable Phospholipids-based Phase Separation Gel Co-loaded with 5-fluotouracil and Magnesium Oxide by Neutralizing Acidic Microenvironment," International Journal of Pharmaceutics, vol. 547, nos. 1–2 (June 1, 2018), pp. 181-9, https://www.ncbi.nlm.nih.gov/pubmed/29864512,

35. A.J. Berry. "Pancreatic enzyme replacement therapy during pancreatic insufficiency," Nutrition in Clinical Practice, vol. 29, no. 3 (June 2014), pp. 312–21, https://www.ncbi.nlm.nih.gov/pubmed/24687867.

36. Ralph W. Moss. "The Life and Times of John Beard, D.Sc. (1858–1924)," Integrative Cancer Therapies, vol. 7, no. 4 (December 1, 2008), pp. 229–251, http://journals.sagepub.com/doi/10.1177/1534735408326174. Also: John Beard. The Enzyme Treatment of Cancer And Its Scientific Basis, http://www.newspringpress.com/beard.html.

37. N.J. Gonzalez and L.L. Isaacs. "Evaluation of pancreatic proteolytic enzyme treatment of adenocarcinoma of the pancreas, with nutrition and detoxification support," Nutrition and Cancer, vol. 33, no. 2 (1999), pp. 117–24, https://www.ncbi.nlm.nih.gov/pubmed/10368805.

38. L. Herszényi, L. Barabás, I. Hritz, et al. "Impact of Proteolytic Enzymes in Colorectal Cancer Development and Progression," World Journal of Gastroenterology, vol. 20, no. 37 (October 2014), pp. 13246–57, https://www.ncbi.nlm.nih.gov/pubmed/25309062.

39. J. Beuth. "Proteolytic Enzyme Therapy in Evidence-based Complementary Oncology: Fact or Fiction?" Integrative Cancer Therapies, vol. 7, no. 4 (December 2008), pp. 311–6, https://www.ncbi.nlm.nih.gov/pubmed/19116226.

40. A.Q. Yu and L. Li. "The Potential Role of Probiotics in Cancer Prevention and Treatment," Nutrition and Cancer, vol. 68, no. 4 (May–June 2016), pp. 535–44, https://www.ncbi.nlm.nih.gov/pubmed/27144297.

41. A. de Moreno de Leblanc, C. Matar, E. Farnworth, et al. "Study of immune cells involved in the antitumor effect of kefir in a murine breast cancer model," Journal of Dairy Science, vol. 90, no. 4 (April 2007), pp. 1920–8, https://www.ncbi.nlm.nih.gov/pubmed/17369232.

42. G. Block. "Vitamin C and Cancer Prevention: The Epidemiologic Evidence," American Journal of Clinical Nutrition, vol. 53, supplement (1991), pp. 270S–282S, https://www.ncbi.nlm.nih.gov/pubmed/1985398.

43. P. Seyeon, A. Seunghyun, S. Yujeong, et al. "Vitamin C in Cancer: A Metabolomics Perspective," Frontiers in Physiology, vol. 9 (June 19, 2018), p. 762, https://www.frontiersin.org/articles/10.3389/fphys.2018.00762/full.

44. T. Byers. "Anticancer Vitamins du Jour—The ABCED's So Far," American Journal of Epidemiology, vol. 172, no. 1 (July 1, 2010), pp. 1–3, https://www.ncbi.nlm.nih.gov/pmc/articles/PMC2892535.

45. D. Feldman, A.V. Krishnan, S. Swami, et al. "The Role of Vitamin D in Reducing Cancer Risk and Progression," Nature Reviews: Cancer, vol. 14, no. 5 (May 2014), pp. 342–57, https://www.ncbi.nlm.nih.gov/pubmed/24705652.

46. C.F. Garland, F.C. Garland, E.D. Gorham, et al. "The Role of Vitamin D in Cancer Prevention," American Journal of Public Health, vol. 96, no. 2 (February 2006), pp. 252–61, https://www.ncbi.nlm.nih.gov/pmc/articles/PMC1470481.

Chapter 4: Avoid the Most Toxic Foods on the Planet

1. Sam Apple. "An Old Idea, Revived: Starve Cancer to Death," New York Times Magazine (May 12, 2016), pp. MM64, https://www.nytimes.com/2016/05/15/magazine/warburg-effect-an-old-idea-revived-starve-cancer-to-death.html.

2. Zawn Villines. "How Do Free Radicals Affect the Body?" Medical News Today (accessed July 9, 2018), https://www.medicalnewstoday.com/articles/318652.php.

3. Bootie Cosgrove-Mather. "FDA: Too Much Benzene in Some Drinks," CBS/Associated Press (March 19, 2006), https://www.cbsnews.com/news/fda-too-much-benzene-in-some-drinks.

4. Deborah Mitchell. "This Is Why Sodium Benzoate Is So Scary," Naturally Savvy (accessed July 9, 2018), http://naturallysavvy.com/eat/this-is-why-sodium-benzoate-is-so-scary.

5. N. Zengin, D. Yüzbaşıoğlu, F. Unal, et al. "The Evaluation of the Genotoxicity of Two Food Preservatives: Sodium Benzoate and Potassium Benzoate," Food and Chemical Toxicology, vol. 49, no. 4 (April 2011), pp. 763–9, https://www.ncbi.nlm.nih.gov/pubmed/21130826.

6. "Do Food Preservatives Cause Cancer?" Cancer Council (accessed July 9, 2018), https://www.cancercouncil.com.au/86049/cancer-information/general-information-cancer-information/cancer-questions-myths/food-and-drink/food-preservatives-do-not-cause-cancer.

7. Luke Yoquinto. "The Truth About Food Additive BHA," Live Science (June 1, 2012), https://www.livescience.com/36424-food-additive-bha-butylated-hydroxyanisole.html.

8. "Artificial Sweeteners and Cancer," National Cancer Institute (accessed July 9, 2018), https://www.cancer.gov/about-cancer/causes-prevention/risk/diet/artificial-sweeteners-fact-sheet.

9. Sarah Kobylewski and Michael F. Jacobson. "Food Dyes: A Rainbow of Risks" (Washington, D.C.: Center for Research in the Public Interest, 2010), https://cspinet.org/resource/food-dyes-rainbow-risks.

10. Press release. "Popular Soda Ingredient Poses Cancer Risk to Consumers," Johns Hopkins Bloomberg School of Public Health (February 18, 2015), https://www.jhsph.edu/research/centers-and-institutes/johns-hopkins-center-for-a-livable-future/news-room/News-Releases/2015/Caramel-Color-in-Soft-Drinks-and-Exposure-to-4-Methylimidazole.html.

11. Markham Heid. "Diet soda and cancer: What you should know," Focused on Health blog/MD Anderson Cancer Center (October 2014), https://www.mdanderson.org/publications/focused-on-health/october-2014/does-diet-soda-cause-cancer.html.

12. A. Konieczna, A. Rutkowska, and D. Rachoń. "Health Risk of Exposure to Bisphenol A (BPA)" Roczniki Panstwowego Zakladu Higieny, vol. 66, no. 1 (2015), pp. 5–11, https://www.ncbi.nlm.nih.gov/pubmed/25813067.

13. Emily Cassidy. "Monsanto's GMO Herbicide Doubles Cancer Risk," Environmental Working Group (October 6, 2015), https://www.ewg.org/agmag/2015/10/monsanto-s-gmo-herbicide-doubles-cancer-risk#.W0eGQfZFxPb.

14. Leah Schinasi and Maria E. Leon. "Non-Hodgkin Lymphoma and Occupational Exposure to Agricultural Pesticide Chemical Groups and Active Ingredients: A Systematic Review and Meta-Analysis," International Journal of Environment Research and Public Health, vol. 11, no. 4 (April 2014), pp. 4449–4527, https://www.ncbi.nlm.nih.gov/pmc/articles/PMC4025008.

15. Press release from Baum Hedlund Aristei Goldman PC, August 13, 2018, https://www.baumhedlundlaw.com.

16. Holly Yan. "Patients: Roundup gave us cancer as EPA official helped the company," CNN (May 16, 2017), https://www.cnn.com/2017/05/15/health/roundup-herbicide-cancer-allegations/index.html?no-st=1534285400.

17. Brittany Cordeiro. "Do GMOs Cause Cancer?" MD Anderson Cancer Center blog (June 2014), https://www.mdanderson.org/publications/focused-on-health/june-2014/gmos-cancer.html.

18. J.F. Ludvigsson, S.M. Montgomery, A. Ekbom, et al. "Small-intestinal Histopathology and Mortality Risk in Celiac Disease," JAMA, vol. 302, no. 11 (September 2009), pp. 1171–8, https://www.ncbi.nlm.nih.gov/pubmed/19755695.

19. Katherine Czapp. "Against the Grain: The Case for Rejecting or Respecting the Staff of Life," Weston A. Price Foundation (July 16, 2006), https://www.westonaprice.org/health-topics/modern-diseases/against-the-grain.

20. V. Marta Blangiardo, C. La Vecchia, and G. Corrao. "Alcohol Consumption and the Risk of Cancer: A Meta-Analysis," National Institute on Alcohol Abuse and Alcoholism/National Institutes of Health (accessed July 12, 2018), https://pubs.niaaa.nih.gov/publications/arh25-4/263-270.htm.

21. Thomas Froehlich. "7 Drinks That May Affect Your Cancer Risk," University of Texas Southwestern Medical School (June 29, 2016), https://utswmed.org/medblog/energy-drink-alcohol-cancer.

22. Julie Grisham. "The Link Between Meat and Cancer: MSK Experts Explain the Headlines," Memorial Sloan Kettering Cancer Center (October 29, 2015), https://www.mskcc.org/blog/link-between-meat-and-msk-experts-explain-headlines.

23. Kellie Bramlet. "Study: How You Cook Meat Can Affect Your Kidney Cancer Risk," MD Anderson Cancer Center (November 9, 2015), https://www.mdanderson.org/publications/cancerwise/2015/11/study-how-you-cook-meat-can-affect-your-kidney-cancer-risk.html.

24. "Milk and Prostate Cancer: The Evidence Mounts," Physicians Committee for Responsible Medicine (accessed July 12, 2018), http://www.pcrm.org/health/health-topics/milk-and-prostate-cancer-the-evidence-mounts.

25. N.S. Scrimshaw and E.B. Murray. "The Acceptability of Milk and Milk Products in Populations with a High Prevalence of Lactose Intolerance," American Journal of Clinical Nutrition, vol. 48, supplement 4 (October 1988), pp. 1079–159, https://www.ncbi.nlm.nih.gov/pubmed/3140651.

26. Jonathan Shaw. "Modern Milk," Harvard Magazine (May-June 2007), https://harvardmagazine.com/2007/05/modern-milk.html.

27. Tim Fitzpatrick. "PCBs (Polychlorinated Biphenyls) are in the Foods You Love," Environmental Chemistry (accessed July 9, 2018), https://environmentalchemistry.com/yogi/environmental/200601pcbsinfood.html.

28. Joe Leech. "Wild vs Farmed Salmon—Can Some Fish Be Bad for You?" Healthline (June 4, 2017), https://www.healthline.com/nutrition/wild-vs-farmed-salmon.

29. Ty Bollinger. "Why Pasteurized Milk Is So Bad for Your health," Truth About Cancer (accessed July 12, 2018), https://thetruthaboutcancer.com/pasteurized-milk.

30. "WHO Plan to Eliminate Industrially-produced Trans-fatty Acids from Global Food Supply," World Health Organization (May 14, 2018), http://www.who.int/news-room/detail/14-05-2018-who-plan-to-eliminate-industrially-produced-trans-fatty-acids-from-global-food-supply.

31. Mark Hyman. "5 Strategies to Prevent and Cure Cancer," Dr. Hyman blog (accessed July 9, 2018), https://drhyman.com/blog/2015/08/07/5-strategies-to-prevent-and-treat-cancer.

32. Lloyd Burrell. "Are Microwave Ovens Safe? (Must Read If You Use a Microwave Oven)," Truth About Cancer (accessed July 10, 2018), https://thetruthaboutcancer.com/are-microwaves-safe.

33. Ibid.

34. Ibid.

35. "Electrical appliances," Powerwatch (accessed July 12, 2018), https://www.powerwatch.org.uk/elf/appliances.asp.

36. Chapter 6: Healing Guides for Common Cancers

37. "What Is Cancer?" National Cancer Institute (accessed April 13, 2018), https://www.cancer.gov/about-cancer/understanding/what-is-cancer.

38. Ibid.

39. Eric Zielinski, D.C., The Healing Power of Essential Oils: Soothe Inflammation, Boost Mood, Prevent Autoimmunity, and Feel Great in Every Way (New York: Harmony Books, 2018).

40. Danielle Delorto. "Avoid Sunscreens with Potentially Harmful Ingredients Group Warns," CNN.com (May 16, 2012), https://www.cnn.com/2012/05/16/health/sunscreen-report/index.html.

41. "Top Sun Safety Tips," Environmental Working Group (accessed April 25, 2018), https://www.ewg.org/sunscreen/top-sun-safety-tips.

42. "Lung Cancer," American Cancer Society (accessed August 2, 2018), https://www.cancer.org/cancer/lung-cancer.html.

43. Ibid.

44. L.L. Marchand, S.P. Murphy, J.H. Hankin, et al. "Intake of Flavonoids and Lung Cancer," Journal of the National Cancer Institute, vol. 92, no. 2 (January 19, 2000), pp. 154–60, https://academic.oup.com/jnci/article/92/2/154/2964983.

45. Julie Langford. "Dietary Influences on Lung Cancer: An Evaluation of the Research and Strategies to Help Counsel Patients," Today's Dietician (accessed August 2, 2018), http://www.todaysdietitian.com/pdf/courses/LanfordLungCancer.pdf.

46. Tina Kaczor, "Soy Intake and Decreased Risk of Lung Cancer Death in Women Survival from lung cancer improves with soy consumption, study says," Natural Medicine Journal, vol. 5, no. 5 (May 2013), https://www.naturalmedicinejournal.com/journal/2013-05/soy-intake-and-decreased-risk-lung-cancer-death-women.

47. "Types of Breast Cancer," BreastCancer.org (accessed August 2, 2018), https://www.breastcancer.org/symptoms/types.

48. The JAMA Network Journals, "Mediterranean Diet Plus Olive Oil Associated with Reduced Breast Cancer Risk," ScienceDaily, September 14, 2015, https://www.sciencedaily.com/releases/2015/09/150914092837.htm.

49. Ana Calado, et al. "The Effect of Flaxseed in Breast Cancer: A Literature Review." Frontiers in Nutrition, vol. 5, no. 4 (February 7, 2018), https://www.frontiersin.org/articles/10.3389/fnut.2018.00004/full.

50. "Nutrition for Breast Cancer Patients and Survivors," Johns Hopkins Medicine (accessed August 2, 2018), https://www.hopkinsmedicine.org/breast_center/treatments_services/nutrition.html.

51. Ibid.

52. Keppi Baranick. "Cruciferous Vegetables and Umbelliferous Vegetables," Health and Beauty by Keppi (February 22, 2011), http://healthandbeautybykeppi.blogspot.com/2011/02/cruciferous-vegetables-and.html.

53. "Nutrition for Breast Cancer Patients and Survivors."

54. Ibid.

55. "10 Natural Cancer Treatments Revealed," Dr. Axe, https://draxe.com/10-natural-cancer-treatments-hidden-cures.

56. Alexander Miller. "Managing Breast Cancer Surgery Side Effects," BreastCancer.org (April 5, 2018), https://www.breastcancer.org/community/podcasts/surgery-side-effects-20180405.

57. Christiane Northrup. "How to Keep Your Breasts Healthy for Life," Christian Northrup M.D. blog (accessed August 8, 2018), https://www.drnorthrup.com/breast-cancer-keep-breasts-healthy-cancer-free.

58. Ibid.

59. "Prostate Cancer," Cancer Research UK (accessed August 2, 2018), https://www.cancerresearchuk.org/about-cancer/prostate-cancer/types-grades.

60. "Lifestyle Therapy for Prostate Cancer: Does It Work?" Harvard Men's Health Watch (posted July 2007), https://www.health.harvard.edu/mens-health/lifestyle-therapy-for-prostate-cancer-does-it-work.

61. "Understanding a Rising PSA After Treatment," Prostate.net (accessed August 8, 2018), http://prostate.net/health-centers/prostate-cancer/living-with-prostate-cancer/understanding-a-rising-psa-after-treatment.

62. C.J. Paller, et al. "A Randomized Phase II Study of Pomegranate Extract for Men with Rising PSA Following Initial Therapy for Localized Prostate Cancer," Prostate Cancer and Prostatic Diseases, vol. 16, no. 1 (March 2013), pp. 50–5, https://www.ncbi.nlm.nih.gov/pubmed/22689129.

63. "10 Ways to Lower Your PSA," Prostate.net (November 17, 2016), https://prostate.net/articles/10-ways-to-lower-your-psa.

64. "Move Over Tomatoes! All Vegetables—Especially the Cruciferous Kind—May Prevent Prostate Cancer," Fred Hutchinson Cancer Research Center News release (January 4, 2000), https://www.fredhutch.org/en/news/releases/2000/01/Veggiesprostat.html.

65. "Calcium Content of Common Foods," International Osteoporosis Foundation (accessed October 25, 2018), https://www.iofbonehealth. org/osteoporosis-musculoskeletal-disorders/osteoporosis/prevention/ calcium/calcium-content-common-foods

66. "Acrylamide and Cancer Risk," National Cancer Institute (accessed August 2, 2018), https://www.cancer.gov/about-cancer/causes-prevention/risk/ diet/acrylamide-fact-sheet.

67. "Colon Cancer," Mayo Clinic (accessed August 8, 2018), https://www. mayoclinic.org/diseases-conditions/colon-cancer/symptoms-causes/ syc-20353669.

68. "Calcium Content of Common Foods," International Osteoporosis Foundation (accessed October 25, 2018), https://www.iofbonehealth. org/osteoporosis-musculoskeletal-disorders/osteoporosis/prevention/ calcium/calcium-content-common-foods

69. "What Can I Eat if I Have Colorectal Cancer?' Dana-Farber Cancer Institute (December 11, 2017), http://blog.dana-farber.org/ insight/2016/03/what-can-i-eat-if-i-have-colorectal-cancer.

70. "Bladder Cancer," MD Anderson Cancer Center (accessed August 8, 2018), https://www.mdanderson.org/cancer-types/bladder-cancer.html.

71. Ray Sahelian. "Bladder Cancer Natural and Alternative Treatment and Prevention, Vitamins, Herbs, and Supplements That May Help," Dr. Ray Sahelian blog (accessed August 8, 2018), http://www.raysahelian. com/bladdercancer.html.

72. Li Tang, et al. "Intake of Cruciferous Vegetables Modifies Bladder Cancer Survival," Cancer Epidemiology, Biomarkers & Prevention, vol. 19, no. 7 (July 2010), http://cebp.aacrjournals.org/content/19/7/1806.long.

73. Ty Bollinger. "Overcoming Bladder Cancer," Truth About Cancer (accessed August 8, 2018), https://thetruthaboutcancer.com/overcoming-bladder-cancer.

74. Thomas J. Guzzo, et al. "Bladder Cancer and the Aluminum Industry: A Review," BJUI International, vol. 102, no. 9 (November 2008), pp. 1058–60, https://onlinelibrary.wiley.com/doi/pdf/10.1111/j.1464-410X.2008.07903.x.

75. G. Thériault, et al. "Bladder Cancer in the Aluminum Industry," Lancet, vol. 1, no. 8383 (April 28, 2984), https://www.ncbi.nlm.nih.gov/ pubmed/6143877.

76. "Parasites that Can Lead to Cancer," American Cancer Society, July 11, 2016, https://www.cancer.org/cancer/cancer-causes/infectious-agents/ infections-that-can-lead-to-cancer/parasites.html.

77. "What Causes Non-Hodgkin Lymphoma?" American Cancer Society (accessed August 8, 2018), https://www.cancer.org/cancer/non-hodgkin-lymphoma/causes-risks-prevention/what-causes.html.

78. Daniel J. DeNoon. "Diet Linked to Non-Hodgkin's Lymphoma," WebMD (March 9, 2004), https://www.webmd.com/cancer/lymphoma/ news/20040309/diet-linked-to-non-hodgkins-lymphoma#1.

79. "Kidney Cancer," Mayo Clinic (accessed August 8, 2018), https://www.mayoclinic.org/diseases-conditions/kidney-cancer/symptoms-causes/syc-20352664.

80. Dennis Thompson, Jr. "Kidney Cancer Diet and Nutrition," Everyday Health (accessed August 8, 2018), https://www.everydayhealth.com/kidney-cancer/kidney-cancer-diet-and-nutrition.aspx.

81. D. Del Pozo-Insfran, et al. "Açai (Euterpe oleracea Mart.) Polyphenolics in Their Glycoside and Aglycone Forms Induce Apoptosis of HL-60 Leukemia Cells," Journal of Agriculture and Food Chemistry, vol. 54, no. 4 (February 22, 2006), https://www.ncbi.nlm.nih.gov/pubmed/16478240.

82. David Lingle. "David Refused Chemo and Healed Leukemia Naturally," Chris Beat Cancer blog (accessed August 9, 2018), https://www.chrisbeatcancer.com/david-refused-chemo-and-healed-leukemia-naturally.

83. E.T. Chang, et al. "Dietary Patterns and Risk of Ovarian Cancer in the California Teachers Study Cohort," *Nutrition and Cancer*, vol. 60, no. 3 (2008), pp. 285–91, https://www.ncbi.nlm.nih.gov/pmc/articles/PMC2365491.

84. American Society of Clinical Oncology. "Uterine Cancer: Risk Factors and Prevention," Cancer.net (accessed August 8, 2018), https://www.cancer.net/cancer-types/uterine-cancer/risk-factors-and-prevention.

85. Roghiyeh Pashaei-Asl, et al. "The Inhibitory Effect of Ginger Extract on Ovarian Cancer Cell Line; Application of Systems Biology," Advanced Pharmaceutical Bulletin, vol. 7, no. 2 (June 2017), pp. 241–49, https://www.ncbi.nlm.nih.gov/pmc/articles/PMC5527238. Also: Jennifer Rhode, et al. "Ginger Inhibits Cell Growth and Modulates Angiogenic Factors in Ovarian Cancer Cells," BMC Complementary and Alternative Medicine, vol. 7, no. 1 (December 20, 2007), p. 1, https://www.ncbi.nlm.nih.gov/pmc/articles/PMC2241638.

86. Ramos do Prado, et al. "Ripening-induced Chemical Modifications of Papaya Pectin Inhibit Cancer Cell Proliferation," Scientific Reports, online (November 29, 2017), https://www.ncbi.nlm.nih.gov/pmc/articles/PMC5707353.

Chapter 7: Kitchen Supplies and Conversion Charts

1. L.B. Biegel, Mark E. Hurtt, Steven R. Frame, et al. "Mechanisms of extrahepatic tumor induction by peroxisome proliferators in male CD rats," *Toxicological Sciences,* vol. 60, no. 1 (March 1, 2001): pp. 44–55, http://dx.doi.org/10.1093/toxsci/60.1.44.

2. Tony Fletcher, David Savitz, and Kyle Steenland. "Probable Link Evaluation of Thyroid Disease," C8 Science Panel (July 30, 2012), http://www.c8sciencepanel.org/pdfs/Probable_Link_C8_Thyroid_30Jul2012.pdf.

3. Antonia M. Calafat, Zsuzsanna Kuklenyik, John A. Reidy, et al. "Serum concentrations of 11 polyfluoroalkyl compounds in the U.S. population: Data from the National Health and Nutrition Examination Survey (NHANES) 1999–2000," Environmental Science & Technology, vol. 41, no. 7 (2007): pp. 2237–42, http://dx.doi.org/10.1021/es062686m.

Chapter 8: Immune-Boosting Juices

1. Deepak Chopra and David Simon. *Grow Younger, Live Longer* (New York: Harmony Books, 2001), p. 20.

2. Josh Axe. "12 Turmeric Benefits—Boosting Mental, Skin and Joint Health," Dr. Axe blog (accessed August 14, 2018), https://draxe.com/turmeric-benefits.

3. S. Suh and K.W. Kim. "Diabetes and Cancer: Is Diabetes Causally Related to Cancer?" Diabetes & Metabolism Journal, vol. 35, no. 3 (June 2011), pp. 195–8, https://www.ncbi.nlm.nih.gov/pmc/articles/PMC3138100/.

4. Bokyung Sung, Hae Young Chung, and Nam Deuk Kim. "Role of Apigenin in Cancer Prevention via the Induction of Apoptosis and Autophagy, Journal of Cancer Prevention (published online December 30, 2016) https://www.ncbi.nlm.nih.gov/pmc/articles/PMC5207605/

5. R. Clark and S.H. Lee. "Anticancer Properties of Capsaicin Against Human Cancer," Anticancer Research, vol. 36, no. 3 (March 2016), pp. 837–43, https://www.ncbi.nlm.nih.gov/pubmed/26976969. Also: "Compound in Chili Pepper Slows Lung Cancer Tumor Growth in Animal Study," American Institute for Cancer Research (October 30, 2014), http://www.aicr.org/press/press-releases/2014/compound-in-chili-pepper-slows-lung-cancer-tumor-growth-in-animal-study.html; and Lynn Griffith, "Capsaicin Found in Chili Peppers Could Slow or Reverse Colorectal and Prostate Cancer," Raw Food World (accessed August 10, 2018), https://news.therawfoodworld.com/capsaicin-found-chili-peppers-slow-reverse-colorectal-prostate-cancer.

Chapter 10: Brain-Protecting Smoothies and Smoothie Bowls

1. Mayo Clinic Staff. "Chemo in," Mayo Clinic, May 16, 2018, https://www.mayoclinic.org/diseases-conditions/chemo-brain/symptoms.../syc-20351060.

Chapter 11: Detoxing Teas and Cleansing Waters

1. B. Hong, et al. "A double-blind crossover study evaluating the efficacy of Korean red ginseng in patients with erectile dysfunction: a preliminary report," Journal of Urology, vol. 168, no. 5 (November 2002), pp. 2070–3, https://www.ncbi.nlm.nih.gov/pubmed/12394711.

2. L. Liu, et al. "Effects of ginsenosides on hypothalamic-pituitary-adrenal function and brain-derived neurotrophic factor in rats exposed to chronic unpredictable mild stress," China Journal of Chinese Materia Medica, vol 36, no. 10 (May 2011), https://www.ncbi.nlm.nih.gov/pubmed/21837980.

3. Z. Sándor, et al. "Evidence Supports Tradition: The in Vitro Effects of Roman Chamomile on Smooth Muscles," Frontiers in Pharmacology, vol. 9 (April 2018), p. 323, https://www.ncbi.nlm.nih.gov/pubmed/29681854.

4. K.S. Yeung. "Herbal medicine for depression and anxiety: A systematic review with assessment of potential psycho-oncologic relevance," Phytotherapy Research, vol. 32, no. 5 (May 2018), pp. 865–91, https://www.ncbi.nlm.nih.gov/pubmed/29464801.

5. N. Maleki-Saghooni, et al. "The effectiveness and safety of Iranian herbal medicines for treatment of premenstrual syndrome: A systematic review," Avicenna Journal of Phytomedicine, vol. 8, no. 2 (March–April 2018), pp. 96–113, https://www.ncbi.nlm.nih.gov/pubmed/29632841.

6. J. Cervini-Silva, M.T. Ramírez-Apan, S. Kaufhold, et al. "Role of Bentonite Clays on Cell Growth," Chemosphere, vol. 149 (April 20-16), pp. 57-61, https://www.ncbi.nlm.nih.gov/pubmed/26849195.

7. A. Robinson, N.M. Johnson, A. Strey, et al. "Calcium Montmorillonite Clay Reduces Urinary Biomarkers of Fumonisin B_1 Exposure in Rats and Humans," Food Additives & Contaminants: Part A, vol. 29, no. 5 (2012), pp. 809–18, https://www.ncbi.nlm.nih.gov/pubmed/22324939.

Chapter 12: Easy, Breezy Breakfasts

1. J. Parker, et al. "Therapeutic Perspectives on Chia Seed and Its Oil: A Review," *Planta Medica*, vol. 84, no. 9–10 (July 2018), pp. 606–12, https://www.ncbi.nlm.nih.gov/pubmed/29534257.

2. F. Thies, et al. "Oats and bowel disease: a systematic literature review," *British Journal of Nutrition*, vol. 112, supplement 2 (October 2014), pp. S31–43, https://www.ncbi.nlm.nih.gov/pubmed/25267242.

Chapter 13: Energizing Lunches and Healing Dinners

1. C. Wasonga and C. Omwandho. "Inhibitory effects of mushroom extracts on progression of carcinogenesis in mice," *Journal of Experimental Therapeutics and Oncology*, vol. 12, no. 3 (May 2018), pp. 231–7, https://www.ncbi.nlm.nih.gov/pubmed/29790315.

2. M. Sangaramoorthy, et al. "Intake of bean fiber, beans, and grains and reduced risk of hormone receptor-negative breast cancer: the San Francisco Bay Area Breast Cancer Study," Cancer Medicine, vol. 7, no. 5 (May 2018), pp. 2131–44, https://www.ncbi.nlm.nih.gov/pubmed/29573201.

3. N. Gupta, et al. "Chickpea Lectin Inhibits Human Breast Cancer Cell Proliferation and Induces Apoptosis Through Cell Cycle Arrest," Protein and Peptide Letters, vol. 25, no. 5 (2018), pp. 492–9, https://www.ncbi.nlm.nih.gov/pubmed/29623820.

4. H. McManus, et al. "Usual Cruciferous Vegetable Consumption and Ovarian Cancer: A Case-Control Study," Nutrition and Cancer, vol. 70, no. 4 (May–June 2018), https://www.ncbi.nlm.nih.gov/pubmed/29693426.

5. R. Vilcacundo, et al. "In vitro chemopreventive properties of peptides released from quinoa (Chenopodium quinoa Willd.) protein under simulated gastrointestinal digestion," Food Research International, vol. 105 (March 2018), pp. 409–11, https://www.ncbi.nlm.nih.gov/pubmed/29433229.

6. A.K. Zaineddi, K. Buck, A. Vrieling, J. Heinz, D. Flesch-Janys, J. Linnseisen, J. Chang-Claude. "The association between dietary lignans, phytoestrogen-rich foods, and fiber intake and postmenopausal breast cancer risk: a German case-control study," Nutrition and Cancer, vol. 64, no. 5 (2012), https://www.ncbi.nlm.nih.gov/pubmed/22591208.

Chapter 15: Comforting Soups and Broths

1. Ann Wigmore. AnnWigmore.org.

Chapter 17: Fun Sides and Savory Snacks

1. From private e-mail correspondence with Donna Schwenk.

CONVERSION CHART

Standard Cup	Fine Powder (e.g., flour)	Grain (e.g., rice)	Granular (e.g., sugar)	Liquid Solids (e.g., butter)	Liquid (e.g., milk)
1	140 g	150 g	190 g	200 g	240 ml
¾	105 g	113 g	143 g	150 g	180 ml
⅔	93 g	100 g	125 g	133 g	160 ml
1/2	70 g	75 g	95 g	100 g	120 ml
⅓	47 g	50 g	63 g	67 g	80 ml
¼	35 g	38 g	48 g	50 g	60 ml
⅛	18 g	19 g	24 g	25 g	30 ml

Useful Equivalents for Liquid Ingredients by Volume				
¼ tsp				1 ml
½ tsp				2 ml
1 tsp				5 ml
3 tsp	1 tbsp		½ fl oz	15 ml
	2 tbsp	⅛ cup	1 fl oz	30 ml
	4 tbsp	¼ cup	2 fl oz	60 ml
	5⅓ tbsp	⅓ cup	3 fl oz	80 ml
	8 tbsp	½ cup	4 fl oz	120 ml
	10⅔ tbsp	⅔ cup	5 fl oz	160 ml
	12 tbsp	¾ cup	6 fl oz	180 ml
	16 tbsp	1 cup	8 fl oz	240 ml
	1 pt	2 cups	16 fl oz	480 ml
	1 qt	4 cups	32 fl oz	960 ml
			33 fl oz	1000 ml 1 L

Useful Equivalents for Dry Ingredients by Weight

(To convert ounces to grams, multiply the number of ounces by 30.)

1 oz	¹⁄₁₆ lb	30 g
4 oz	¼ lb	120 g
8 oz	½ lb	240 g
12 oz	¾ lb	360 g
16 oz	1 lb	480 g

Useful Equivalents for Cooking/Oven Temperatures

Process	Fahrenheit	Celsius	Gas Mark
Freeze Water	32° F	0° C	
Room Temperature	68° F	20° C	
Boil Water	212° F	100° C	
Bake	325° F	160° C	3
	350° F	180° C	4
	375° F	190° C	5
	400° F	200° C	6
	425° F	220° C	7
	450° F	230° C	8
Broil			Grill

Useful Equivalents for Length

(To convert inches to centimeters, multiply the number of inches by 2.5.)

1 in			2.5 cm	
6 in	½ ft		15 cm	
12 in	1 ft		30 cm	
36 in	3 ft	1 yd	90 cm	
40 in			100 cm	1 m

INDEX

ACKNOWLEDGMENTS

Thank you to Sahara Rose for igniting the passion and confidence in me to go forward with this important subject matter: talking about healing cancer and sharing these recipes.

Thank you, Howard Hoffman, for your constant positivity and mastermind! Thank you so much, beautiful Christina, Chubs, and Frank too. So glad you have joined the fam, Frank. Thank you to Paul Lepore for protecting my back over the years! And thank you, cuz Oscar.

Thank you, Monica Rowsom, for your unbelievable generosity in helping me with this project . . . and life!

Thank you, Reid Tracy, for consistent support. Thank you to the brilliant Hay House team: Patty Gift, Nicolette Young (and baby Max Amelia, you were there through the whole process), Lindsay McGinty, Mary Norris, Tricia Breidenthal, and those at work behind the scenes. Thank you to Nick C. Welch for the interior design, and Kathleen Lynch for the cover design. I hope you know the extent of my gratitude and recognize how many people are being healed because of your efforts and talents.

Thank you to my editor, Stephanie Gunning. I love working on books with you, eating chocolate, and drinking green juice. You are a dream come true.

Thank you, Mark Hyman, for generously contributing a foreword to the book and for all the incredible work you do in the world. You give me confidence to continue teaching people about the importance of eating real food.

Thank you, Helen Gray, for calculating the nutrition facts for every single recipe, and not just the standard macronutrients but the extra details that matter so much when it comes to cancer healing and prevention, like how much vitamin C and magnesium a recipe offers us. This will be so helpful to so many people. Thank you for your extra effort.

Thank you, Mae Rose, for helping me to detoxify my body, as well as for taking me in when I was at a physical rock bottom and helping me get my life back on track. Love you forever.

Thank you, Craig and Steph Green. I am at 13 years going strong on green juice and yoga thanks to you guys! JD, thank you for all the great adventures! Also, thank you, Shawn and Shane Chapman.

I am very grateful to the individuals who shared personal cancer stories in this book: Anita Moorjani, your story is so inspiring and crucial to share with the world. You demonstrate that it's never ever too late to heal, even if you have 24 tumors! Jimmy Lechmanski, your story is going to help *so* many people, and especially those who have non-Hodgkins lymphoma or chronic lymphocytic leukemia and are aged 60, 70, 80, and above. Your example is inspiration to never give up. Giving up was never an option for you. Thank you, also, dear Helen. We'll celebrate with a wine and then a tea, heehee! Bill Stewart, your story of healing bladder cancer is powerful. Linda and Sarah Stewart, I am extremely grateful for your generosity, time, and grace with this project. Thank you also to Craig Clemens. CC Webster, thank you for sharing your journey of healing lymphoma and the epic Chemo Brain Buster Smoothie recipe! Pasha Hogan, you shared your incredible breast cancer warrior story with me and provided a delicious recipe for the book. I am grateful. Thank you Lorna Robinson for sharing your cancer treatment story work me and for reminding me the importance of including healthy dessert recipes in the book.

I am also deeply grateful and indebted to those who contributed kick butt cancer-healing recipes: Chris Wark, Kris Carr, Dr. Oz, David Jockers, Dr. Z and Mama Z, Dr. Kelly Brogan, Dr. Mike Dow, Diane Gray (and thank you, Kyle Gray), Donna Schwenk, and Vani Hari.

Thank you too, Fabrizio Manchini. You are one of my favorite people on earth and absolutely so fab! Thank you, Robert Scott Bell, for your support for more than seven years! Thank you so, so much for all your wisdom on colloidal silver and healing using homeopathy.

Thank you, Ty and Charlene Bollinger, and everyone involved in the Truth about Cancer Summit. You launched a platform that gave me and so many others the confidence to talk about cancer when it was the most controversial subject on earth. Now, because of you, the truth is being shared with millions of people and you are helping to save millions of lives.

Thank you to my beautiful friend Maria Marlowe, I love our adventures together.

Thank you, Dr. Daniel Fenster, for giving me a platform to coach people one on one. The most fulfilling thing I could ever do on a Wednesday is work with this team! Thank you, Jan Fenster; how can I say you are one of the nicest people I've ever met—you are goals. Thank you, Dr. Dana Cohen, for your support and guidance. You are amazing. Thank you, Dr. Kay, who told me to keep going even when it looked like rough seas ahead. Thank you for all your good ideas! And thank you to the rest of the Complete Wellness NYC team. Yossie, I am grateful to you for keeping the front together. Jeanette, I am grateful to you for keeping the back together. Krysleen, Pamela, and Stephanie, I wouldn't be able to get all my work done without you! Always so good to see your smiling faces. Thank you, Masae, for massaging me and helping keep my body balanced. Thanks, Dr. H., for helping keep my body in check. Tim Coyle, love our walks to Juice Press haha! Ofelia, you are an inspiration to every single person who meets you. Thank you to the patients at CW.

Thank you to my family for always supporting me. Mum, I am beyond proud of you. To my sisters, Nadine and Caitlin, to my Aunty Tammy and my uncle, to Bernie, to Nanna and Laurie, to my extended family, to Lauren, to Sav, to Steven, to Rock, and especially to Carol Lucas—thank you so very much.

Thank you, Dr Buttar. You are so strong and so full of love! Thank you, Mary Gonzalez, for your grace and beauty. I love your presence so much. Thank you, Heather Dean, for teaching me tools to get control over my mind. Thank you to my awesome friends Roxxe Ireland, Heidi Williams, Jill DeJong,

Kristy Rao, Marci and Eric Schnell, Max Goldberg, Malia Kulp and Maia Monasterios, Brenda Vongova and Sarah Deanna, my angels. Thank you, Geney Kim, my Aussie Taz angel! I am excited for more GigiLili adventures with you. Thank you, Gi, for changing my life by reminding me to think outside the box. Thank you, John and Kevin, and Bill in spirit—heehee! I love our adventures and hope there are many more to come! Thank you, Natalie Jill. I love you! Let's make a dessert recipe again soon! Thank you, Rodney Habib, for kicking my butt and reminding me to pay attention to Facebook—homes! Thank you, Mary Mucci! I have loved doing all our Long Island Naturally segments on News 12 over the years! It's always so fun to work with you! Thank you, Lori Harder, for having me on your podcast to discuss the important issue of cancer. Thank you, AJ, for your love, support, wisdom, teachings, and prayers. Thank you for your support, Dr. Jess Peatross; you are a dream-come-true kind of doctor!

Thank you to the Vitacost team. It is a genuine pleasure working with you and I am so grateful that you make organic living much more affordable for me and millions of others! Thank you, Katie, Alisha, Rebecca, Thomas, Terri, Guy, Elyssa, and Katelyn. Thank you to the Explore Cuisine team! I love that my diet can now safely include pasta once again! Thank you for making such gluten-free deliciousness, Joe, Erika, Jim, Elizabeth, Alex, and Greg. Thank you to the Sawtooth team. Thank you to the Sunbutter team: Justin, Shane, Wyatt, and Nadine. Thank you to the Hu Kitchen team! Jordan and Rita, I love the chocolate tasting we do at expos! Thank you to the Nutiva team. John Roulac, I always smile so big when I think of you! Thanks for all your insight! I love working with you, Madalyn, Virginia, Anne, Steven, and Dan. Thank you to the Sovereign silver team, Scott, Darlene, Ami, and Karen. Theo, you are a legend! Thank you to the Redmond Salt team. Thank you, Darryl Bosshardt, for all the education and wisdom you have given me on bentonite clay. I am honored to be a clay disciple. Thank you, Jason R Eaton.

Thank you to the staff at Candle Cafe. Thank you, Bart, Joy, and Benay. I love you guys so much . . . and the crepe and chocolate peanut butter dessert. Thank you to Juice Press, for existing. Thank you, Daniel, Jeff, Marcus, Leah, and Michael. Without Juice Press I don't know where I would spend a third of my time—lol! Thank you, Jo Park, for coming on board the Earth Diet team!

Also, thank you so much to my Northfork fam: Peter Rowsom, Alexander, Andrea Rowsom, Larry and Trisa, Jim Lechmanski, Kim Andersen, Laura Arena, Cindy Bumble, and Laura McCarthy. Thank you, DK, for helping me put together an epic webinar. Special thanks belong to Daryl Gioffre, Drew, and Adam Weiss. Thank you #5. Thank you, Joyce Walker Robertson, for the mostly heavenly organic bed. I had the best night's sleep—ever—while writing this book. Thank you, Susan Misuraca, for your dedication over the years and helping TED grow. Thank you to the Earth Diet health coaches.

I am forever grateful for the presence of the late Wayne Dyer and Louise Hay in my life and the growth that they initiated in me. Thank you to everyone I am forgetting who has influenced my thinking in any way that has contributed to this book from the time I began writing to the time it was launched. My thank you pages are always so long, but I get a lot of help and support and so I want to acknowledge these people who are giving to me which keeps me going.

Thank you, God. The beautiful work You have done in my life is immeasurable. I am in awe, wonder, and gratitude every day wondering what You will do next. Thank You for the lessons and for teaching me how I can be of service to others. Thank You for showing me how food can heal. Thank You for my life and for forgiving me. With You, God, anything is possible.

And lastly, thank YOU, dear reader. If you have ever thought something positive for me, prayed for me, told one of your loved ones about my books or healing recipes, please know that I am sending you great energy right now!

ABOUT THE AUTHOR

Liana Werner-Gray is a natural food and healing chef. She is a passionate advocate for healthy diet and lifestyle, and author of two best-selling books about wholesome nutrition, *The Earth Diet* and *10-Minute Recipes*. Liana is the Resident Health and Nutrition Coach at Complete Wellness NYC. Since 2009, she has been lecturing and teaching internationally about the benefits of consuming natural whole food, visiting schools, corporations, churches, libraries, and police departments, including the NYPD, to educate people on making healthier choices. Her commitment to this cause is personal. Liana lost both grandparents to cancer and her mother is a breast cancer survivor.

Liana and her work have been featured on NBC, ABC, CBS, and Fox television networks, *The Wendy Williams Show,* and News 12 NY, among other programs; on iHeart Radio and WABC; in print publications, including *Woman's Own* and *The Sun* (UK); and in lifestyle blogs such as Yahoo Beauty, Bustle, and Pop Sugar. She has contributed her articles to Mind Body Green, Huffington Post, Food Matters, and Heal Your Life. As a speaker, she has lectured for online events like the Keto Edge Summit and TEDx Orient; and she has appeared onstage at the I Can Do It Conference and the Truth About Cancer Live.

Liana was born in Perth, Australia, raised in Alice Springs and Arno Bay, and now resides in New York City. Visit her at LianaWernerGray.com.

Hay House Titles of Related Interest

YOU CAN HEAL YOUR LIFE, *the movie,* starring Louise Hay & Friends
(available as a 1-DVD program, an expanded 2-DVD set,
and an online streaming video)
Learn more at www.hayhouse.com/louise-movie

THE SHIFT, *the movie,* starring Dr. Wayne W. Dyer
(available as a 1-DVD program, an expanded 2-DVD set,
and an online streaming video)
Learn more at www.hayhouse.com/the-shift-movie

———◆———

CHRIS BEAT CANCER: *A Comprehensive Plan for Healing Naturally,*
by Chris Wark

CRAZY SEXY KITCHEN: *150 Plant-Empowered Recipes to
Ignite a Mouthwatering Revolution,* by Kris Carr

MEDICAL MEDIUM LIFE-CHANGING FOODS: *Save Yourself
and the Ones You Love with the Hidden Healing Powers
of Fruits & Vegetables,* by Anthony William

OUTSIDE THE BOX CANCER THERAPIES: *Alternative Therapies That
Treat and Prevent Cancer,* by Dr. Mark Stengler and Dr. Paul Anderson

THE TRUTH ABOUT CANCER: *What You Need to Know about
Cancer's History, Treatment, and Prevention,* by Ty M. Bollinger

———◆———

We hope you enjoyed this Hay House book. If you'd like to receive our online catalog featuring additional information on Hay House books and products, or if you'd like to find out more about the Hay Foundation, please contact:

Hay House, Inc., P.O. Box 5100, Carlsbad, CA 92018-5100
(760) 431-7695 or (800) 654-5126
(760) 431-6948 (fax) or (800) 650-5115 (fax)
www.hayhouse.com® • www.hayfoundation.org

———

Published in Australia by:
Hay House Australia Pty. Ltd., 18/36 Ralph St., Alexandria NSW 2015
Phone: 612-9669-4299 • *Fax:* 612-9669-4144 • www.hayhouse.com.au

Published in the United Kingdom by:
Hay House UK, Ltd., Astley House, 33 Notting Hill Gate, London W11 3JQ
Phone: 44-20-3675-2450 • *Fax:* 44-20-3675-2451 • www.hayhouse.co.uk

Published in India by: Hay House Publishers India,
Muskaan Complex, Plot No. 3, B-2, Vasant Kunj, New Delhi 110 070
Phone: 91-11-4176-1620 • *Fax:* 91-11-4176-1630 • www.hayhouse.co.in

———

<u>Access New Knowledge.</u>
<u>Anytime. Anywhere.</u>

Learn and evolve at your own pace
with the world's leading experts.

www.hayhouseU.com

Free e-newsletters
from Hay House, the Ultimate
Resource for Inspiration

Be the first to know about Hay House's free downloads, special offers, giveaways, contests, and more!

 Get exclusive excerpts from our latest releases and videos from *Hay House Present Moments*.

 Our *Digital Products Newsletter* is the perfect way to stay up-to-date on our latest discounted eBooks, featured mobile apps, and Live Online and On Demand events.

 Learn with real benefits! *HayHouseU.com* is your source for the most innovative online courses from the world's leading personal growth experts. Be the first to know about new online courses and to receive exclusive discounts.

 Enjoy uplifting personal stories, how-to articles, and healing advice, along with videos and empowering quotes, within *Heal Your Life*.

Sign Up Now!

Get inspired, educate yourself, get a complimentary gift, and share the wisdom!

Visit www.hayhouse.com/newsletters to sign up today!

 HAY HOUSE

HAYHOUSE RADIO *radio for your soul®*

 HAYHOUSE online learning